The Whole Way to
Natural
Detoxification

Clearing Your Body of Toxins

JACQUELINE KROHN, MD, MPH

FRANCES TAYLOR, MA

JINGER PROSSER, LMT

Hartley & Marks
PUBLISHERS

Published by
HARTLEY & MARKS PUBLISHERS INC.
P. O. Box 147   3661 West Broadway
Point Roberts, WA   Vancouver, BC
98281   V6R 2B8

LIBRARY OF CONGRESS CATALOGING-IN-PUBLICATION DATA

Krohn, Jacqueline, 1950–
    The whole way to natural detoxification : clearing your body of
toxins / Jacqueline Krohn, Frances Taylor.
        p.   cm.
    Includes bibliographical references and index.
    ISBN 0-88179-127-X
    1. Toxicology—Popular works. 2. Health. 3. Alternative medicine.
I. Taylor, Frances A., 1938–   . II. Title.
RA1213.K76   1996   96-22512
615.9—dc20   CIP

DESIGN AND COMPOSITION BY THE TYPEWORKS
COVER DESIGN BY BRIGHT IDEAS
SET IN SABON   PRINTED IN THE U.S.A.

NOTE TO THE READER

This book is meant to be a source of information for those who are interested in learning about how detoxification can help to cleanse and balance the body and lead to better health. Every person has different problems based on age, sex, lifestyle, health status, genetics, diet, psychological state, and spiritual maturity. Our intent is to share our experience and offer guidelines to help you to become more informed about detoxification and your health. In cooperation with your physician you can then take the necessary steps to maintain optimum health. This book is sold with the understanding that the publisher is not engaged in rendering medical or other professional services. If medical or other expert assistance is required, the services of a competent professional should be sought.

The Whole Way to
Natural
Detoxification

DEDICATION

To those health care practitioners in all medical disciplines who:

- Have shed the shackles of dogma
- Have the courage to look beyond the "accepted and standard" treatment
- Think independently
- Treat on the cutting edge of medicine
- Hold the good of their patients as their foremost concern

CONTENTS

FOREWORD

Everyone recognizes that our planet is increasingly polluted, but few recognize that humans are the final resting place for many of the toxic substances and materials to which we are exposed. Even fewer know what can be done to reduce the body's burden of toxins, or xenobiotics, through a process known as detoxification. The population of the earth is faced with increasing risks from toxic chemicals and physical forces, and now, more than ever, humans may be facing a race between knowledge and extinction.

Dr. Krohn has put together a comprehensive book outlining the many sources of toxic injury to our bodies, the mechanisms of injury and, most importantly, directions on how these injuries can be treated. With an understanding rooted in science, the authors introduce the many simple techniques which can help to cleanse, balance, and prevent exposures to toxins.

Dr. Krohn outlines the development of detoxification from early history up to modern times. Historically, humans developed simple but effective methods to reduce their body's burden of pollutants; many of which are still in use today. Science now confirms the efficacy of such modalities as sauna detoxification used by earlier cultures. By combining the past with the present knowledge of biochemistry, toxicology and nutrition, we now have multiple alternative programs offering safe, simple, effective ways to reduce our body burden of toxins.

Dr. Krohn is to be congratulated for her contribution in educating the public about the dangers in our environment—but more importantly, for showing us how to prevent and treat illness through natural detoxification. Knowledge is our first line of defense in a toxic world.

Allan D. Lieberman, MD
Medical Director
Center for Occupational and Environmental Medicine
Charleston, South Carolina

PREFACE

In working with our patients, we discovered that nearly every one of them had toxins of some sort in their bodies. Some had numerous toxins and were laboring under such an overwhelming load that their health would be permanently damaged without some type of cleansing. Others were mildly affected by only a few toxins.

There are numerous substances and situations that can be toxic to an individual. We have attempted to list all of those that most people might encounter. Readers should be able to identify those toxins that might be affecting them.

The methods of obtaining cleansing, detoxification, and balance are many and varied. We have endeavored to present a broad spectrum of possibilities and methods, including some that are considered alternative by standard medicine.

Every discipline of medicine and healing has some techniques that are of merit. The discerning individual will examine these techniques and incorporate them into an overall health program.

Quality of life can be dramatically increased by cleansing toxins from the body. It is our hope that readers of this book who suffer from toxic overload will find ideas, information, and inspiration for improving their health.

Jacqueline Krohn, MD, MPH, C.Hom.
Frances A. Taylor, MA, C.Hom.
Jinger Prosser, LMT, C.Hom.
Los Alamos, New Mexico
1996

ACKNOWLEDGMENTS

Our thanks and gratitude to:

The many health care practitioners, both past and present, whose genius and courage enabled the development of the techniques presented in this book.

Our office staff who gave us support and encouragement and who, as always, stepped in to do the extra work necessary to enable us to continue seeing patients in addition to writing this book.

Susan Powell and Cappy Hanson for their talent and industry at the computer.

Carol Richter and Jeanette Meadows for their hours of painstaking proofreading.

Erla Mae Larson for her contributions and suggestions, as well as for sharing her knowledge of nutrition over the years.

Our families, who again have allowed us the hours it took to write this book.

Sue Tauber, in whose mind the idea for this book originated.

Steven Carter, our editor, for his editing expertise and his efforts on our behalf.

Elizabeth McLean, our copy editor, who so capably helped organize and put the polishing touches on the book.

Susan Juby and the staff of Hartley & Marks who have so ably produced this final presentation of our book.

Introduction

From the beginning of time, humans have interacted extensively with their physical world. It has provided them with air to breathe, water to drink, food for nourishment, materials for shelter, substances for maintaining their well-being, and beauty for their enjoyment. For thousands of years, the relationship of ancient people with their earth was a clean and nurturing one. Except in extreme circumstances, the earth was not toxic, and they were not damaged by their world.

Unfortunately, ancient people sometimes damaged their world. They overhunted and stripped the land of its vegetation, cutting down trees for shelter and firewood. When the land was depleted and would no longer support them, they moved to another area.

As civilization developed and population increased, people began to congregate in cities. In these ancient cities pollution became a problem. Garbage was thrown into the streets. No provisions were made for sanitation, and drainage water and sewage ran down the middle of city streets. The streets were deep in mud, and animals wallowed in the mud. Drinking water became contaminated, and people contracted diseases. Indoor fires and poor ventilation in the small dwellings of the masses fouled the air in many homes. Houses were shared with domestic animals who ate the scraps that were thrown

on the floor. Rodents were rampant, spreading infectious diseases. The health of people was adversely affected.

The Industrial Revolution dramatically increased another type of pollution. Industrial wastes were not disposed of properly, and no attempt was made to protect workers from harmful exposures on the job. Both adults and children worked long hours under toxic conditions. People's health suffered further from these new toxins.

The "Chemical Revolution" that has occurred since World War II and the ever increasing industrialization in all parts of the world have multiplied our exposures to harmful substances to incalculable levels. Our bodies have had no previous experience with these chemicals and therefore have no efficient mechanism to metabolize or eliminate them. Our bodies have been unable to adapt quickly enough to the changes in exposure. Today the health of people is affected adversely on a daily basis.

While industry and science have made incredible progress, we have paid a price for it. Our air is no longer clean, the soil is contaminated, our water supply contains high levels of toxic chemicals and microorganisms, the purity of our food cannot be guaranteed, and its quality is dangerously low. Without proper cleansing, preventive measures, and a careful lifestyle, our bodies can be assaulted and overwhelmed by toxic substances.

Toxins

What is a toxin? *Dorland's Medical Dictionary* defines a toxin as a poison that is a protein or a conjugated protein substance produced by plants, some animals, and pathogenic bacteria; a toxicant is a poisonous agent. Another useful definition for a toxin is xenobiotic, which means a foreign chemical not produced by the human body. Dr. Elson Haas of Marin, California, defines a toxin as "any substance that creates irritating and/or harmful effects in the body, undermining our health or stressing our biochemical or organ functions." In this book, the term toxin will refer to anything that can be harmful or hazardous to the body, or that affects the balance of the body.

There are many sources of toxins in our world, including toxic metals, solvents, pesticides, herbicides, agricultural and industrial chemicals, terpenes, foods, microorganisms, noise, radiation, water, air, plants, altitude, weather, temperature, excess of body chemicals, emotional trauma, and cumulative life experiences.

Our exposures to toxins can be both external and internal. Pollution is responsible for many external exposures. The exposures may be serious contamination, such as industrial pollution, or they may be as simple as exposure to cleaning supplies, perfume, or cigarette smoke. Any of these exposures can cause a variety of symptoms in the sensitive person. These symptoms can include headaches, muscle pain, fatigue, mental confusion, emotional upset, poor coordination, skin rashes, neurological problems, and vision disturbances.

Our bodies absorb and then excrete the water-soluble chemicals to which we are exposed. The fat-soluble chemicals are absorbed, but not excreted. They accumulate in our fat cells and cell membranes and become internal toxins. When the body is under stress, it releases these chemicals from the fat to circulate in the bloodstream. Later, these chemicals will return to the fat cells and cell membranes, to be released another time. The constant release and return of these chemicals continues indefinitely unless we take action.

Our bodies also create internal toxins in response to various conditions, often producing excess metabolic products that become toxic to the body. For example, injury, anesthesia, and pollution cause the body to produce free radicals that are toxic to the tissues. The symptoms caused by these internal toxins include headaches, fatigue, memory loss, mental confusion, lack of mental acuity, "flulike" symptoms, mucous membrane irritation, skin problems, iritis (inflammation of the iris of the eye), and musculoskeletal pains. Internal toxins can also cause gastrointestinal symptoms such as nausea, vomiting, and diarrhea.

CLEANSING AND BALANCING METHODS

Despite all our exposures to these toxins, both external and internal, it is possible to enjoy good health. Lifestyle management, cleansing techniques, balancing methods, and preventive measures make it possible to obtain and maintain good health.

When we think of cleansing our bodies, most of us think of detoxification. The term "detoxification" means to diminish or remove the toxic quality of a compound, and indeed, within the body there are mechanisms that do just that. Toxic compounds are changed by chemical reactions in the body into less toxic compounds that can be excreted from the body. In some ways, the term "depuration" may be more accurate for describing other methods of cleansing the body. The definition of depuration is to remove a toxic contaminant, or to purify. We have elected to use the term detoxification for all cleansing processes discussed because it is more commonly used, both by the lay person and in the medical world.

In this book the terms cleansing, balancing, and detoxification are used interchangeably. Balancing enables detoxification; detoxification cleanses; cleansing leads to balance. This interaction in the body helps to restore and maintain health.

Among the cleansing and balancing methods discussed are the following:

- *Water*: Internal consumption of water, and various types of baths can aid in cleansing the body and restoring health.
- *Detoxification baths*: Can be taken in your own bathtub to remove toxins from your body.
- *Saunas*: An excellent method in a detoxification program.
- *Diet*: Macrobiotics, rotation diets, other specialized diets, and fasting will balance and cleanse the body.
- *Nutrients*: Help cleanse the body and supply the necessary building blocks for tissue repair.
- *Herbs*: May be used for cleansing and for treating health problems.
- *Homeopathic remedies*: Can be used to treat and balance many conditions that prevent optimum health.
- *Allergy extracts*: Special types help the body to release stored toxins and prevent subsequent accumulations.
- *Chelation*: Can remove such toxins as heavy metals and atherosclerotic plaque.
- *Exercise*: Imperative to detoxifying the body, even at nonstress levels.

- *Bodywork*: Various forms can facilitate release of toxins as well as the cellular memory of toxic events.
- *Acupuncture/acupressure*: Excellent balancing techniques.
- *Electromagnetic*: Various methods to balance the body electromagnetically and to protect from electromagnetic disturbances are imperative for good health.
- *Compresses/packs/poultices*: Aid the body by drawing out toxins.
- *Oxygenation*: Increasing oxygen levels in the body will help detoxify the body.
- *Organ cleansing*: Mild organ cleansing procedures are useful for restoring the body to better health.
- *Breathing*: Various techniques of manipulating and exercising this life force can help cleanse the body.

Challenge to Health

There are many ways of detoxification but, for complete health, the whole person must be addressed: mind, body, emotions, and spirit. Healing is a cleansing and rebalancing process that must take place in all of these areas. Once we take steps to cleanse and balance our bodies, we need to maintain our new level of health; thus, methods of prevention are also important.

We are the guardians of our own health—it is our most precious gift. Without good health our adaptability declines, our quality of life suffers, and our enjoyment of life is mediocre. Cleansing and balancing the body to restore health is a learning experience, even an adventure, when we accept the challenge to pursue the best health and therefore the best possible quality of life.

PART ONE

Approaches to Detoxification

I

Historical Approaches to Cleansing

Because primitive humans were unable to explain their illnesses, they developed the philosophy that disease was a spiritual matter caused by supernatural forces. For many centuries, medicine was a mixture of magic, superstition, and religion. Medicine men were the first physicians, but this role was taken over by priests long before the birth of Christ.

The ancient Greeks separated medicine from religion and formulated the earliest principles of scientific medicine. Their medicine began as a skill and became a trade. By the end of the sixth century they had developed the doctrine of the humors, which formed the basis of ancient medical pathology.

Cleansing Methods

For centuries, it was believed that an equilibrium between the four humors—blood, phlegm, yellow bile, and black bile—must be achieved for health to be maintained. Early medical treatment of illness sought to re-establish humoral harmony through diet, internal medicine, purging, vomiting, bleeding, cupping, and other techniques, all of which were cleansing and balancing treatments.

One might expect that as time went by each culture would develop its own unique program of medical treatment. This was not the case. The recorded history of all cultures and countries shows almost identical techniques, with some local variations. Many of these treatments evolved concurrently.

BLOODLETTING

Bloodletting was perhaps the favorite of the ancient treatments. The purpose of bloodletting was to cleanse and balance the humors by removing "bad blood." Bleeding was used as a cleansing technique in the case of abscesses; swelling of the spleen; fever; diseases of the mouth, eye, and head; headaches; and gynecological disorders. In the case of hemorrhage, whether from a ruptured blood vessel, wound, or childbirth, bleeding was used as a balancing treatment. The most common method of bleeding was to open a vein to divert the blood from the problem area or to use leeches, a milder method of bloodletting.

At first, ancient physicians performed all of the bloodletting. When the university schools of medicine were organized around 1000 A.D., bloodletting became the task of the barber-surgeons. Both bloodletting and surgery were considered beneath the university-trained physicians, and surgeons and barber-surgeons were beneath them in status. Below them were the apothecaries and bath house keepers who frequently rented the leeches to their clients.

Cupping was also a favorite bloodletting method. A small piece of hemp (tow) was burned in a cup. As soon as it had burned out, the cup was placed over a cut on lightly greased skin. Suction from the cup caused it to fill with blood.

Bloodletting began centuries before the birth of Christ and remained popular into the 19th century. It is still practiced today, even in North America, but on a very reduced scale, and for more practical reasons. Leeches are valuable for removing blood from bruises and black eyes, and for removing the congestion from around a reattached amputated limb.

COUNTER-IRRITATION

Another method of balancing the humors by drainage was to cause a chronic inflammatory re-action in the form of a running sore. This sore could be maintained for long periods of time, and the humors could be continuously released from the body. For treatment of asthma and paralysis, counter-irritation was as popular as bloodletting.

The blister was the simplest method of counter-irritation and was sometimes produced by direct application of a cautery, a hot instru-ment, in a variety of shapes.

ENEMAS

Enemas were used without exception by all cul-tures. Not only were enemas used as a cleansing procedure, but also as a standard beginning treatment for almost every illness, injury or health problem, including diarrhea. Many early physicians required that an enema be adminis-tered before bleeding, and medication was sometimes administered in the enemas. The Egyptians and Greeks routinely used an enema for treating wounds received in battle. Even to-day, some cultures still use the enema as a vital part of treatment for all conditions.

CATHARTICS

Because constipation was considered a disease rather than a symptom, cathartics were used even more frequently than the enema to cleanse the digestive tract. A cathartic (or purgative) is a substance that causes an active movement of the bowels.

There are four types of cathartics:

- *Stimulant*: cascara, senna, castor oil
- *Saline*: salts such as Epsom and Glauber's salts
- *Bulk-forming*: absorb moisture and swell up, such as psyllium seed, bran
- *Lubricant*: mineral oil

These types of cathartics have been used for cen-turies, but because of their toxicity several of the favorites used by the ancients are now obsolete.

EMETICS

An emetic is a substance that induces vomiting. Nearly all the ancient civilizations routinely used emetics in addition to cathartics and ene-mas for cleansing treatments. An active emetic, such as white hellebore, was supposed to recall the humors from the innermost recesses of the body. Until this century, it was felt that emetics and purgatives:

- cleansed the body of harmful accumulations
- increased the appetite
- promoted digestion
- cooled the system
- destroyed wind

Emetics were standard treatment for gastric disturbances, and they were used as routine treatment for most medical conditions. Emetics were kept ready for the "ease, comfort, and hap-piness" of the patient! With our better under-standing of physiology and digestion, we now realize that these measures are too harsh, and in some instances can be fatal. Digestion is better aided by proper diet and nutrition, and cleans-ing can be accomplished by milder methods.

BATHS

Numerous types of baths have been used by all civilizations to wash away illness and to purify and cleanse the body. The original baths were in rivers, seas, lakes, and pools. Springs were considered to be divine, with special powers for healing and fertility.

The temperature of the medicinal bath varied with its medical purpose and the disease for which it was being used. For centuries, cold baths, cooling compresses, and cooling diets were used to treat fevers in all civilizations. Tepid or warm baths have a sedative effect and were used to calm hysterical and agitated, mentally ill patients.

The most popular was the hot bath, even in ancient Egypt. A hot bath is clinically analgesic, but is also stimulating to the nervous system. The Greeks and Romans frequented bath houses in which both hot and cold baths were available. In medieval Europe, there were no baths in private homes and the general public went to bath houses, not for cleanliness, but for their health. Bleeding, cupping, and massage were available at the bath houses, along with various tonics and herbal remedies.

The hot bath was important because it caused sweating, which was considered therapeutic as well as cleansing. According to ancient tradition, there were three kinds of sweat: the sweat of illness, toil, and bathing.

MASSAGE

Some form of massage has been practiced by humans since the beginning of time. Some massages were no more than an oil rub. Others involved deeper work to relieve muscle tension and to help eliminate waste matter from the muscles. Massage also served as a mechanical cleanser, pushing out waste products, particularly in those suffering from constipation.

Massage has been described with many different terms, such as passive exercise, therapeutic manipulations, stroking and kneading, rubbing, and mechanotherapy. As medical theory and practice have expanded, bodywork has kept pace with these developments. During this century there has been an explosion of techniques, practitioners, and discoveries of new ways in which the hands can be used to affect human physiology. Regardless of the technique used, massage helps to cleanse and balance the body.

ACUPUNCTURE

Organized medicine began in China in the first millennium B.C. and by the end of the first millennium A.D. was contemporary with Ayurvedic medicine in India and Hippocratic medicine in Greece. Although the exact origin of acupuncture in China is not clear, the first written reference to acupuncture dates to 90 B.C. It is probable that the technique is older.

Acupuncture involves inserting, into the skin, fine metal needles one-half to several inches in length. Some needles are inserted gently and others are inserted with great force and at different depths. The needles may then be heated, twirled, or vibrated. They are left in place for varying amounts of time, depending on the condition being treated.

The points where the needles are inserted are called acupuncture points, which are located on meridians that run the length of the body. These meridians are energy pathways and control certain physical conditions. The Chinese believe that all disease or pain is the result of imbalance in the energy flow along these meridians in the body. Inserting acupuncture needles at the appropriate points restores and balances the energy by diminishing an excess and replenishing a deficiency. Order and harmonious balance is restored in the chi, or life force, that circulates through all the organs of the body.

FASTING

True fasting is complete abstinence from food and beverage. Primitive humans began to fast in an attempt to placate the divine powers who were supposedly unhappy with them. As time went by, fasting became part of religious and purification rituals. Hippocrates and other early physicians felt that fasting dried the body and balanced the humors. Although fasting was occasionally prescribed as a cleansing treatment, most early physicians preferred the emetic, cathartic, and bleeding approaches to cleanse and balance the body.

Early Medications

Early medications in most cultures were plant remedies. Flowers, fruits, roots, barks, leaves, juices, oils, and resins from the plants were used. Many plants were believed to have specific applications for balancing a particular humor or element.

The Chinese claim to have used herbal remedies for over 10,000 years to balance their five elements of fire, metal, earth, water, and wood. Ancient East Indian literature listed 760 plants as having medicinal properties. They, too, were endeavoring to balance their five elements. However, history points to the Egyptians as being the first to use plant remedies.

Mineral remedies were also used, particularly in Egyptian and Hindu pharmacies. In most cultures, mercury was considered the "king of metals" and was given both externally and internally.

Many cultures, especially in the ancient East, felt that water had cleansing and cooling properties, and purified both body and soul. Water was employed for its own medicinal properties and also as a vehicle for other remedies.

Medicines were classified according to their function, such as emetic, purgative, laxative, tonic, and aphrodisiac, for a total of 35 different classifications. Medications were prescribed in several forms, including infusions, decoctions, mixtures, pills, salves, syrups, pastes, plastics, poultices, powders, ointments, suppositories, tinctures, and fumigations. Preparation of these various forms of medication was governed largely by astrology.

Treatment with all medications was an attempt to cleanse, purify, or balance the humors or elements of the body. Although most ancient remedies are not in use today, some medicinal herbs are still given for the same conditions. Modern scientific research into the medicinal actions of these herbs continues to document the effectiveness of many of these "folk remedies."

It's a Question of Balance

Early civilizations looked on disease and health problems as a matter of imbalance or disequilibrium in the body. For centuries, this was the major concept of pathology in medicine, and all treatment was designed to cleanse and effect a balance in the body.

Even though Western medicine no longer believes in the four humors, Chinese and Ayurvedic medicine continue to use the concept of balance between five elements as necessary to health. Today, this concept can still be applied; health can be viewed as a question of balance. However, we now balance other factors to restore and maintain health.

To have good health, we must be balanced:

- *Allergically*: Allergic reactions imbalance the body by causing an increase in antibodies, an activation of cells of the immune system, and tissue inflammation from the release of chemicals in an attempt by the body to heal itself.
- *Biochemically*: Life is possible because hundreds of biochemical reactions take place in our bodies each second. Toxic exposure can interrupt these processes, causing poor health or even death. There must also be acid-alkaline balance in the body, which needs to stay within an optimal range for the detoxification pathways to function properly.
- *Electrically*: Electron transfers take place in biochemical reactions of the body. Our

bodies contain both alternating and direct electrical fields of current. An electrical imbalance in the body causes acute sensitivity to weather changes as well as symptoms when exposed to electrical equipment or appliances.

- *Emotionally*: Emotional health depends on a balance in the emotions. Love must be given and received. Anger and anxiety must be expressed and relieved.
- *Energetically*: The breakdown of organic molecules releases energy that is used by the cells as they perform their tasks. An imbalance in this energy makes it impossible for the body to perform its work and maintain body temperature.
- *Environmentally*: A healthy body requires an environmental balance. A safe home and workplace with minimal environmental stresses and toxins is necessary.
- *Enzymatically*: Enzymes are essential for the biochemical reactions that take place in the body. A deficiency or an excess of any enzyme affects the efficiency, speed, and balance of these reactions.
- *Hormonally*: Hormones play a major role in metabolism, circulation, water and electrolyte balance, reproduction, and stress. An imbalance can greatly reduce or even stop these processes in the body.
- *Magnetically*: Our brains produce a steady magnetic field. We project a magnetic field out into the space around our bodies. A magnetic imbalance affects our biological cycles, such as the sleep cycle.
- *Mentally*: Mental health depends on a balance between work and play to keep the mind healthy. Too much work or too much play can adversely affect the mind, which in turn adversely affects the body.
- *Microbiologically*: Our bodies contain normal microbiological flora that aid in body functions, such as digestion. A defi-

ciency or an overgrowth of these organisms, or an infection by pathogenic organisms, can cause an imbalance and illness.

- *Nutritionally*: The body must have a certain optimum, balanced amount of nutrients for proper functioning and good health. A continued deficiency of any one vitamin, mineral, or amino acid can lead to serious health problems.
- *Psychologically*: Psychological health depends on the proper balance between emotions and the mind. An imbalance of any of these health factors listed can ultimately affect psychological health.
- *Spiritually*: Spiritual balance is necessary for health. The soul, as higher being, must be nurtured by prayer, worship, or meditation, depending on the beliefs of the person. To neglect this aspect can cause a serious imbalance in the body.
- *Structurally*: The skeleton always comes to mind when thinking of body structure. Certainly it must be healthy and balanced to keep the body aligned properly. However, all of the cells of the body must also be structurally correct and in balance for good health.

The human body is constantly undergoing biological change and shift, subject to both internal and external stimuli. During these shifts, it tries to maintain a balance—an equilibrium or homeostasis.

Picture a moving, well-balanced mobile formed from all of the above-mentioned elements of good health. The slightest touch on one part of the mobile causes all of the remaining parts to move. The parts readjust to conform to a different but stable position to re-establish balance. Larger changes to a part of the mobile cause more active movement of the other parts and a longer time is needed to achieve a balance.

As the mobile settles, the parts will be in slightly different positions, but balance is re-established.

All the body functions on which our health depends are linked in a carefully balanced and monitored equilibrium. Our level of health and flow of vital energy can be measured by how well our body systems adapt, maintain their flexibility, and rebalance after a stress. Some changes occur rapidly, in seconds or minutes. Others may take days or years to occur.

If the tension created by an imbalance remains, the healing process is impeded. When our functions become rigid, unadaptable, unable to change, and imbalanced, a disease pro-cess usually results. Unraveling the complicated imbalance and finding the multiple causative factors is often a difficult and slow process. Any or all of the metabolic functions listed above can be involved.

The balance of the body is affected by continual changes and adjustments in both internal and external factors: weather, temperature, humidity, moods, emotional trauma, diet, environmental exposures, food, water, air, thoughts, illnesses, radiation, toxins, hormones, allergic reactions, microorganisms, altitude, noise, spiritual influences, response to events and other individuals, and cumulative life experiences.

2

Contemporary Approaches to Detoxification

Current Medical Disciplines

As the practice of medicine evolved over the centuries, many different schools of thought and methods of practice developed. Several medical ideologies exist today. In some instances, these ideologies work in harmony but, sadly, there is often conflict and competition among them. Most people are unaware of the differences in medical disciplines and what each has to offer. Every person should have enough knowledge to be able to make an informed decision about the type of practitioner with whom the responsibility for health care will be shared.

Many different cleansing/detoxification/balancing techniques are discussed in later chapters. In order to better understand these therapy modalities, it is necessary to understand the philosophy of the medical discipline offering that therapy.

ALLOPATHY

The standard medical practice is considered by many to be allopathy. Although medicine is often described as the art of healing, the status of allopathy is believed to be firmly rooted in medicine as a science. Physicians with an MD degree are allopaths, and the majority of medical schools in North America are allopathic. There are two general divisions in allopathy: medicine and surgery. The medicine division is descended from the original university-educated physicians. Surgery's historical roots come from the barber-surgeons. Both medicine and surgery have many different types of specialties:

Medicine	*Surgery*
Internal medicine	Surgery
Cardiology	Orthopedics
Gastroenterology	Urology
Pediatrics	Ear, nose, and throat
Geriatrics	Obstetrics and
Dermatology	gynecology
Immunology	Anesthesiology
Epidemiology	Opthalmology
Allergy	
Neurology	
Psychiatry	
Radiology	
Pathology	

Because of the specialties, allopathic practices tend to be rather compartmentalized, focusing on parts of the body or particular body systems, and often without considering the mental or spiritual aspects that are always involved in both health and illness.

Allopaths treat disease with medications that produce effects different from those that the disease produces. Many allopaths use only pharmaceuticals, and most use minimal, if any, nutritional therapy. They receive approximately

10 to 20 hours of nutritional instruction in medical school and feel the least prepared in this area. Very few allopaths ask their patients about their dietary habits or attempt to correct health problems with diet.

For traumas, acute bacterial infections, and medical emergencies, allopathic medicine is very effective, but it does not handle viral infections, degenerative diseases, serious cancers, mental illness, or functional illness nearly as well.

Allopathic medicine defines health primarily as the maintenance of a certain level of measurable values and vital signs. These include normal values for blood pressure, body temperature, pulse, respiratory rate, visual acuity, auditory threshold, electrolyte balance, height, and weight. These values are determined by lab tests, and in general, allopathic medicine relies on technology.

According to allopathy, a person is healthy when a set of balanced parameters is displayed corresponding to his or her age and environment. The body and its functions must display no abnormalities; dysfunctions in the life processes are considered to be disease.

Allopathy has little to offer for detoxification treatments. Practitioners do use chelation therapy for lead poisoning, but most do not acknowledge its value for atherosclerosis. Some physical therapy treatments offer minimal detoxification possibilities. Allopathic use of drugs for most treatments introduces more chemicals to bodies that are already laboring under a toxic load and are unable to process additional chemicals. While some allopaths suggest special diets and exercise, which can be cleansing, these are not primary constituents of allopathic practice.

Some allopaths have augmented their practices with techniques that are not part of traditional allopathic procedure. Environmental medicine physicians, having received additional hours of training in nutritional, homeopathic, herbal, and many other therapies, treat environmentally ill patients using cleansing and balancing methods.

OSTEOPATHY

The basic theory of osteopathy has altered little since its inception in mid-19th century. Osteopathy accepts the interrelationship of all parts of the body and its inherent capacity to resist disease and to repair itself. Osteopathic philosophy of disease considers that strains or dislocations in the skeletal system affect the body's structural integrity and result in disease. Osteopaths use manipulation to correct this problem.

Osteopaths are often primary care physicians. Although they prescribe drugs and perform surgery, they also use manipulation. Osteopaths combine broad medical knowledge with their manipulation techniques. Sixteen osteopathic medical colleges grant DO degrees, and osteopathic pharmacology and medical specialties are the same as allopathic pharmacology and medical specialties. Osteopaths and allopaths take the same state board exams (medical licensing exams).

Osteopathic manipulations balance the skeleton, restore nerves, increase lymph and blood circulation, and relieve muscle spasms, thus causing cleansing. Although it depends on the practitioner, osteopathy places more emphasis on diet and exercise, which are valuable cleansing techniques. Many osteopathic physicians have additional training in alternative methods of treatment.

CHIROPRACTIC

Chiropractic derives from the Greek words *cheir,* meaning hand, and *praktikos,* meaning practical. Chiropractors receive a DC degree, but cannot prescribe drugs or perform surgery. Their license permits them to use spinal manipulation. Modern chiropractic has added diagnostic techniques including X-ray and applied kinesiology. Much emphasis is placed on exercise, diet, and nutritional supplementation. Chiropractors incorporate treatments with heat and ice, massage, electrical stimulation, traction, ultrasound, and trigger-point therapy (locating and working with the specific points on the body that cause the tension/pain).

Chiropractic offers several cleansing modalities. Manipulation treatments both balance and cleanse. Their knowledge of nutrition enables chiropractors to recommend many cleansing and balancing nutrients. Trigger-point therapy and electrical stimulation also cause the release of toxins.

HOMEOPATHY

Homeopathy is a medical system developed 200 years ago by German physician Samuel Hahnemann (1755–1843). Hahnemann was critical of the harsh, suppressive, conventional medical therapies of the day. He developed the law of similars, "let likes be cured with likes," based on his experiences and the writings of Hippocrates and Paracelsus. Hahnemann chose the word homeopathy to describe this medical system. The Greek root *homoios* means similar, and the root *pathos* means suffering or disease. The law of similars states that a substance that causes symptoms in healthy persons can help cure a sick person who has similar symptoms.

Hahnemann discovered that the body's responses to illness are an effort to heal itself. He realized that these efforts to heal were not always strong enough to complete the healing process, and he concluded that treatment should stimulate the symptoms developed by the body in response to illness. Hahnemann invented a method to choose the right catalyst to complete the healing process.

Each homeopathic substance or medicine, called a remedy, is listed in a book called a *Materia Medica,* with all of its characteristics and symptoms. An index to the *Materia Medica* is known as a *Repertory.* In a *Repertory,* symptoms are listed by body systems. Remedies effective for treating each symptom are listed.

To cure a patient, Hahnemann found he had to choose the remedy that most closely fit the patient's symptoms. The main symptom is im-

portant in choosing a remedy. How the symptom is affected by various modalities such as heat, cold, and motion is important in choosing the remedy. Emotional symptoms may be as important or more important than physical symptoms. An important principle of homeopathy is the individualization of the homeopathic remedy to the person's physical and emotional characteristics.

Hahnemann found that what was being treated was the "vital force." The vital force refers to a person's overall, interconnected energetic and defense processes that aid in self-healing. The vital force guides the homeopath to determine whether or not a remedy is working. Hahnemann realized that he was practicing "energy medicine" as the body seemed to "resonate" with the remedy used.

Initially Hahnemann used small doses of a remedy, but found that many people developed toxic symptoms. He then began to dilute substances and found that the more diluted substances had fewer side effects and were more able to cure. He called this "potentization." Soluble remedies are diluted in water or alcohol. If the remedy is insoluble, it is ground (triturated) in powdered lactose (milk sugar) and then put into solution. Once in solution, all remedies are succussed, not stirred, by hitting them firmly against a leather surface. Remedies diluted in a 1-to-9 ratio are known as a decimal potency and labeled as X. If this 1-to-9 remedy is diluted in the same proportions thirty times, it is known as a 30X potency. Some common potencies used are 6X and 12X. Remedies diluted 1 to 99 are known as centesimal, or C potencies; common C potencies are 6C and 30C. The remedies have to be both diluted and succussed to be effective. The more diluted remedies have a higher potency, act deeper, act longer, and require fewer doses to effect a cure.

Homeopathy spread throughout Europe and then the United States. The survival rate of patients treated by homeopathic remedies in 1900 was two to eight times that of the conventional medical care of that era. Homeopathy was used in cholera, typhoid, scarlet fever, and yellow fever epidemics. The first national medical association in the United States was the American Institute of Homeopathy, founded in 1844.

Partly in response to the growth of homeopathy, a rival medical group, known as the American Medical Association (AMA), formed to slow the development of homeopathy. In 1855, the AMA ruled that orthodox physicians would lose their membership in the AMA if they consulted with a homeopathic physician or a "nonregular" practitioner. Homeopathy offered an integrated, coherent, systematic basis for its practice, and it threatened orthodox medicine of the day.

In the early 1900s, there were 22 homeopathic medical schools and more than 100 homeopathic hospitals in the United States. The homeopathic medical schools were on a par with the education offered at the orthodox medical schools of the day. This all changed in 1910 when Abraham Flexner, working for the Carnegie Endowment for the Advancement of Teaching, and in cooperation with leading members of the AMA, reported on the "unscientific basis" of some medical schools. His report placed the highest value on those medical schools with a full-time teaching faculty who taught a pathophysiological analysis of the human body. Only graduates of the schools that received a high rating were allowed to take the medical licensing exams.

The homeopathic colleges were given poor ratings by the Flexner Report. As a result, the homeopathic schools converted to more orthodox medical schools based on "pure science" and the theory that germs (microorganisms) cause disease. With this change in curricula, graduates of homeopathic schools were not as skilled at homeopathic prescribing as were earlier graduates.

Pain-killing drugs and antibiotics that seemed to work magically became the most used medi-

cines. Orthodox physicians were able to see and treat patients in a shorter period of time. Drug companies, which controlled the major medical journals and what was published in them, were antagonistic toward homeopathy. By 1950, all homeopathic medical schools in the United States were closed or no longer teaching homeopathy.

In the last 20 years, homeopathy has regained popularity and is used widely in Europe, India, and Britain. In Britain, 42% of physicians refer patients to homeopaths and India has more than 100 homeopathic medical colleges. There are now several academies in the United States where a homeopathic education may be obtained.

Today there is a variety of homeopathic philosophies, ranging from the classical homeopaths, who use only one remedy at a time, to those who use combination remedies, which are mixtures of low potency doses of the most commonly used remedies for a given condition.

Homeopathy begins the healing response. Remedies are small potentized doses from the plant, mineral, or animal kingdom. The remedies stimulate the immune response, increase overall resistance to infection, and increase a person's vital force. Homeopathic remedies are significantly safer than conventional drugs.

Acute symptoms are treated first, fundamental or chronic symptoms are treated next, and constitutional remedies are given last. Constitutional remedies are used for strengthening the immune system. A common mistake in homeopathic prescribing is to give the constitutional remedy before the acute and fundamental problems have been treated. As with all medical treatment, discussing and understanding your planned treatment fully with a well-trained practitioner is essential.

Once a person takes the correct homeopathic medicine, he or she will feel better in many ways. If the person wakes up refreshed, this indicates that the vital force is improved and that the medicine chosen is the correct one. Sometimes one dose of one remedy is enough to bring about a cure, while other times a series of remedies are used to heal a person.

There are over 2000 homeopathic remedies, but a small group of remedies called polycrest remedies are the most frequently used. These remedies will help symptoms related to many different body systems. Some of these remedies are:

- *Arsenicum album*
- *Calcarea carbonica*
- *Graphites*
- *Ignatia*
- *Lachesis*
- *Lycopodium*
- *Natrum muriaticum*
- *Nux vomica*
- *Phosphorus*
- *Pulsatilla*
- *Sepia*
- *Silica*
- *Sulfur*
- *Thuja*

Homeopathic remedies can be used for detoxification. Some examples include the use of a remedy after radiation, surgery, chemotherapy, insect or snake bites; and for diarrhea, emotional trauma, and strengthening the liver.

In subsequent chapters, homeopathic remedies are suggested as treatment for many different toxic exposures. Any given remedy may be used for more than one condition or problem. The remedy that best fits the person and his or her symptoms should be used. At times, research in the homeopathic literature is necessary in order to choose the proper remedy. Seek the help of a qualified homeopathic practitioner.

HOMOTOXICOLOGY

In an attempt to synthesize medicine, the German physician Hans-Heinrich Reckeweg proposed the concept of homotoxicology in 1955. It is considered by some to be a "marriage" between allopathy and homeopathy. It is based on the assumption that the body is a dynamic system that constantly adjusts to the environment to remain in a state of balance. Reckeweg considered disease to be the body's struggle against endogenous (internal) and exogenous (external) homotoxins (substances toxic to humans), and

an attempt to compensate for homotoxically related toxic damage.

Reckeweg described five interlinked subsystems of the body's defense that combat and render toxins harmless:

- production of antibodies
- use of neuronal adaptation hormones
- toxin defense by the nervous system
- detoxification by the liver
- detoxification by the connective tissue (The connective tissue is a deposition and drainage system. It receives waste from the cells and transfers or deposits it through the lymphatic system.)

Homotoxicology relates disease patterns to their localization, and their degree to a network of humoral and cellular schemes of tissue and disease. Reckeweg felt that treatment should involve as few side effects as possible because the body is already damaged. His treatments were designed to give rapid, optimum relief with no inhibition or suppression of symptoms. Suppression of symptoms prevents the body from eliminating the homotoxins. Homotoxicological remedies stimulate and regulate the self-healing capabilities of the body, and avoid any damage resulting from the therapy.

For treatment, Reckeweg used individual homeopathic remedies, organ and tissue preparations, nosodes (remedies made from diseased tissue or microorganisms), trace elements, catalysts, and homeopathically prepared allopathic drugs. For syndromes, Reckeweg used combination homeopathic remedies that cover a broad range of possible causes of the problems and functional disorders, including constitutional circumstances and environmental influences. Homotoxicology offers many of the same cleansing and balancing techniques as homeopathy.

NATUROPATHY

Naturopathy had its beginnings in treatment that included clean air, food, and water. It was first brought to the United States in 1892. In 1902 a group of German homeopathic physicians enlarged the treatment methods to include herbs, homeopathy, and physical therapy. The name naturopathy is a combination of the words nature and homeopathy. At one time there were as many as 45 naturopathic medical schools in the U.S. These schools were affected by the Flexner Report, as were homeopathic and chiropractic schools. By 1955 there were only two schools left, and by 1978, just one.

Today there are four accredited naturopathic medical colleges in North America: the National College of Naturopathic Medicine in Portland, Oregon; Bastyr University of Natural Health Sciences in Seattle, Washington; the Southwest College of Naturopathic Medicine in Scottsdale, Arizona; and the Canadian College of Naturopathic Medicine in Toronto, Ontario. Graduates of these schools are trained to be primary care physicians and are granted an ND degree. Several states currently provide licensing for naturopathic physicians.

Naturopathic physicians receive training in clinical nutrition, physical medicine, homeopathic medicine, botanical medicine, naturopathic manipulations, psychological medicine, cleansing protocols, and minor surgery. They may elect to do further training in naturopathic obstetrics, acupuncture and Oriental medicine, and Ayurvedic medicine.

The philosophy of naturopathy includes the following principles of healing:

- To first do no harm
- To recognize the healing power of nature
- To treat the whole person
- To identify and treat the cause of illness
- To realize that prevention is the best cure
- To teach the principles of healthy living and preventive medicine.

Naturopathy offers several treatment possibilities for detoxification and balancing, using herbs, homeopathic remedies, and extensive diet and nutritional therapy, with the emphasis on natural healing.

VIBRATIONAL MEDICINE

Vibrational medicine is energy medicine. Dr. Richard Gerber of Livonia, Michigan, defines vibrational medicine as a healing philosophy that treats the whole person—the mind, body, and spirit—by delivering measured amounts of frequency-specific energy to the human multidimensional system. It seeks to heal the physical body by balancing the higher energetic systems.

Traditional medicine is based on the Newtonian concept of the human body as a complex machine; vibrational medicine, based on the Einsteinian viewpoint, considers the human body to be a multidimensional organism made up of physical systems that are interrelated with complex regulatory energetic fields. Vibrational medicine techniques direct healing energy into these energy fields.

Vibrational healing methods include homeopathy, flower essences, gem therapy, sound therapy, some types of bodywork, acupuncture, color therapy, and other techniques. All of these therapies affect and heal the body on an energetic level. Vibrational medicine cleanses and balances the body at the deepest cellular level.

Traditional medicine also uses some energy techniques. The use of electromagnetic fields to stimulate fracture healing, radiation to treat cancer, and electricity to alleviate pain are all energy modalities.

Methods of Detoxification

This discussion of the Hubbard method is included because it was one of the first detoxification programs developed. It marked the beginning of interest and focus on cleansing and detoxifying the body. The Hubbard method is still used in some detoxification centers today, very much as it was originally designed. Its effectiveness is undisputed and the principles involved have now been applied to other methods of cleansing that are the emphasis of this book.

Consult a health care professional before beginning any detoxification program. The detoxification process can trigger unpleasant symptoms, particularly if the body burden of toxins is high, or if the liver is unable to handle the increased load of released toxins.

THE HUBBARD METHOD OF DETOXIFICATION

In the 1960s, L. Ron Hubbard, the founder of an applied religious philosophy known as Scientology, and scientists from the Environmental Protection Agency (EPA), began to research the effects of recreational drugs, including alcohol, on the body in an effort to find methods that would help people cleanse the harmful effects of drugs. In 1977, the program was called "The Sweat Program," and it took months to complete. People in the program began to report the excretion of substances in their sweat that smelled or tasted like medications, anesthetics, diet pills, food preservatives, and pesticides. They also reported sensations of old sunburns, past illnesses, and physical and emotional conditions from the past.

By 1979, the scientists had developed the "Purification Program." It is a long-term detoxification program, designed to assist in releasing and flushing accumulated toxins from the tissues as well as in rebuilding impaired tissues and cells. Health Med, a group in California, has used the Hubbard method of detoxification on over 3000 patients with good rates of success.

Because this program was so successful, the details of the Purification Program were published. It is a precise program of exercise; sauna; adequate fluid intake and replacement; a regimented schedule; certain vitamins, minerals, and oils; and a diet with appropriate, lightly cooked fresh vegetables. People with heart disease, kidney disease, or anemia, and pregnant women should not participate in the program.

The Purification Program begins with exercise (running is recommended) to loosen deep-seated toxins. Exercise causes cell wastes to be eliminated more rapidly and the circulation to go more deeply into muscle tissue to pick up deposited wastes. Exercise is followed immediately by sweating in a sauna at 140° to 180°F to flush out the toxins. The treatment ratio is 20 to 30 minutes of exercise for each 4 to 4½ hours of sauna time. A proper schedule is very important; the ratio of exercise time to sauna time must be maintained. The sauna, vitamins, and minerals must be taken at the same time each day and adequate sleep is essential while a person is on the program.

They recommended using a blend of cold-pressed soy, walnut, peanut, and safflower oils with lecithin to replace the bad oils in the body with good oils. These oils are polyunsaturated and need to be refrigerated to prevent rancidity. The amount of oil recommended is 2 tablespoonfuls to ½ cup a day, but each person needs to find his or her individual dose. If the oil shows up in the stool or sweat, intake should be reduced.

People who lose weight slowly or who have had heavy drug or alcohol use do better with evening primrose oil. The standard dose is 3 capsules, twice a day, up to 12 capsules a day.

The scientists used a calcium-magnesium formula containing two parts calcium gluconate (1 teaspoon) to one part magnesium carbonate (½ teaspoon), mixed with apple cider vinegar (1 tablespoon) and dissolved in ½ cup of boiling water and ½ cup lukewarm water. Calcium must have an acidic base to work in the body. They felt that calcium and magnesium would balance vitamin B_1, thiamine.

Niacin, vitamin B_3, is an important cornerstone of the program. Niacin stimulates the cardiovascular system and causes vasodilation of skin capillaries. This causes the skin to flush, especially in areas of old sunburn. This hot flush, accompanied by prickly, itchy skin, can last up to one hour. This is not an allergic reaction. If one continues to take niacin, the flush disappears at a given dose, then returns with less intensity at a graduated higher dose. Niacin seems to release drugs or chemicals from the tissue. It causes an initial drop in blood fatty acids, leading to the release of more fats along with their toxins. Exercise and sweating then flush the chemicals out of the body.

Niacin dosing is very important, and only the short-acting form is used. Most people start with 100 milligrams (mg) a day of niacin, taken in one dose, with food. When there is minimal flushing and other symptoms have disappeared or diminished, the niacin dosage is increased, along with vitamin C and B-complex doses. People increased their niacin dose by 100 mg until they reached 1000 mg daily, then increased the dose by increments of 300 to 500 mg. The most effective method was to use niacin tablets of 100 mg until the 1000 mg of niacin was reached, then to use niacin in the powder form. People were able to take 5000 mg of niacin a day at the end of the program.

CAUTION: See the discussion on niacin under Nutritional Therapy, chapter 14.

Toxins and drugs cause nutritional deficiencies in vitamin C, B$_1$, niacin, and B-complex vitamins. Because drug and chemical residues persist in the body for a long time, they can continue to deplete these vitamins while stored. The scientists recommended the following daily regimen.

- *Niacin*: beginning with 100 mg a day
- *Vitamin B-complex*: 2 tablets each containing 50 mg of most of the B vitamins
- *Vitamin B$_1$*: 250 to 500 mg a day
- *Vitamin A*: 5000 IU (International Units)
- *Vitamin D*: 400 IU

- *Vitamin C*: 250 to 1000 mg, depending on the person's tolerance
- *Multi-mineral*: 1 to 2 tablets a day
- *Cal-Mag formula*: 1 glass

The scientists theorized that the endocrine system needed minerals to work properly and they recommended large quantities of minerals to replace those lost by sweating. Their mineral formulation contained chelated calcium, magnesium, iron, zinc, manganese, copper, potassium, and iodine.

The scientists recommended a Program Case Supervisor to monitor a participant's program daily. The participant keeps a daily report form. The program is considered completed when the person does not feel the effects of past drugs or chemicals, and feels and looks better. People finished the program in an average of 18 to 20 days at five hours per day. At the end of the program, the vitamins, minerals, oil, vegetables, and Cal-Mag are continued at the minimum recommended daily requirements in balanced amounts.

The Hubbard program has been incorporated into many detoxification programs offered today. It represented a breakthrough in treatment as it showed that toxins can be eliminated rather than stored in the body indefinitely.

CURRENT SAUNA DETOXIFICATION PROGRAMS

Most of today's sauna detoxification facilities use a regimen of exercise, sauna, shower, and massage. These specialized units have added to the use of nutritional supplements and aids to detoxification. These units are built of environmentally safe materials and specialize in treating environmentally ill patients rather than patients detoxifying from recreational drugs.

Patients are assisted by programs that promote the mobilization, or release from tissues, then the elimination of xenobiotics, which are chemicals that are foreign to the body. The specific nutrients, vitamins, and minerals that aid detoxification will be discussed more fully in Detoxification Pathways, chapter 3.

Elimination of Xenobiotics   In the current sauna detoxification programs, xenobiotics are eliminated in the urine, feces, breath, tears, skin, and sweat. The following are some of the substances used to aid the elimination process.

- *Sodium potassium bicarbonate*: Helps eliminate toxins in the urine as well as aiding in electrolyte balance.
- *Chlorella*: A single-celled algae that helps eliminate toxins in the feces. The cell wall of chlorella binds to toxic metals, making them easier to remove from the body. It also aids in removing toxic chemicals. In addition, it enhances immune function and has antibacterial and antiviral properties.
- *Psyllium seed*: A bulking agent that helps eliminate toxins and xenobiotics by binding them in the feces so they are not absorbed back into the bloodstream.
- *Activated charcoal*: Helps eliminate toxins and xenobiotics in the feces and adsorbs many times its weight in toxins.

Two of the first special sauna detoxification units in North America are located in Texas and South Carolina. Dr. William Rea of Dallas, Texas, has treated over 20,000 environmentally sensitive patients. His detoxification unit was the first environmentally safe unit constructed in the U.S. Dr. Rea has helped to develop many of the current modalities of the sauna detoxification programs.

Dr. Allan Lieberman of North Charleston, South Carolina, also uses a similar sauna program in his detoxification unit. He reported in 1993 that of 80 environmentally ill or acutely chemically sensitive patients who underwent sauna detoxification at the Center for Environmental Medicine:

- 71% reported improvement in chemical sensitivity
- 21% reported no change in chemical sensitivity
- 8% reported chemical sensitivities became worse

Both the Hubbard method and the current detoxification programs are very effective in reducing the body burden of chemicals and toxins resulting from industrial accumulation or overwhelming exposures. Unless the body is relieved of its xenobiotic burden, it cannot heal. See Recommended Sources and Organizations for a listing of detoxification units. Several of these units have been constructed using environmentally safe materials.

Even if you are unable to go to one of these detoxification units, it is still possible for you to detoxify with the help of a local health care practitioner. Many of the methods discussed in this book can be utilized at home, and some health clubs have saunas that are clean enough to use. While detoxification will not be as rapid, over a period of time you will detoxify.

PART TWO

The Body

3

Detoxification Mechanisms and Pathways

How We Become Toxic

Toxins, defined here as any substance or condition that is harmful to the body, include:

- food
- water
- air
- noise
- chemicals
- heavy metals
- plants
- organisms
- radiation
- electromagnetic fields
- weather
- geopathic stress
- excess of body chemicals
- emotional trauma
- cumulative life experiences

A person's susceptibility and response to toxins varies with age, gender, genetic factors, nutritional status, other diseases, exposure pattern, and behavioral/lifestyle factors. People who have lowered immune defenses or impaired body defense mechanisms (the skin, the lungs, and the gastrointestinal tract) are more likely to be affected by toxins.

Responses to toxins also vary with the nature of the toxin. There is more documented information regarding the effects of chemicals foreign to the body, called xenobiotics, than for other toxins. The body responds to some toxins and detoxifies them in the same way that it detoxifies xenobiotics; other toxins are removed from the body by different mechanisms.

ECOGENETICS

Ecogenetics refers to the genetically determined differences in susceptibility to the toxic effects of xenobiotics. People have different varieties of genes that control detoxification enzymes. Geneticists theorize that as people are exposed to more chemicals, more individuals with chemical susceptibility will be identified. The observed genetic varieties probably represent only a small fraction of the diversity that will be identified.

GENETIC ENZYMATIC DEFECTS

Genetic factors play a role in detoxification, but the efficiency of the detoxification enzymes, other host susceptibilities, and environmental factors play an additional role. A person's susceptibility to chemicals can be caused by one or more of about 50 inherited enzymatic defects. These defects are rare and most have been identified from studying the metabolism of pharmaceutical drugs; they have not been studied in relation to environmental pollutants.

The metabolism of some drugs has been found to be controlled by one gene. Further investigation will probably show that one gene can control the metabolism of many drugs.

ENZYME METABOLISM

One enzyme that metabolizes drugs and chemicals is debrisoquine hydroxylase. It is controlled by one gene, which has different forms (polymorphism). Individuals with slow rates of debrisoquine hydroxylation (poor metabolizers) are found more frequently in European populations than Asian populations.

Parkinson's disease and lung cancer in smokers have been associated with slow metabolism of debrisoquine hydroxylase. In several epidemiologic studies, Parkinson's disease was associated with pesticide use. One may postulate that patients who cannot metabolize and rid their bodies of pesticides may be more susceptible to Parkinson's disease.

Another detoxification enzyme metabolizes S-carboxymethyl cysteine. Many people with food sensitivities are poor metabolizers of this chemical. Vitamin C has increased the activity of this enzyme in a few food-sensitive patients. This may partially explain why large doses of vitamin C are helpful for some allergy patients.

The genetically governed slow metabolism of other enzymes has caused peripheral neuritis (inflamed nerves in hands and feet), increased risk of bladder cancer, and emphysema in some people. Many of these enzymes are also part of the cytochrome P-450 family, a major detoxification system (see below).

Detoxification Mechanisms

The Environmental Protection Agency (EPA) estimates that approximately 500,000 chemicals are in use today, and each year more than 5000 new chemicals are added. Our bodies are exposed to many of these chemicals daily.

We have detoxification mechanisms to rid ourselves of toxins and chemicals. The skin, lungs, gastrointestinal tract, kidneys, and liver are the organs of detoxification, eliminating foreign chemicals, drugs, as well as compounds that the body produces, such as hormones, vitamins, cholesterol, and fatty acids.

Many chemicals that the body absorbs tend to remain in the tissues for long periods of time. Most of these chemicals are lipophilic, that is, they dissolve readily in fat, which is one of the main components of cell membranes. These lipophilic chemicals are complex and difficult for the body to break down and excrete.

Detoxification Pathways

The detoxification process in the body is composed of two phases, known as Phase I and Phase II. These phases are two different biochemical processes that enable the body to eliminate xenobiotics. Fat-soluble (lipophilic) chemicals, which accumulate in the body, are converted to water-soluble substances, which can then be excreted. These detoxification processes occur in the highest concentrations in the liver, but also occur in the skin, lungs, and intestines.

PHASE I DETOXIFICATION

Phase I detoxification changes nonpolar, non-water-soluble chemicals into relatively polar (electrically charged) compounds with the help of enzymes by adding a polar group or a reactive group. These changes are a type of chemical reaction known as biotransformation. Some typical changes are:

- eliminate a sulfur group and add an oxygen group (desulfuration)
- eliminate a halogen group and add an oxygen group (dehalogenation)
- lose an electron (oxidation)
- gain an electron after an atom of oxygen is added to the molecule (reduction)

The Phase I enzymes are known as the cytochrome P-450 monooxygenase system, and the mixed-function amine oxidase system. The cytochrome P-450 system is the major system.

Many forms of cytochrome P-450 are involved in Phase I reactions. The highest concentration of cytochrome P-450 occurs in the liver, and it is the site of the most active metabolism. Cytochrome P-450 has also been found in the intestines, adrenal cortex, testes, spleen, heart, muscles, brain, and skin. The lungs and the kidneys are secondary organs of biotransformation, having about one-third of the liver's detoxification capacity.

The action of detoxification enzymes depends on the presence of various minerals. For example, alcohol dehydrogenase, which converts alcohols (such as ethanol) to aldehydes, depends on an adequate supply of zinc to function properly. In the next step in alcohol metabolism, aldehyde oxidase changes the aldehyde into an acid that can be excreted in the urine. Aldehyde oxidase depends on an adequate supply of molybdenum and iron.

Usually, these enzymatic reactions decrease chemical toxicity. However, unless there is a balance with Phase II, toxic or reactive chemicals can form during Phase I metabolism, and these metabolites are more toxic than the original compound. This is known as bioactivation. Teratogens (causing fetus malformation), mutagens (causing cell mutation), and carcinogens (causing cancer) have been identified that can adversely affect the liver and other areas of the body. For example, benzo[a]pyrene, a chemical in coal tar and cigarette sidestream smoke, is biologically inert until it is converted by the mixed-function oxidases into a metabolite that can then initiate cancer-causing activity. Many compounds form dangerous reactive free radicals, chemicals with an unpaired electron that can cause tissue damage. (See Free Radicals, chapter 9, for further discussion.) Some people are at risk for cancer from a buildup of these free radicals.

Because of the possibility of more toxic compounds forming in the case of an imbalance between Phase I and Phase II, it has been suggested that biotransformation is a more appropriate term than detoxification when describing Phase I and Phase II. When the more toxic compounds form, it is not a detoxification process, but biotransformation. However, we have consistently used the term detoxification because it is more frequently used in the literature describing the Phase I and Phase II reactions.

Phase I of the detoxification pathway can be measured with a caffeine metabolism test. Phase II can be evaluated by the ingestion of acetaminophen (Tylenol) and aspirin, and measuring the percent recovery of conjugation products of these compounds. A known quantity of caffeine is ingested, and saliva samples are obtained twice after the caffeine has been ingested. Rapid clearance of caffeine shows enzyme induction (increased production), either from xenobiotic exposure or toxins within the body. Low caffeine clearance indicates that cytochrome P-450 activity in the liver is abnormal. Patients with low caffeine clearance would have difficulty eliminating xenobiotics.

The following nutrients aid in Phase I detoxification, and many of them are used in sauna detoxification programs. For more information on the specific nutrients listed below, see Nutritional Therapy, chapter 14.

- *Alpha-ketoglutaric acid*: Helps to detoxify ammonia. Addition of an ammonia group to this acid forms glutamic acid, which is then transformed to glutamine, providing the major pathway for removing ammonia from the body.
- *Choline*: When combined with an acetyl group helps increase intestinal peristalsis (contractions during digestion); this in turn aids in elimination of toxins. Cytochrome P-450 enzymes are dependent on choline.
- *Fatty acids*: Speed up transit time of the stool, averting buildup of toxins and reducing toxic load for the liver.
- *Lecithin*: Used with oils. Its action allows safe transport of fats through the bloodstream.

- *Methionine*: Because of its sulfur content helps to remove heavy metals from the body; adds a methyl group to xenobiotics that aids in their excretion from the body; precursor for other sulfur amino acids.
- *Milk thistle*: Helps to detoxify the liver of alcohol and various pollutants.
- *Recommended oils*: The body exchanges these oils for contaminated fat, which is eliminated through bile excretion and feces. The oils also decrease plasma cholesterol, encouraging fecal excretion.

Phase I Vitamins

- *Beta-carotene*: Converted in the body to vitamin A, which helps to protect the lipid portion of the cell membrane. It promotes the healthy intestinal mucosa necessary for absorption of other nutrients. Vitamin A is also necessary for the conversion of alcohols to aldehydes.
- *Vitamin B_1*: Thiamine pyrophosphate, the coenzyme form of thiamine (the form most easily utilized by the body), is necessary for moving an aldehyde group from one molecule to another. It is needed for the enzyme necessary for glutathione regeneration.
- *Vitamin C*: Increases antioxidant protection and is necessary for electron transport. The action of cytochrome P-450 is dependent on vitamin C.
- *Vitamin E*: Antioxidant that prevents the formation of peroxides, and the oxidation of vitamins A and K, and fat-soluble hormones. Vitamin E helps to prevent an overactive cytochrome P-450 enzyme system, which can be a source of free radicals.

Phase I Minerals

- *Copper*: Activates several enzymes. It is in superoxide dismutase.

- *Iron*: Contained in cytochrome P-450.
- *Magnesium*: Necessary for glutathione synthesis, ammonia detoxification, and oxidative phosphorylation (produces ATP, the main source of energy for the body).
- *Manganese*: In the enzymes superoxide dismutase and glutathione synthetase.
- *Molybdenum*: In aldehyde oxidase, which helps change aldehydes to acids that are excreted in the urine.
- *Sulfur*: All glutathione enzymes contain sulfur.
- *Zinc*: In alcohol dehydrogenase, a Phase I enzyme.

PHASE II DETOXIFICATION

In Phase II detoxification, chemical groups are added, or conjugated, to the chemical. The chemical is now water-soluble and can be excreted through the kidneys. Major conjugation reactions include:

- *Acetylation*: Addition of acetyl Co-A to form a mercapturic acid conjugate. Chief degradation pathway for aromatic (aryl) amines, sulfur amides, and aliphatic amines.
- *Acylation*: Peptide conjugation using acyl Co-A and amino acids, taurine, glycine, and glutamine.
- *Gluconation (Glucuronidation)*: Addition of a sugar group, using glucuronic acid; the major conjugation reaction for xenobiotics and body chemicals.
- *Methylation*: Addition of a methyl (CH_3) group, and using the amino acid methionine.
- *Sulfonation*: Adds inorganic sulfate to hydroxyl groups for detoxification and requires high energy.

Phase II of the detoxification pathway can be evaluated by ingestion of acetaminophen and aspirin, and measuring the recovery of the products of glutathione conjugation, sulfation, glucuronidation, and glycine conjugation.

The following nutrients aid in Phase II detoxification, and many of them are used in sauna detoxification programs. For more information on the specific nutrients listed below, see Nutritional Therapy in chapter 14.

- *Cysteine*: Detoxifies pesticides, plastics, hydrocarbons, and other chemicals.
- *Garlic*: Aids in detoxification because of its high sulfur content; very helpful in removing heavy metals.
- *D-Glucarate*: Helps in major conjugation reaction in converting xenobiotics to polar water-soluble compounds.
- *Glycine*: Stimulates the production of glutathione. It also aids in the detoxification of benzoic acid and phenol.
- *L-glutathione (reduced form)*: An antioxidant that conjugates with metabolites of xenobiotics to increase their water solubility, enabling excretion by the kidney.
- *N-acetyl cysteine*: Converted by the body to cysteine, which along with vitamin C detoxifies pesticides, plastics, hydrocarbons, and other chemicals.
- *Taurine*: Helps peptide conjugation of xenobiotics.

Phase II Vitamins

- *Folic acid*: The coenzyme form is an intermediate carrier for methylation.
- *Vitamin B_1*: Needed for glutathione regeneration. Provides energy for conjugation.
- *Vitamin B_2*: Necessary for the enzyme glutathione reductase.
- *Vitamin B_3*: Essential for recycling glutathione.
- *Vitamin B_5*: Pantothenic acid is bound to coenzyme A, a carrier of acetyl groups.

This combination is essential in acetyl conjugations of several classes of chemicals. It is also important in transamination processes.
- *Vitamin B_6*: Required for the metabolism of methionine for glutathione. A deficiency of B_6 slows conjugation.
- *Vitamin B_{12}*: The coenzyme form participates in reactions in which methyl groups are transferred.

Phase II Minerals

- *Germanium*: Helps with toxic metal detoxification. It raises glutathione levels for Phase II detoxification, increases oxygen utilization at cell levels, and is a free-radical scavenger.
- *Magnesium*: Necessary for glutathione production and is a mineral activator for many detoxification enzymes. Methyltransferase requires magnesium.
- *Manganese*: Required for glutathione production, as well as for enzymes necessary to detoxification pathways.
- *Molybdenum*: Helps in the synthesis and use of sulfur amino acids, is a component of detoxification enzymes, and is necessary for utilization of vitamin C at cell level.
- *Selenium*: Is in glutathione peroxide.
- *Sulfur*: In the form of sulfates, with the enzyme sulfotransferase, enables the conjugation process of sulfonation. This process results in products that are less toxic and more easily excreted than the original compound.
- *Zinc*: In enzymes necessary for conjugation.

Dr. Jeffrey Bland, of HealthComm in Washington State, studied patients with chronic fatigue. Patients had different speeds of metabolism during Phase I and Phase II. Dr. Bland found that 55% of patients were fast/fast metabolizers (normal), 30% were slow/slow metabolizers, and 15% were fast/slow metabolizers during Phase I/Phase II, respectively. Patients with fast/slow enzymatic systems are at most risk for problems.

Fast/slow patients are at risk for cancer from a buildup of the free radicals formed during Phase I detoxification. Free radicals are chemicals with an unpaired electron that can cause tissue damage. (See Free Radicals, chapter 9 for further discussion.)

4

Organs of Protection and Detoxification

Toxins can enter the body in three ways:

- absorption through the skin
- inhalation through the respiratory tract into the lungs
- ingestion through the mouth into the gastrointestinal tract

The skin, lungs, and intestines have developed some protective mechanisms and methods of detoxification, although the liver is the major organ of detoxification for the body.

The Skin

The skin consists of two layers. The outer layer, the epidermis, is made of epithelial cells. The inner layer, the dermis, is composed of connective tissue.

THE EPIDERMIS

This outer layer of protective skin is approximately 1 millimeter thick and is replenished every 14 days. Called the stratum corneum, the layer is pigmented and varies in thickness in different areas of the body, determining how easily chemicals can penetrate the skin. An exception is the palm of the hand, where the stratum corneum is thicker than in other areas of the body, yet absorbs chemicals more readily.

New skin cells form in the basal cell layer, entirely replacing itself approximately once a month. Melanocyte cells produce melanin pigment, which determines skin color. Melanin also protects against ultraviolet injury, sunburn, and skin cancer. Melanin absorbs ultraviolet and visible light, and quenches free radicals.

Epidermal cells produce lipids and a protein called keratin. Lipids, which include cholesterol and free fatty acids, help protect the skin against water loss and help the stratum corneum cells stick together properly. The epidermis produces vitamin D_3 with the aid of sunlight.

THE DERMIS

A tight junction transports substances between the epidermis and the thicker dermis. The dermis consists of the proteins collagen and elastin. They make the skin elastic and give it strength.

The dermis also contains the eccrine and apocrine sweat glands, sebaceous glands, and hair follicles. Eccrine sweat glands are distributed over the body's surface, helping to regulate its temperature. Sebaceous glands are located near hair follicles. They secrete sebum, a lipid mixture that has some antibacterial and antifungal properties. Sebum helps the body excrete lipid-soluble toxins.

HOW TOXINS ENTER THE SKIN

Solvents can easily penetrate the skin because of their lipid (fat) solubility. Caustic chemicals, such as acids and alkaline solutions, can also penetrate the skin. Once a chemical has penetrated the stratum corneum, it moves through the epidermis into the dermis. Then the rich blood supply of the dermis readily transports the chemical into the bloodstream.

The amount of toxins that the skin absorbs is determined by several factors:

- The thickness of the stratum corneum affects how rapidly a chemical is absorbed.
- Oily solutions usually penetrate the skin more readily. The stratum corneum acts like a lipophilic membrane and absorbs lipids or fats readily.
- To be absorbed, a toxin must also be somewhat water-soluble. Toxins that are only lipid-soluble or only water-soluble are poorly absorbed.
- When the skin is wet, water-soluble chemicals penetrate more easily.
- Organic solvents are rapidly absorbed across the skin.
- At higher environmental temperatures, the skin absorbs more.
- Thin plastic against the skin, such as wearing gloves, increases absorption.
- Some toxins are absorbed directly through hair follicles.
- Chemicals penetrate injured skin more easily than intact skin.

Drugs, steroid hormones, and xenobiotics can be metabolized by the skin as it contains the enzyme cytochrome P-450. The skin converts chemicals into more water-soluble forms, which can then be excreted from the body more readily.

PROTECTIVE DEVICES

Barrier creams do not usually block absorption of toxins through the skin. Rubber gloves may be useful, but some chemicals and microorganisms can penetrate the gloves.

The Lungs

As we breathe, oxygen enters the respiratory tract and travels to the lungs. The lungs supply oxygen to the cells of the body, then expel the metabolic byproduct carbon dioxide.

The upper air passage of the respiratory tract consists of the nose, the pharynx, the hypopharynx, and the larynx, which houses the vocal cords. The lower air passage stretches from the vocal cords through the trachea to the bronchioles.

Air enters the upper passage, then traverses the trachea. The trachea is surrounded by rings, which can be felt in the neck. This area is the narrowest cross-section of the entire airway. The trachea branches into the right and left mainstem bronchi behind the ribcage. One bronchi enters each lung. The bronchi then divide into two to three more branches, called bronchioles. The bronchioles lead to air sacs called alveolar sacs or alveoli. Their total surface area is estimated to be 70 square meters.

Inhaling brings oxygen into millions of alveoli. Oxygen molecules diffuse across a single-cell membrane to the capillaries. Oxygen then combines with hemoglobin in the red blood cells and is carried to the rest of the body. Exhaling diffuses carbon dioxide molecules from the capillaries into the alveoli and expels them from the body through the bronchial tubes.

HOW TOXINS AFFECT THE LUNGS

Three diseases affect the bronchial tube system of the lungs: asthma, bronchitis, and emphysema. Asthma is characterized by attacks of difficulty in breathing. Bronchitis is inflammation of the bronchial tubes. Toxins can trigger both asthma and bronchitis, which are reversible in their early stages. The toxins in cigarette smoke can cause both chronic bronchitis and emphysema. Emphysema ruins lung elasticity by destroying the walls separating the alveoli from one another, creating tiny craters. Other alveoli become permanently enlarged. Emphysema is irreversible.

The lungs have the greatest exposure to the environment. Gases, small solid particles, and liquid aerosols can easily enter the lungs and be deposited in three ways: impaction, sedimentation, and diffusion.

Impaction In impaction, large particles continue in straight paths through the airway passages. Most larger particles land on the surface of the nose and throat area (nasopharynx) or at the branching of the larger airways. These particles become embedded in mucus or trapped by nasal hairs and are eliminated by sneezing, swallowing, or blowing the nose. The nose and throat remove particles greater than 20 microns in diameter. The nasopharynx removes 95% of particles 5 microns or larger.

Sedimentation Medium-sized particles, 1 micron (the size of a cell) to 5 microns in diameter, are deposited in the lungs by sedimentation. They settle more slowly than the larger particles. The medium-sized particles land in the mucus layer of the more distant (peripheral) airways. These particles are eventually moved up in the mucus and exhaled or swallowed. If the particles do reach the air sacs (or alveoli) or smaller airways, they can become trapped permanently and may damage the lungs.

Diffusion The smallest aerosol particles, less than 0.1 micron in diameter, are deposited in the lungs by diffusion. Many small particles are exhaled immediately, while those that are trapped can cause lung disease, known as pneumoconiosis. Two types of pneumoconiosis are asbestosis, caused by asbestos fibers, and silicosis, caused by silica dust.

Gases Gases are absorbed differently in the respiratory tract, depending on their solubility, flow rate, and duration of exposure. Some gases dissolve in the fluid that lines the epithelium, which are the cells that line the respiratory tract. Most absorption of gases takes place in the upper air passages.

The nose absorbs gases more readily if the air flow increases. This may account for some of the increased absorption of gases that people have when they are physically active. It is also possible that during the exposure the gas may alter the lining fluid so that absorption increases.

PROTECTIVE DEVICES

The lungs protect themselves against environmental pollutants with filters, epithelial barriers, enzyme systems, and immune responses. Filters include mucus and cilia. The mucociliary system traps pollutants and moves them out of the lungs. A person can then sneeze and cough out the irritants.

Mucus is produced by glands that are located in the area beneath the epithelial lining cells. Certain cells contain cilia, which are hairlike projections that beat in a synchronized fashion about 1000 times per minute. This motion helps to move particulate matter out of the lungs. However, cilia cannot transport particles if no mucus is present. Influenza virus can paralyze these cilia, thus leading to secondary bacterial infections. Some people have a condition known as immotile cilia syndrome, and they are prone to sinus and respiratory tract infections.

Lungs also have epithelial barriers. Alveolar macrophages, a type of white cell, ingest particles, and kill bacteria and viruses, which they then present to lymphocytes. The lymphocytes, another type of white cell, destroy them. The alveolar macrophages also contain aryl hydrocarbon hydroxylase, a type of enzyme that detoxifies chemicals.

In addition, an enzyme system helps to protect the lungs. When particles are inhaled, inflammatory enzymes, known as proteases, are released. These proteases can damage the lung cells or the connective tissue in the lungs. Specific proteins known as antiproteases protect the alveoli. These antiproteases combine with proteases to inactivate them. Cigarette smoke destroys the balance between proteases and antiproteases maintained by the lungs, shifting the balance to the activity of the proteases. The most common antiprotease is alpha-1-antitrypsin. People with a deficiency of this antiprotease are prone to emphysema.

The lungs contain enzymes from the mixed-function oxidase family (cytochrome P-450), enabling them to metabolize drugs and xenobiotics to more water-soluble chemicals, which can then be excreted by the kidneys.

The lungs also have antioxidants to counteract free radicals. Some antioxidant enzymes found in the lungs are superoxide dismutase, glutathione enzymes, and catalase. In addition, alveolar lining fluid, containing transferrin, ceruloplasmin, and glutathione, protects the lungs from oxidant stress. Vitamin E, an antioxidant found in cell membranes, protects the lungs against toxic lipid peroxides produced by the cell membranes of the lungs when attacked by organisms. Fluid lining the alveoli from patients who smoke cigarettes can be deficient in vitamin E.

Finally, the lungs have immune responses to protect them against inhaled organisms. Lymphocytes in the lungs produce immunoglobulins (antibodies), and they cross from the blood into the lungs. Immunoglobulins IgA, IgG, and IgE have all been found in the respiratory tract. IgA neutralizes many viruses, and it seems to prevent antigen absorption across the lung cells. T-lymphocytes help protect the lungs against microbes and tumor cells. T-lymphocytes also release lymphokines, molecules that activate and stimulate macrophages (white blood cells that ingest foreign material).

The Gastrointestinal Tract

The gastrointestinal (GI) tract includes the mouth, pharynx, esophagus, stomach, small intestine, large intestine, and rectum. The other portion of the gastrointestinal system is made up of glandular organs that secrete substances into the gastrointestinal tract. These glands include the salivary glands, liver, gallbladder, and pancreas. The function of the gastrointestinal system is to process the food we eat into a form that the circulatory system can distribute to the cells of the body.

The GI tract is a tube that runs through the body from the mouth to the anus. In adults, this tube is approximately 15 feet long. The lumen, which is the interior of this tube, is connected with the outside world in that, technically, its contents are outside the body. For example, millions of bacteria populate the large intestine. Most are helpful, but if these bacteria should leave the intestine and enter the body, they are harmful and can be lethal.

Food is taken into the mouth where it is mixed with saliva, which contains an enzyme that begins processing the food. This enzyme, amylase, aids in digesting carbohydrates. The saliva moistens and lubricates the food particles so they may be swallowed easily. It also dissolves some of the molecules of the food particles so they can react with receptors in the mouth to cause the sensation of taste.

The pharynx and esophagus serve as a pathway to deliver the food from the mouth to the stomach. The spontaneous movement of these two parts of the gastrointestinal tract controls the process of swallowing.

The stomach mixes the food with hydrochloric acid, pepsin, gastrin, and mucus. The pepsin processes protein, and gastrin stimulates the release of hydrochloric acid. These materials break the food down into even smaller particles, and the resulting mixture is known as chyme. In addition to breaking down the particles of food, the hydrochloric acid also kills almost all the bacteria that enter the body with the food. Some do survive and subsequently begin to live and multiply in the large intestine.

The stomach also stores food while it is being partially digested. It then delivers fluid and partially digested food to the small intestine in amounts that allow for maximum digestion and absorption.

The last stages of digestion and absorption take place in the small intestine. Enzymes from the pancreas break down chyme into monosaccharides, fatty acids, and amino acids. These substances then cross the layer of epithelial cells that line the intestinal wall and enter the blood and lymph.

A small volume of water, minerals, and undigested material passes into the large intestine. This material is temporarily stored and acted upon by the intestinal bacteria. The large intestine concentrates the material by removing water. The concentrated material is then eliminated from the body through defecation when the rectum becomes distended. The eliminated material is called feces and consists of a small amount of food that was not digested or absorbed, and bacteria, which contribute to the bulk of the feces.

The gastrointestinal tract is an important route for the absorption of toxins. The intestines are affected by bacteria; viruses; yeasts and parasites; food and plant ingredients; and toxins in food, water, and the environment. The mucosal surface of the stomach and intestines is 200 times that of the body surface area, making it a major route for exposure of the body to toxins.

HOW TOXINS ENTER THE GI TRACT

Toxins enter the body through the stomach. Toxins may be ingested in food or water, or they may be swallowed from the nasopharynx. Absorption depends on the amount ingested, the lipid solubility, molecular size, and pH of the toxin. Digestive enzymes, hydrochloric acid, and bile acids also affect the absorption and metabolism of a toxin.

Xenobiotics are absorbed into the gastrointestinal tract by diffusion, active transport, and pinocytosis (absorption of liquid by cells). Absorption depends on the degree of xenobiotic water solubility, the degree of ionization, and the size of the molecule.

Most foreign chemicals are not metabolized in the intestinal tract. To be absorbed, chemicals must be made soluble before they come into contact with the intestinal mucosa. The intestinal absorption is affected by gastric emptying time, intestinal motility, the size and condition of the surface area of the small intestine, blood flow to the intestine, diet, genetic factors, and age. A poorly nourished person can be more easily affected by toxins.

Chemicals are usually absorbed slowly from the GI tract, but the amount absorbed depends on how fast the chemicals move through it. The faster the chemical moves, the less is absorbed.

PROTECTIVE DEVICES

The GI tract has various defense mechanisms against bacteria, viruses, yeasts, parasites, and toxins. It is protected by enzymes, mucus, normal intestinal bacteria, intestinal secretions, and the innermost layer of epithelial cells. Digestion, metabolism, detoxification, secretion, elimination, and the normal turnover of cells can affect organisms and toxins.

In the stomach, pepsin and hydrochloric acid can affect chemicals and toxins. The intestines contain bile acids and various enzymes, such as proteases, lipases, and glucuronidases, which can affect chemicals and toxins. Unabsorbed chemicals reach their highest concentration in the colon (large intestine).

In the intestines the first barrier to the absorption of chemicals is the unstirred water layer. It is a layer of immobile fluid that coats the intestinal mucosa. This unstirred water layer has a mucus layer and an acid microlayer that is rich in protons (particles with a positive charge). It acts as a barrier to the chemical penetration of the mucosa. Chemicals often diffuse through the unstirred water layer more slowly than they would penetrate a cell membrane. The unstirred water layer delays the absorption of nonpolar chemicals, which do not have an electrical charge and are lipophilic. Pesticides, dyes, and food additives are examples of nonpolar chemicals.

The second barrier to the absorption of chemicals is gastrointestinal mucus. Mucus protects the intestinal mucosa from physical and chemical injury, and acts as a lubricant. Cells in the esophagus, stomach, small intestine, and large intestine all produce mucus. Mucus consists of 95% water with the remainder consisting of salts, proteins, nucleic acids, and mucins. Mucins, made up of carbohydrates, lipids, and proteins, give mucus its viscous, gel-like texture. Mucus is sticky and can trap large molecules, such as metals. It can also trap parasites and bacteria, and can bind viruses, helping to eliminate them.

The third barrier to absorption of chemicals is the acid microclimate layer, consisting mostly of protons. This layer has a 5.9 pH, which is acidic, compared to the 7.3 pH of the small intestine, which is mildly alkaline.

The ileum, the third part of the small intestine, has a low population of bacteria. However, beyond the ileocecal valve, where the large intestine joins the small intestine, the bacterial concentration increases dramatically. More than 400 species of bacteria reside in the colon. Intestinal bacteria metabolize drugs and other chemicals.

Bacteria may metabolize chemicals in a manner completely opposite to the body's metabolism. While detoxification enzymes in humans convert fat-soluble chemicals to water-soluble chemicals, bacteria often do the reverse, converting water-soluble chemicals to fat-soluble chemicals.

DETOXIFICATION

Both Phase I and Phase II detoxification systems are found in the GI tract. Phase I changes the chemicals so that Phase II can add a small molecule (see chapter 3). The GI tract has the same biotransformation enzymes as the liver, but metabolism in the GI tract is slower than that of the liver. The GI tract can transform a xenobiotic to either a less toxic chemical or a more toxic chemical.

The mixed-function oxidase system is most active in the duodenum, the first part of the small intestine. The activity decreases from the duodenum to the colon. The mature enterocytes, the lining cells of the intestine, contain the largest amount of cytochrome P-450 activity.

When people go on starvation or semi-starvation diets, the activity of many of the metabolic enzymes decreases. Herbicides can decrease or increase enzymatic activity. Iron deficiency and selenium deficiency can reduce cytochrome P-450 activity. Cruciferous plants (cabbage, cauliflower, broccoli) increase the activity of the mixed-function oxidase system in the liver and the small intestines. Enzyme activity in a portion of the small intestine called the jejunum has been found to be lower in females than in males. The very young and the very old seem to have less detoxification enzyme activity.

Cells lining the intestinal walls can secrete xenobiotics into the intestines. Strong acids and digitalis compounds are secreted from the bloodstream into the intestinal lumen. Lipophilic toxins can be excreted faster if a person is given cholestyramine (a resin drug, which is used to lower cholesterol levels) or paraffin. Activated charcoal can bind poisons, so that they can be excreted from the intestines.

Intestinal cells are shed very rapidly, and they are some of the most actively dividing cells in the body. Up to 100 cells per hour are formed in the intestines, and billions of cells are shed every day. Metals and lipophilic chemicals seem to be excreted from the intestines by the shedding of epithelial cells.

IMMUNE RESPONSES

Antibodies (IgA) are secreted into the intestines, and lymphocytes are released from clusters found in Peyer's patches (lymphoid nodules) in the intestines. Approximately one-quarter of the cells in the intestinal mucosa are lymphocytes. All parts of this system work together to protect the GI tract.

The Liver

The liver is a dome-shaped gland that fits under the diaphragm, and it is the largest gland in the body. It has six main functions:

- storage of carbohydrates, vitamins, and minerals
- metabolism of hormones, endogenous wastes, and foreign chemicals
- synthesis of blood proteins
- formation of urea
- metabolism of fats, proteins, and carbo-hydrates
- formation of bile and gamma globulin
- assimilation and storage of fat-soluble vitamins

The liver consists of five lobes composed of cells called lobules, held together by alveolar tissue.

The central vein, on the side of the liver, drains away waste products from several liver lobules. The cells of the lobule closest to the central vein are known as centrilobular hepatocytes (liver cells). Cytochrome P-450 is mostly concentrated in these centrilobular cells.

On the other side of the liver, the hepatic artery and portal vein are known as the periportal system. It supplies oxygen and nutrients to the liver cells. The cells of the lobule closest to the portal artery are called periportal hepatocytes.

Periportal liver cells have the highest concentration of oxygen and nutrients because the liver is the first organ to receive nutrients absorbed by the GI tract. Periportal cells also have higher concentrations of glutathione and transaminase enzymes, which are the enzymes that are tested in the standard blood chemistry test. These cells have the highest exposure to xenobiotics.

The liver is situated to receive a majority of the venous blood from the lower body, the kidneys, the spleen, and the gastrointestinal tract.

BIOTRANSFORMATION OF CHEMICALS

The liver is the main organ for biotransformation of chemicals. It can remove chemicals absorbed into the blood, regardless of how the chemical entered into the body. However, the liver is susceptible to tissue injury from the toxic effects of chemicals.

Some chemicals induce liver metabolism while others inhibit the activity of cytochrome P-450. Chemicals can cause inhibition in three ways:

- competitive binding to and metabolism by cytochrome P-450
- inhibition of heme or cytochrome P-450 synthesis
- inactivation or destruction of cytochrome P-450 or the endoplasmic reticulum

Inhibition of cytochrome P-450 can lead to the toxicity of other chemicals. If they are not metabolized, these chemicals build up in the body. For example, theophylline is a drug used to control asthma and is in the same family as caffeine. It can build up to toxic levels if the patient is given erythromycin simultaneously. Erythromycin inhibits the cytochrome P-450 enzyme system from breaking down the theophylline. Erythromycin and antifungals such as keto-conazole can also inhibit the breakdown of Seldane, an antihistamine. High levels of Seldane can cause heart rhythm disturbances. For further discussion on the liver, see Organ Cleansing in chapter 17.

The Kidneys

Paired organs that are the principal excretory organs in all vertebrates, the kidneys lie in the back of the abdominal wall, one on each side of the backbone. They are bean-shaped, and on the concave side of each one is an area called the hilus, where the renal artery enters and renal vein exits.

The kidneys filter the blood and drain wastes, mostly breakdown products of protein metabolism. In addition, they regulate acid-base (pH) balance, calcium metabolism, electrolyte balance, and extracellular volume (circulating fluid outside the cells). The kidneys play a role in vitamin D metabolism, regulate blood pressure by the renin-angiotension pathway, and eliminate foreign chemicals from the body.

The kidneys have a higher blood flow than even the brain, liver, or heart, and receive 25% of the body's total blood volume, causing high exposure to chemicals in the blood. They reabsorb and redistribute 99% of the volume of this blood, and 0.1% of the blood filtered becomes urine.

Approximately 10% of the normal resting oxygen consumption of the body is used by the kidneys.

STRUCTURE OF THE KIDNEY

The kidney consists of the outer cortex and the inner medulla. The cortex receives 85% of the total renal blood flow and is composed of nephrons, which are excretory units. Each kidney has over one million nephrons. The nephron has three parts:

- The vascular or blood circulation component composed of interconnected capillaries.
- The glomerulus, the filtering agent of the kidney. Most proteins are too large to pass through the pores of the glomeruli. If a substance is completely bound to a protein, it is not eliminated from the body. Some of the partially protein-bound substances are excreted.
- The tubules reabsorb 98% to 99% of the salts and water of the glomerular filtrate. Seventy-five percent of the glomerular filtrate fluid is reabsorbed in the first part of the tubular system. The kidney concentrates the urine in the last tubule, the collecting duct, with the aid of a hormone known as antidiuretic hormone, or vasopressin.

The nephron tubular element joins the ureter, a collecting duct, which exits from the same side of the kidney as the renal vein and artery. The ureter carries the urine to the bladder, which is a balloon-shaped chamber that is folded when empty. As urine enters the bladder, its walls of smooth muscle unfold to the volume needed to contain the urine. When the bladder becomes distended with urine, receptors are stimulated to contract the bladder. The urine then flows under voluntary control through the urethra, and out of the body.

DETOXIFICATION

Phase II detoxification converts fat-soluble non-polar substances into more polar substances. This makes them less fat-soluble and less likely to be reabsorbed by the kidney tubules. They are then available for excretion.

Some chemicals (ammonia, for example) are secreted by the tubules and move from the peritubular capillaries into fluid in the lumen of the tubule. They are then eliminated from the body in the urine.

Tubule cells are also capable of catabolizing (breaking down) certain organic compounds taken up from either the peritubular capillaries or the tubular lumen. This catabolism causes their elimination even though they have not actually been excreted in the urine.

The kidneys have a transport system for both positively and negatively charged chemicals. In the transport system, chemicals may compete for a given chemical pathway, or one may inhibit the excretion of the other.

Other Routes of Excretion

The hair, sweat, fingernails and toenails, and breast milk are minor routes of excretion. Hair can be used to estimate the amount of toxic exposures. Chronic lead poisoning is better estimated by hair lead levels than by blood lead levels.

Breast milk contains 3% to 5% fat, and lipophilic chemicals can be excreted in breast milk. Polychlorinated biphenyls (PCBS) and DDT have been found in breast milk. Cow's milk containing the same amount of DDT as is frequently found in breast milk would be banned by the FDA. Toxic metals, such as lead, can also be excreted in breast milk.

The Environmental Protection Agency (EPA) states that the average American breast-fed baby ingests nine times the permissible level of dieldrin, a cancer-causing pesticide, and ten times the maximum allowable level of PCBS. PCB has been found to cause birth defects and cancer in animals in the parts per billion range. During lactation, stores of body fat are mobilized, which then release their stored toxins into the bloodstream. Women who have more stored toxins probably release more toxins into their breast milk.

In spite of these possible toxins in breast milk, breast feeding is still preferable to bottle feeding because it decreases the possibility of autoimmune disease, reduces ear infections, and decreases respiratory disease. Women who plan to nurse their babies should avoid toxic exposures and undergo detoxification procedures before pregnancy, if possible. Women who are pregnant should under no circumstances undergo detoxification while pregnant, but try to live and eat as cleanly as they can.

Cow's milk also has been found to be contaminated with such chemicals as dieldrin, heptachlor epoxide (a metabolite of a pesticide), lindane (pesticide), and DDT. Infant formula that is composed of cow's milk can also contain this contamination.

Tears are another minor route of excretion for the body. Both emotional and irritant tears contain three chemicals known to be released by the body during stress. These are adrenocorticotropic hormone (ACTH), the most reliable indicator of stress; leucine-emhyphalin, an endorphine that probably modulates pain sensation; and prolactin, a hormone that regulates milk production in mammals.

PART THREE

Types and Sources of Toxins

5

External Toxins: Food, Water, Air, and Noise

External Toxins

External toxins are found in our world's air, food, and water. Indoor and outdoor air pollution, toxins found in food and water, xenobiotics (foreign and synthetic chemicals), toxic metals, and poisons produced by plants or microorganisms are all external toxins. Other external elements, including radiation, electromagnetic fields, and weather, can also be toxic and will be discussed in the following chapters. Even emotional trauma can be considered an external toxin when people are subjected to abuse.

Foods

Contaminants and additives cause food to be toxic. Food contaminants include microorganisms and the toxins they produce, pesticides, and various other chemicals. Additives are chemicals that can be legally added to food.

CHEMICAL CONTAMINATION

Food can be contaminated by:

- natural and synthetic organic chemicals, and radioactive substances
- diffusion of small amounts of chemicals through the environment, large-scale industrial accidents, or waste disposal
- pesticides used on crops
- irrigation water used on crops

- exposures during food processing
- toxic metals from sewer sludge used as fertilizer
- herbicide and chemical fertilizer residues

The Food and Drug Administration (FDA), the Food Safety Inspection Service of the U.S. Department of Agriculture (USDA), and the Environmental Protection Agency (EPA) monitor food contamination in the U.S. The FDA analyzes 234 food items for pesticides, toxic chemicals, industrial chemicals, and radionuclides, but this amounts to only 1% of the food sold. Only half of the pesticides used can be detected by current testing methods. Imported foods are analyzed for pesticides banned in the United States. The Global Environment Monitoring System (GEMS) analyzes food contamination from countries around the world.

Pesticide Residues   Pesticides are regulated in the U.S. by the FDA, the USDA, and the EPA. Unfortunately, the 600 active pesticides registered before 1984 have not been adequately tested. If new evidence is found that a pesticide already in use is more dangerous than it was thought, the EPA initiates a Special Review. This process can take 12 years or more, during which the pesticide can still be used. The reregistration process is very slow, and by 1991 less than 2% of the older pesticides had been re-evaluated.

The United Nations Food and Agriculture

Organization (FAO) and the World Health Organization (WHO) have developed Acceptable Daily Intakes (ADI), which are levels of pesticides that can be ingested over a lifetime and do not seem to create a significant risk. The EPA has established a standard known as reference doses (RfDs), which have a safety factor of 100% in the calculations. The RfDs and ADIs do not always agree. None of these regulatory agencies have modified their calculations to account for the synergistic effects of pesticides or chronic health problems. The RfDs were established several decades ago and have not been updated.

The sale of pesticides, which include insecticides, herbicides, and fungicides, increased by five times from 1985 to 1990. Although DDT was banned in the United States in 1973, all people in the United States have residues of DDT or its metabolite DDE in their fat tissue. DDT can still be found in the fatty tissue of such foods as meat, fish, poultry, and in dairy products because it persists in the soil. Organophosphate insecticide residues may be found in grains and cereals.

U.S. manufacturers are allowed to continue to produce pesticides that are banned, unregistered, or restricted as long as the pesticides are exported. Third World countries then use these pesticides, and up to 70% of the foods grown with the use of these unregistered or restricted pesticides is imported back into the United States.

Polycyclic Aromatic Hydrocarbons About 100 polycyclic aromatic hydrocarbons (PAHS) have been found in foods. These chemicals are mutagenic (they change DNA) and/or carcinogenic. Food that has contact with petroleum and coal tar products is contaminated with PAHS. All charbroiled and smoked foods contain PAHS, and seafood may contain PAHS because of bioaccumulation from polluted water. In some countries an association between consuming foods high in PAHS and gastrointestinal cancer has

been demonstrated. Polycyclical aromatic hydrocarbons have been found in the body fat, liver, adrenal glands, and ovaries.

Industrial Chemicals Polychlorinated biphenyls (PCBS) were banned by the EPA in 1977 because of widespread environmental contamination and persistence. PCBS are still found in freshwater fish from contaminated streams; 20% of the fish in the United States is contaminated. Fish is used to feed domestic animals; meat, milk, eggs, and poultry have been found to be contaminated with PCBS. Research has shown that a high percentage of people have PCBS in their fat tissue.

Dr. Russell Jaffe of the Serammune Lab in Reston, Virginia, reports significant levels of chloroform, carbon tetrachloride, and trichloroethylene in 16 nonorganically grown common foods. Chloroform levels were highest in cheese, butter, potatoes, and tea. The levels of carbon tetrachloride were higher in butter and olive oil. Butter, beef, and tea contained the highest levels of trichloroethylene.

TOXIC METALS

Arsenic, cadmium, lead, and mercury have been found in food and all are potentially very toxic.

Arsenic is found in foods contaminated by pesticides, in the form of lead and calcium arsenate. Seafood contains the largest amount of arsenic. Arsanilic acid is used as a growth additive in cattle and poultry feeds, and may enter the food chain in this way.

Cadmium enters the food chain through root crops and leafy vegetables fertilized with contaminated sludges. Fish and organ meats concentrate cadmium. Cadmium is poorly absorbed, and is stored in the liver and kidneys. Cadmium has also been found in breast milk, thereby linking old pollution to new generations.

Food accounts for 55% to 85% of a person's lead exposure. Lead solder in cans is a major contributor. Infants and children absorb more lead from food than do adults.

Fish and other seafood may be contaminated with methylmercury. This most toxic form of mercury is deposited in the brain. Mercury exposure can be detected in blood and hair, but blood concentrations of mercury are more accurate for recent exposures.

FOOD PACKAGING MATERIALS

Polyvinyl chloride, which is made from vinyl chloride, a known carcinogen, and acrylonitrile, a suspected carcinogen, are found in containers for margarine and cooking oil, food packaging films, bottle closure liners in soft drinks, and the liner in foil-wrapped candies. The United States has no monitoring of dietary exposure to vinyl chloride. Acrylonitrile was used as a fumigant for foods until 1978. The amount of acrylonitrile in the average American diet has not been estimated.

FOOD ADDITIVES

At least 2800 substances are used as food additives. In 1958, the Generally Recognized as Safe (GRAS) list was generated. Substances on the GRAS list are those for which no complaints have been filed about an illness related to their ingestion. Once a substance is listed as GRAS, it is not subject to specific regulations, other than for the manufacturer to use appropriate processes.

The FDA did not start to review the scientific literature on the GRAS substances until 1969; by 1987 fewer than 500 substances had been reviewed. The Delaney Clause is part of the Food Additives Amendment and states that "no additive shall be deemed safe if it is found to induce cancer when ingested by man or animal." The FDA ignores potential cancer-causing additives if they are associated with what they consider an insignificant risk to the population eating the food.

In 1960, the Color Additives Amendment was added to the United States Food, Drug, and Cosmetics Act. Food colors are rigorously tested before they can be certified by the FDA. Only seven synthetic colors are allowed to be added to food. One of these, tartrazine (Yellow No. 5), has been found to cause allergic reactions, especially in people sensitive to aspirin. High doses of approved synthetic colors cause cancer in animals.

The following additives represent 95% of the total quantity of food additives used in the United States: sucrose, corn syrup, dextrose, salt, black pepper, caramel, carbon dioxide, citric acid, modified starch, sodium bicarbonate, yeasts, and yellow mustard. The best way to avoid food additives is to eat fresh, unprocessed, organically grown food.

TOXINS IN FOOD

There are two main causes of food poisoning: toxins excreted by organisms in the foods, and the transfer of organisms in food to humans, where they then grow.

Organisms   The most common cause of food poisoning is *Staphylococcus aureus*, which produces six exotoxins (toxins loosely associated with the bacterial cell). Boiling kills the bacteria but will not destroy the heat-stable toxin. Staphylococcal food poisoning causes nausea, vomiting, diarrhea, gastrointestinal pain, dizziness, and headache. Symptoms appear from 1 to 11 hours after ingestion of the contaminated food and last for 24 to 48 hours. The most common foods contaminated are meats, cooked ham, milk, and cream-filled bakery goods. Staphylococcal toxins develop in foods at temperatures between 42°F and 130°F. To avoid food poisoning, foods must be refrigerated well before the incubation time (less than four hours). Food that has been frozen, reheated, and refrozen favors the growth of staphylococcal bacteria.

The toxin produced by *Clostridium botulinum* is one of the most notorious. It triggers a disease called botulism, which paralyzes the eye, throat, laryngeal, and respiratory muscles. Paralysis of the voluntary muscles, as well as dry mouth, constipation, and urinary retention are other symptoms. Symptoms appear from 12 hours to 10 days after ingestion. The mortality rate in the past has been as high as 60% to 80%, but is now less than 10%. Boiling food for 5 minutes or heating at 176°F for 30 minutes will destroy the toxin.

C. botulinum grows in anaerobic, low-acid food preparations, usually during storage and causing no change in the color or taste of the food. Home-canned foods, smoked fish, and occasional faulty, commercially canned foods have caused outbreaks of botulism. Infants have developed botulism from honey; it is recommended that infants less than one year of age not be fed honey.

Foods may also introduce bacteria into the body where they then multiply. The most common infections, from *Salmonella*, cause fever, nausea, abdominal cramps, diarrhea that may be bloody, headache, dizziness, and vomiting. Some people have died from this type of food poisoning. Symptoms appear 4 to 24 hours after ingestion. A larger number of organisms causes symptoms to appear more rapidly. *Salmonella* may be found in eggs, poultry, baked goods, milk and milk products, vegetables, dried coconut, and cocoa. Insects, poultry, rodents, and even humans can be carriers.

A recent well-publicized outbreak of an *Escherichia coli* infection was caused by contaminated beef from fast-food hamburgers. The beef had been contaminated by cattle feces at the slaughterhouse, and undercooking allowed live organisms to be consumed. The resulting infections produced serious symptoms in these individuals as well as three deaths. *E. coli* is normally a beneficial bowel bacteria. However, the strain of *E. coli* in the cattle feces was a pathogenic mutant strain, one of many being produced by feeding antibiotics to animals. These mutant strains are antibiotic-resistant and very difficult to treat. U.S. Federal meat in-

spection rules have now been changed to zero tolerance for feces and ingesta (food from the stomach) on meat.

Proper food handling is the key to avoiding this type of food poisoning; food must be thoroughly cooked to destroy the organisms, as well as promptly refrigerated to prevent their growth. Careful handling of raw meats and proper cleansing of such utensils as knives and cleavers is also critical.

Another occasional source of food poisoning is shellfish, which can contain a paralysis-causing toxin produced by dinoflagellates, a marine protozoan. The toxin is called paralytic shellfish poison, and it depresses respiration and affects the heart, causing complete cardiac arrest. As little as 4 mg of this toxin can be fatal to a human. Shellfish, such as mussels and clams, accumulate the protozoa from seawater, and death may result when they are ingested by humans.

Always be aware of local closures before harvesting shellfish yourself or purchasing from a vendor.

Mycotoxins Toxins produced by molds are called mycotoxins. The *Aspergillus* genus of mold, including *A. flavus* and *A. niger,* produce several aflatoxins, the best known mycotoxins. The molds grow on cereal grains, rice, apples, milk, peanuts, corn, nuts, and oil seeds. Aflatoxins can be potent liver toxins and carcinogens for most species.

Ergot alkaloids are another type of mycotoxin, produced by *Claviceps purpurea* while growing on rye. This mycotoxin causes central nervous system disorders called ergotism. When harvesting was delayed during World War II, many grains in Siberia were contaminated by *C. purpurea*. People consuming this grain suffered gastrointestinal symptoms, internal hemorrhage, and skin rashes. About 10% of the people who ate infected grain died.

Spoilage of Foods Fresh or raw foods normally carry a bacterial population. The type and amount depend on the food, the pH, handling, temperature, and the time from harvest or slaughter to use. Bacteria destroy cell walls in the food. Enzymes released from cutting and bruising, or from destruction of normal inhibitors further contribute to deterioration of the food. Spoilage of fresh food is usually obvious, and the consumer can avoid these foods. Fish and dairy products are the most sensitive foods.

Fish is caught, pitchforked, packed in ice for up to ten days, loaded onto scales, and then onto carts. Fish readily decompose by breakdown from both enzymes and bacteria. As they age, fish develop a fishy odor caused by trimethylamine. When the fish spoils, it smells like hydrogen sulfide (or rotten eggs).

HORMONES AND DRUGS IN FOOD

Cows, pigs, and chickens are fed hormones and drugs to help them gain weight faster and to mask signs of disease. The majority of pigs have pneumonia when they are slaughtered. Cattle develop pneumonia when they are shipped by trucks that are not heated or cooled.

In Puerto Rico, there was an outbreak of early puberty in four- to five-year-old girls. When the children eliminated milk, poultry, and beef (which contained growth hormones) from their diet, most of the symptoms disappeared.

Livestock eat more than half of the antibiotics produced in North America each year. Antibiotic-resistant bacteria develop in the animals and can then be passed to humans, causing new mutant strains of bacteria.

FOOD ALLERGY

Food allergies can cause a toxic type of reaction. There are two types of food allergies that are mediated by special antibodies called Immunoglobulin G (IgG), and Immunoglobulin E (IgE). IgE-mediated food allergies cause life-threatening anaphylaxis, with swelling of the throat, tightness of the chest, and low blood pressure. The IgE reactions occur from minutes to several hours after ingesting food.

IgG-mediated food allergies account for about 85% of food allergies. A delayed reaction can occur as long as 24 hours after consuming the food. IgG food allergies can cause chronic headaches (often migraine), chronic indigestion and heartburn, fatigue, depression, failure to thrive, joint pain, recurrent abdominal pain, canker sores, chronic respiratory symptoms such as wheezing or bronchitis, bedwetting, and bowel symptoms such as diarrhea or constipation.

Eating too much food, or the same food repeatedly, can also be toxic. Overeating can be a sign of food addiction and usually leads to obesity. It also stresses the digestive system, causing it to work overtime and use enormous amounts of energy. Overeating also tends to wear out enzyme systems, as does eating the same foods over and over. This leads to improper food processing by the body, and food allergies.

CLEANSING, BALANCING, AND PREVENTIVE TECHNIQUES

Healthy Eating Tips To enjoy optimum health, everyone should incorporate the following practices into daily eating habits.

AVOID

- All refined sugar and any foods or mixtures that contain refined sugar, including sucrose, dextrose, corn syrup, brown sugar, turbinado, and nutritive corn sweetener. Refined sugar:
  - disturbs glucose metabolism
  - causes tooth decay
  - depletes minerals, B vitamins, and vitamin C
  - can lead to elevated cholesterol, blood pressure, and triglycerides
  - causes hyperactivity and irritability

- interferes with white cell immune function
- weakens muscles and contributes to fatigue
- is addictive
- creates an added load for the pancreas and adrenal glands
- Caffeine (regular coffee, regular tea, dark carbonated drinks, chocolate, cocoa, aspirin compounds). Caffeine:
  - is addictive
  - disturbs glucose metabolism and elevates blood sugar levels
  - disrupts the function of endocrine glands and the liver
  - constricts blood vessels and causes cell degeneration
  - increases triglycerides, cholesterol, and blood pressure
  - demands extra minerals, particularly potassium
  - contributes to fibrocystic breast disease
  - weakens muscle, induces fatigue, interferes with immune function
  - causes nervousness and loss of sleep
  - is linked to peptic ulcers
  - contributes to diabetes, hypoglycemia, allergies
  - exhausts adrenal glands
  - interferes with mineral absorption
  - causes headaches when stopped suddenly and can cause morning headaches that are relieved by a dose of caffeine
- Alcohol in all forms. Alcohol:
  - has a toxic effect on the liver during its metabolism
  - is addictive
  - increases blood pressure, triglycerides, and cholesterol
  - causes degeneration and cell death
  - depletes B vitamins and vitamin C

- demands extra minerals, especially zinc, magnesium, and manganese
- interferes with glucose metabolism
- causes fatigue and weakened muscles
- lowers immune function
- High salt intake. It:
  - is linked to high blood pressure, which can lead to stroke or heart attack
  - creates an imbalance with potassium metabolism
- Artificial sweeteners, colors, and flavors, and preservatives. These substances:
  - damage cells
  - can be carcinogenic
  - are non-nutritional
  - cause allergic reactions
- Chemical additives, including MSG (monosodium glutamate), BHA, BHT, nitrates, and nitrites. These substances:
  - damage cells
  - can be carcinogenic
  - are non-nutritional
  - add to the possibility of high blood pressure (MSG)
  - affect liver and kidney function (BHA and BHT)
  - are allergenic
- Processed foods and mixes. They:
  - contain chemicals and toxins added as preservatives and stabilizers
  - are high in sodium and low in nutrition
  - can be high in sugar and salt
  - are likely to contain several common food allergens
- Refined carbohydrates, such as white flour and white rice. They:
  - lack fiber
  - lack nutrition
  - contain chemical residues
  - have been bleached
- Fruits and vegetables that have been waxed, sprayed, fumigated, or dyed.

These foods:
- contain toxic chemicals that may be carcinogenic
- are permanently covered with insoluble waxes and oils
- are permanently colored with dyes

DO EAT
- Whole grains. They:
  - contain fiber
  - contain vitamins and minerals needed for enzyme formation and cell repair
- Fresh instead of frozen foods, frozen instead of canned.
  - fresh means fewer additives
  - frozen foods are purer than canned
  - more vitamins and minerals are retained in fresh and frozen foods
- Fruit juices instead of soft drinks or fruit-flavored drinks. Fruit juices:
  - contain more vitamins
  - contain less sugar
  - contain no chemicals or synthetic ingredients
- Whole vegetables and fruit instead of juices. These foods:
  - contain natural enzyme activity that help with digestion
  - provide adequate fiber
  - provide healthful snacks
- Foods high in fiber, such as oat bran and all beans. These foods:
  - are effective for lowering cholesterol
  - aid in digestion
- Low-fat meals. They:
  - aid in countering obesity and high cholesterol
  - may protect against heart disease and cancer
- Natural foods. They:
  - are a good source of fiber
  - should be eaten raw when possible, as cooking destroys vitamins, enzymes, and some minerals
- Only foods that will spoil and eat them *before* they do. This:
  - will lower intake of added preservatives and chemicals
  - can avoid microorganisms and enzyme changes that accompany food spoilage
- Organically grown fruits and vegetables. They:
  - have none of the harmful chemicals found in pesticides and chemical fertilizers
- Good quality meats and poultry. These:
  - should be free of antibiotics and hormones
  - should be from animals fed good-quality grains, not contaminated with pesticides
- Fresh fish. It:
  - must be as fresh as possible, with no bruises or drying
  - should be rinsed before use, as many fish are dipped in formaldehyde to preserve them
  - should have been caught in water uncontaminated by industrial waste

Treating Food Poisoning
- Vitamin C, both orally and intravenously, will help clear food poisoning.
- "Magic Brew" will help control nausea and headaches. To make Magic Brew:
  1 teaspoon sea salt
  1 teaspoon baking soda
  Mix in 1 quart of tolerated water and sip as needed. It may be more soothing if cold.
- Rosemary, sage, and thyme can help prevent food poisoning. Food poisoning can be treated with catnip, mint, chamomile, echinacea, goldenseal, mullein, and burdock.

HOMEOPATHIC REMEDIES

- *Arsenicum album*: food, pesticide, and chemical poisoning
- *Baptisia tinctoria*: poisoning from bad water
- *Nux vomica*: too much spicy food or alcohol, coffee headache, or fat poisoning
- *Zingiber*: diarrhea from bad food or water
- *Chamomilla*: coffee headache
- *Ipecacuanha*: food poisoning
- *Argentum nitricum*: sugar poisoning
- *Pulsatilla*: fat poisoning, spoiled fish
- *Natrum phosphoricum*: problems with acids, alcohol, citrus, sweets
- *Lycopodium*: poisoning from shellfish

Water

We drink water, cook with it, bathe in it, and inhale it in aerosols or as vapors. When it is contaminated, water becomes a toxin. Water can be contaminated with chemicals or microorganisms at the source, at the local utility, and in the home. Water is generally analyzed only for dissolved oxygen, fecal coliform bacteria (bacteria found in the intestines), suspended sediment, dissolved solids, and phosphorus.

Chemicals that can pollute drinking water include solvents, pesticides, metals, cleaning preparations, and septic tank degreasers.

Water can be polluted by the activities around chemical manufacturing, steel mills, sewage treatment plants, forest management, highway building, mining, hazardous waste disposal sites, dam construction, and water redirection/channelization. Runoff from lawns, paved areas, pastures, feedlots, and mine tailing sites also contributes to pollution. In 1988, the most common cause of polluted water in the U.S. was nutrients from fertilizers, phosphates from detergents, and sediments composed of suspended silt from fields, construction sites, and strip-mined lands.

DRINKING WATER

Drinking water quality depends on the quality of the raw or untreated water, the number of additives used in the water treatment plant, and contaminants added in transit to the tap. Raw water, from groundwater or surface sources, can be contaminated with naturally occurring substances in rocks, such as asbestos, radioactivity, and metals. Because of the large volumes of water in rivers, these surface waters are usually not very contaminated. They are more likely to contain biological contaminants and natural organic pollutants than groundwater.

The source of groundwater is precipitation; it is stored by nature in water-bearing rocks called aquifers. Aquifers can be contaminated by underground gasoline tanks, leaking septic systems, poorly located landfills, mine tailings, agricultural runoff, oil field operations, and industrial waste storage tanks. Aquifers near the coast can be contaminated with saltwater. It is difficult to trace contamination in an aquifer, and once contamination has occurred it cannot be reversed. Groundwater moves very slowly, and there is no way to dilute or mix the water to decrease the contamination.

Groundwater is the water source for about half the people in North America. The volume of groundwater is second only to that of the oceans and seas. The use of groundwater has increased in the past 30 years, and approximately 75% of American cities use groundwater for some or all of their water. In some parts of the country, groundwater is used with little or no treatment.

A study done in the 1980s by the EPA found that 10% of community wells and 4% of rural wells contained at least one pesticide above the minimum limits of the EPA. One to two percent of the wells were contaminated with nitrates (from fertilizer runoff), which can cause methemoglobinemia, a change in red blood cells that prevents them from carrying oxygen. Babies are more sensitive to the effects of methemoglobin than adults. Nitrates are also precursors to nitrosamines, which are known carcinogens.

Water Contamination Water is moved from groundwater and surface sources to storage areas for treatment, where it can be contaminated. Copper sulfate may be added to control the growth of algae. Aluminum, in the form of alum, is added to the water to precipitate and to remove organic material. Most of the alum precipitates out with the organic material, but even a minute amount of aluminum is very toxic for people with kidney disease.

Chlorine or other disinfectants may be added to the water to kill microorganisms. However, sometimes the level of microorganisms increases in the water after it leaves the treatment plant because of breaks in the pipes and growth on the inside surfaces of the pipes. Although chlorination does not kill viruses or protozoa (such as *Giardia lamblia*), it is the major method used to disinfect water in North America. Chlorine can react with naturally occurring organic materials in the water, such as decaying leaves, to form trihalomethanes (THMs). Trihalomethanes are suspected to be carcinogens, so other chemicals, such as ozone, chlorine dioxide, and chloramine, are sometimes used to disinfect the water. People who have used chlorinated water all of their lives have a higher incidence of bladder cancer than those who have used unchlorinated water.

Corroded pipes between the treatment plant and the consumer can leak lead, cadmium, iron, zinc, and nickel into the water supply. Asbestos is also a potential contaminant.

Fluoride is added to drinking water in some areas to prevent tooth decay. There is controversy over the toxicity of fluoride and whether it can cause other diseases.

Water in the home can be contaminated with lead from pipes or from lead solder used to join copper pipes. Corrosion of pipes, fittings, and solder adds still more lead to the water. Water with an acidic pH leaches more lead from the pipes. Flushing out the tap in the morning for three to five minutes before collecting the water, and using only cold water for drinking and cooking ensures a lower lead content. Infants and children are more susceptible to the effects of lead. Lead can affect the formation of blood, the gastrointestinal tract, the kidneys, and the central nervous system.

The levels of such chemicals as arsenic, cadmium, chromium, fluoride, lead, mercury, nitrate, selenium, uranium, radium, radon, and trihalomethanes are all regulated under the Safe Drinking Water Act.

- Exposure to inorganic arsenic is associated with skin cancer, lung cancer, and neurological disease. The most common source of arsenic contamination is water drainage through mineral formations that contain natural arsenic ores.
- Cadmium in drinking water comes from the corrosion of galvanized pipes. Cadmium can cause kidney disease and lung cancer.
- Inorganic mercury is discharged into the water table and rivers from solid waste treatment plants and water seepage through natural mineral deposits. Bacteria then convert it to organic mercury, which can cause brain damage.
- Nitrates in groundwater come from seepage from septic systems and runoff from fertilizer and feed lots. Sometimes natural organic matter can be a source of nitrate contamination.
- Selenium comes from water seepage through natural mineral formations. It can cause stomach and intestinal problems.

- Uranium is found in groundwater and surface water. Up to 13% of communities in the United States have uranium in the water supply.
- Radium is found in igneous rocks and sand aquifers. Occupational radium exposure has been associated with bone cancer.
- Radon is a gas that dissolves in water and is found naturally in groundwater. Radon in homes is associated with lung cancer, but the amount in water is much less than the exposure people receive from air.

CLEANSING, BALANCING, AND PREVENTIVE TECHNIQUES

Clean drinking water is an absolute necessity for good health and body cleansing.

- Adequate water intake is necessary to flush toxins and waste materials from cells.
- Nutrients must be kept in solution, available for cell nourishment and repair.
- Adequate fluid levels are necessary for ions in the body to flow and maintain electrical equilibrium.

Obtaining safe water can be a problem because of the various possibilities for contamination. Well water is no longer as safe as it once was because of contamination of deeper water tables. Also, some well water contains so many dissolved minerals that sensitive people cannot tolerate it. Bottled water may not always be a dependable safe source.

Frequently, additional purification treatment is required at home. Treatment possibilities are:

- *Boiling water*: Destroys organisms and removes chlorine and volatile chemicals. Heavy metals and nitrates remain in the water. Do not use aluminum pots to boil water because this will add aluminum to the water.

- *Filtering water*: Removes many contaminants. Portable, single-faucet, and whole house filters are available. Carbon block filters remove pesticides, organic chemicals, bad taste and odor, some organisms, and chlorine. They do not remove heavy metals, salts, minerals, nitrates, or fluorides.
- *Distillation*: Removes salts, asbestos, organisms, minerals, heavy metals, and nitrates. It does not remove chlorine or organic chemicals.
- *Reverse osmosis*: Removes particulate matter, some organic chemicals and pesticides, asbestos, heavy metals, fluorides, and chlorine compounds. It does not remove chlorine, all organisms, all chemicals, or all pesticides.
- *Hydrogen peroxide*: Purifies water by killing organisms, but it will not remove chemicals. Add seven drops of 35% hydrogen peroxide per gallon of distilled water. This method is also acceptable for the water of pets.

Use safe water for drinking, cooking, brushing teeth, and washing fresh food. Some sensitive people may require safe water for hand washing and bathing.

Never drink spring, stream, lake, or river water when you are on a camping or hiking trip, especially standing water or water that flows through cow lots or pastures. Much of the natural water in the United States is now contaminated with *Giardia lamblia*. *Giardia* is a microscopic parasite that causes bloating, abdominal cramps, diarrhea, and sometimes vomiting. If not treated, a *Giardia* infection can persist for years.

There are three ways water can be purified on a hiking or camping trip, or even when city traveling.

- *Boiling*: Water must be boiled from five to ten minutes, then cooled to a comfortable drinking temperature. This is time-consuming, and finding fuel can be a problem.

- *Iodine crystals or tablets*: The easiest and least expensive way to purify water. This method absolutely kills microorganisms, but the resulting taste of the water is not good.
- *Filters*: Portable ceramic water filters are effective for removing organisms. Most pumps can process a quart of water in one to two minutes. The filters are bulky and can be expensive. However, the extra effort required to carry the filter and use it is worthwhile.

Air

Air pollution can come from indoor and outdoor sources. Of the two, indoor air pollution may be more important because people spend more time indoors. Air pollution can cause short-term effects, long-term or chronic effects, lung cancer, and other respiratory and nonrespiratory symptoms. Acute or short-term effects generally last a few hours to days; asthma is an acute effect. Chronic effects last over a longer period of time, usually for years. Emphysema is a type of chronic effect.

OUTDOOR AIR POLLUTION

Air pollution consists of gases and particulate matter. Carbon monoxide makes up almost half of air pollutants. Other gases include sulfur oxides, nitrogen oxides, photochemical oxidants, and hydrocarbons. Volatile organic compounds, metals, asbestos, and radionuclides are also found in the atmosphere.

The main sources of pollution are:

Natural	Manmade
• smoke from forest fires	• transportation
	• fuel combustion
• dust from soil	• industrial processes
• dust from volcanoes	• waste disposal

Transportation pollution comes from automobiles, trucks, buses, planes, boats, and trains. Internal-combustion-engine exhausts emit carbon monoxide, nitrogen oxides, unburned fuel, soot, fuel additives, lead, and hydrocarbons. Fuel combustion sources emit sulfur, nitrogen oxides, and particulate pollutants. Industrial processes may emit soot, metal, organic vapors, and mineral residues. Waste disposal sites may emit carbon monoxide, nitrogen oxides, hydrocarbons, solvents, volatile organic chemicals, aldehydes, toxic metals, and smoke.

Carbon Monoxide Carbon monoxide is an odorless, colorless gas released when any material burns. Two-thirds of carbon monoxide comes from the gasoline burned in vehicles. It enters the bloodstream through the lungs and displaces oxygen from its binding site on the hemoglobin in the red blood cells. Overexposure to carbon monoxide can lead to death from lack of oxygen.

Metals Arsenic, cadmium, chromium, copper, lead, mercury, and nickel have been found in air. Mercury, cadmium, and nickel come from smelters. Arsenic is emitted from coal and oil furnaces. Chromium is released from chrome-plating operations. Smoke from refuse incineration contains copper. Lead is in the soil, air, and water from leaded gasoline, paint, and lead solder in pipes.

Nitrogen Oxides Nitrogen forms several oxides that are emitted from burning coal, oil, and gasoline. During combustion, nitric oxide is produced and then is changed chemically to nitrogen dioxide. Because half the nitrogen dioxide in air comes from transportation sources, concentrations are higher in urban areas than in rural areas. Nitrogen oxides can damage the mucous membranes of the eyes, upper respiratory tract, tracheobronchial tree, and alveoli. Nitrogen dioxide disrupts some enzyme systems, and it is likely that it causes lipid peroxidation, which is destruction of the lipid cell membrane by free radicals.

Particulate Matter   Particulate matter in the air mostly consists of small carbon and dust particles. Particulate matter can be released from natural sources, such as forest fires, soil, and volcanoes, or by industrial sources, such as fuel combustion, transportation, and solid-waste emissions. The small particles are more likely to be inhaled into the lungs. Toxic gases can be attached to these particles and are deposited into the lungs, causing damage to the lung tissue.

Photochemical Oxidants   Photochemical oxidants are produced by the action of sunlight on hydrocarbons and nitrogen oxides in the air. Ozone, aldehydes, and acrolein can be produced. Ozone is a major chemical in smog and is a product of reactions, triggered by sunlight, between volatile organic compounds and nitrogen oxides. The speed of the reaction increases when temperature and sunlight levels are high. Some nitrogen dioxide is converted to nitric acid, which contributes to acid rain. Ozone is irritating to the mucous membranes of the eyes and respiratory tract, and has been shown to cause pulmonary edema.

Sulfur Dioxide   Sulfur dioxide is the stable oxide produced when fossil fuels containing sulfur, mostly coal, are burned. Coal and oil power plants, pulp and paper mills, and refineries are the main sources. Sulfur dioxide is a heavy, colorless, pungent gas that can become sulfuric acid when oxidized. Sulfur dioxide is an irritant to the eyes, skin, and respiratory system and can damage the walls between alveoli in the lungs. Chronic exposure to sulfur dioxide can cause chronic bronchitis and emphysema.

Volatile Organic Chemicals   Volatile organic chemicals (VOCs) generally result from incomplete combustion. They are released from incinerator plants, hazardous waste sites, and use of industrial and household solvents. The plastic and semiconductor industries release VOCs. Benzene, carbon tetrachloride, chloroform, formaldehyde, methylene chloride, perchloroethylene, trichloroethylene, toluene, and vinyl chloride are VOCs that have been found in the earth's atmosphere. Volatile organic chemicals are a precursor to smog, and many are known or suspected carcinogens.

AIR QUALITY STANDARDS

In 1973, the World Health Organization developed a worldwide program to monitor air pollution in order to identify and avoid dangerous levels. The program became a part of the United Nations's Global Environmental Monitoring Systems (GEMS). The EPA has set primary safety standards for various pollutants. However, standards for many toxic chemicals have not been set.

Air quality standards measure six pollutants—total suspended particulates, sulfur dioxide, carbon monoxide, nitrogen dioxide, ozone, and lead. In the United States, the levels of these pollutants, except ozone, have declined over the last ten years. Many violations of the ozone levels have occurred in large cities, in particular Los Angeles.

CLEANSING, BALANCING, AND PREVENTIVE TECHNIQUES

Natural events, such as forest fires, dust storms and volcano eruptions, contribute to outdoor air pollution. Nothing can be done to prevent these phenomena. However, we do have some measure of control over other contributors to outdoor air pollution.

Prevention of outdoor air pollution is of paramount importance and extremely difficult to accomplish. The following techniques would help lower pollution levels:

- control emission from cars, trucks, and trains so that the exhaust emitted contains low levels of pollutants
- control factory and refinery emissions
- control industrial and household solvent use
- control wood burning in homes by limiting burning days when air pollution is high

When we are outdoors and the pollution is high, wearing a mask is helpful. Using an air cleaner in our cars is also a method of reducing pollution. Both the mask and the auto model air cleaner should remove particulate matter and chemicals.

INDOOR AIR POLLUTION

In the last few years, it has become evident that indoor air pollution levels may be higher than those outside. Urban populations spend at least 80% of their time indoors, and the most susceptible population groups, such as the elderly and infants, spend even more time indoors. Indoor air pollutants may come from outdoor air, from materials in the building itself, or from human activity. Paint, tobacco smoke, carpets, furniture, plastics, pesticides, cleaning materials, air fresheners, and personal and household products are all sources of indoor air pollution. However, the indoor levels of ozone, sulfates, aerosols, sulfur dioxide, and lead are 20% to 80% lower than outdoors.

Radon   Radon is an indoor air pollutant that comes from the outdoors. Many rocks contain uranium deposits, which are a source of radon. High radon levels have been found in the United States in Pennsylvania, New England, Colorado, and New Mexico. Radon can enter houses through cracks in the foundation, through util-

ity service lines as they enter the house, from drinking water, or from building materials with a high radium concentration. Kits are available to measure radon levels in a home. Home owners can decrease radon levels by improving the house ventilation or sealing cracks in the floor. Radon decays to radioactive products that are suspected causes of lung cancer. The EPA suggests that a radon level greater than 4 picocuries per litre is unsafe.

Construction and Building Materials   Since the energy crisis in 1973–74, new buildings are more airtight and more insulation is being added to older buildings. New offices use mechanical ventilation rather than relying on open windows. The number of air exchanges in buildings has been reduced to 0.5 per hour. By the 1980s, complaints regarding indoor air pollution mushroomed.

Many building materials off-gas volatile chemicals. Concrete, stone, plywood, particleboard, insulation adhesives, paints, and carpets are sources of indoor air pollutants. Stone and cinder block may contain radon. Particleboard and plywood off-gas formaldehyde from bonding agents. Carpets also off-gas formaldehyde and paints may contain toluene and formaldehyde.

The Environmental Protection Agency (EPA) is studying the exposure of people to volatile organic compounds (VOCs) and pesticides. For 11 chemicals (including benzene, carbon tetrachloride, chloroform, tetrachloroethylene, styrene, and trichloroethylene) measured in cities and rural areas, the indoor air exposures were higher than outdoor exposures. Pesticide exposure came from indoor sources.

The EPA found that levels of volatile organic compounds in new buildings were 100 times greater than those found outdoors. Over a period of time, these levels gradually decreased to two to four times that of outdoor levels. These VOCs came from the building materials.

Human Activities Human activities add to indoor air pollution. Carbon monoxide, nitrogen dioxide, nitrogen oxide, carbon dioxide, sulfur dioxide, volatile organic compounds, and particulates are products of combustion of natural gas, fuel oil, coal, and heating systems. Gas stoves, hot-water heaters, and dryers also contribute to the problem.

Room deodorizers, disinfectants, detergents, cleaning compounds, floor waxes, mothballs, perfumes, pesticides, and any perfumed chemical add to indoor air pollution. Fabric softener dryer sheets contribute both to indoor and outdoor pollution if the dryer is vented to the outside.

Inhalants Pollens, dust, dust mites, animal dander, insect parts, and mold are commonly found in indoor air. Because we inhale them, they can cause health problems.

Molds are frequent residents of heating, ventilation, and air-conditioning units. Their spores can travel on air currents throughout a building. They grow anywhere there is dampness, particularly in bathrooms, laundry rooms, and kitchens. Mold may be found behind tile and under linoleum. Water leaks are always accompanied by mold growth.

Dust and dust mites can cause allergies; dust mites trigger asthma in sensitive people. Dust is organic dirt because it contains minute plant fibers, food remnants, pollen, mold spores, insect fragments, danders, fabric fibers, soot, paper and paint fragments, and other microscopic fragments. Suspect a dust problem if you are worse:

- indoors, better outside
- when the furnace is running
- when housecleaning is in progress
- in the morning and improve during the day
- when you first go to bed

Dust mites are microscopic insects that live in dust and feed on skin scales shed by humans. They are harmful only to sensitive people who inhale their airborne feces. They colonize in mattresses, carpets, stuffed toys, and upholstered furniture and thrive in humid climates.

Some pollen is in indoor air. Because it is microscopic, pollen can come into the house through open doors and windows. It can also be brought into the house on clothing, shoes, and on pet fur.

Tobacco Smoke Tobacco smoke is a major contributor to indoor air pollution. In a 1975 study, all adults (even nonsmokers) tested by a urine test had evidence of tobacco smoke exposure. Tobacco smoke consists of mainstream smoke, the smoke drawn through the tobacco during active smoking, and sidestream smoke, which comes from burning tobacco. The sidestream smoke contains a higher concentration of gases and particulates than does mainstream smoke. Four thousand different chemicals and particulates have been identified in sidestream smoke, and include carbon monoxide, ammonia, acetaldehyde, formaldehyde, hydrogen cyanide, nitrogen dioxide, nicotine, benzo[a]pyrene, phenols, and cadmium.

Sick-Building Syndrome In sick buildings, a large percentage of workers complain of nonspecific symptoms of eye, nose, and throat irritation; headaches; fatigue; drowsiness; dizziness; and decreased concentration. Symptoms typically improve over the weekend or vacation time and worsen on return to work. Most cases of sick-building syndrome are in new buildings or buildings remodeled to be more energy-efficient. Studies of these buildings have not shown any chemicals to be elevated above limits set by the EPA. At first, the symptoms of workers in sick buildings were thought to be caused by hysteria.

In most cases, the cause of the sick building is not identified, yet volatile organic compounds are thought to play a role. Ventilation systems have often been found to be inadequate to meet the needs of the number of people in the buildings or to handle new sources of chemicals, such as copy machines and computers. Also, pesticides, deodorizers, and scents are sometimes added to ventilation systems for dispersal throughout the building.

Building-related illness refers to those illnesses that have an identified cause. These illnesses include hypersensitivity pneumonitis (inflamed lungs caused by an allergy to mold or bird droppings), asthma, Legionnaire's disease, influenza, and carbon monoxide poisoning.

CLEANSING, BALANCING, AND PREVENTIVE TECHNIQUES

We have much more control over indoor pollution than over outdoor pollution. Although we may not be able to control indoor air pollution in the workplace or where we shop, we certainly can control it in our homes. It is imperative that we have environmentally clean, safe homes.

The following should be considered for controlling indoor air pollution:

- Carefully select the building materials used in the construction or repair of your home. Plywood, particleboard, and chipwood all have high formaldehyde content.
- Use less toxic paints. Some companies will leave the mold retardants or fungicides out of the paint for you.
- Select your carpets and drapes carefully. Some less toxic carpets are on the market now, although hardwood, brick, or tile floors are still best. Washable 100% cotton drapes are the least toxic.
- Hardwood, glass, or metal furniture is the safest furniture. Upholstery can add to indoor air pollution both from the fabric and the padding.
- Select unscented and safe cleaning supplies. Most cleaning can be accomplished with hot water, baking soda, and lemon juice.
- Use unscented personal care products, and do not wear perfumes or aftershaves.
- Do not use pesticides or store them in your house.
- Do not use commercial air deodorizers, air fresheners, or disinfectants.
- Have your house checked for radon, and if the levels are high, instigate repairs to lower the levels.
- Do not use fabric softeners, and wash your clothes in unscented detergents or use ceramic laundry discs. One-half to one cup of baking soda in the rinse water will substitute for fabric softener.
- Do not use pesticides or insecticides in your home or on your lawn.
- Do not smoke and do not allow anyone else to smoke in your home or car.
- Use electric cooking stoves, dryers, hot-water heaters, and furnaces to avoid the presence of gas, coal, or oil combustion products in your home.
- Keep your home clean and vacuumed to avoid accumulation of dust and dust mites, animal dander, insect parts, mold, and pollens.
- Control dampness in order to control molds. (See Organisms, chapter 7, for further discussion of molds.)
- Use an air cleaner to remove both chemicals and particles.

In the workplace, proper ventilation will help reduce odors from copiers and computers. It will also reduce the chemical levels in the building. An individual air cleaner in your work area will help to reduce your exposures. Do not allow coworkers to smoke in your area. (See also chapter 10.)

Homeopathic remedies will help cleanse from exposure to pollution.

- *Sulphuricum acidum*: pollution in general
- *Ignatia*: exposure to perfumes
- *Arsenicum album*: chemical poisoning

Take bowel tolerance levels of vitamin C daily to help cleanse the body of pollution chemicals and to help prevent damage from toxic exposures. Also take antioxidant nutrients (see Nutritional Therapy, chapter 14).

Noise

Noise, which may be described as unwanted sound, is considered a toxic pollutant. It is found in both urban and rural environments and is a cause of stress. Sound consists of an air pressure wave. Any object that vibrates causes waves of compressed and expanded air that induce vibration on the parts of a human ear. The ear perceives it as a sound, depending on the frequency (how rapidly the source is vibrating) and the pressure of the sound (loudness).

Sound pressure varies over a range of more than 1 million units. A logarithmic scale, known as the decibel (dB) scale, is used to identify sound pressure. The human ear responds logarithmically, not linearly, and loudness doubles when noise increases by 10 dB. According to the EPA, almost half of the U.S. population is frequently exposed to sound levels greater than 55 dB, such as on land next to airports and freeways. In this century, noise has increased 2 dB per decade.

Sound	Decibel level
Whisper	25
Conversation	60
Vacuum cleaner	70–85
Hair dryer	80
Gas lawnmower	95
Rock concert	110–120

Noise at 70 dB can wake a sleeping person. In the 80 dB range, noise can damage hearing over time. Over 80 dB can cause ringing in the ears, a feeling of pressure, and muffling of sound. Continued exposure can cause hearing loss. The normal pain threshold for noise is 110 dB, and permanent deafness is caused by 135 dB. Sounds of 140 dB can instantly destroy hearing.

EFFECTS OF NOISE

Noise can cause hearing loss; interfere with speech; interrupt communication; and interfere with sleep, leisure, and other activities. The EPA has chosen 45 dB indoors and 55 dB outdoors (averaged over a 24-hour period) as the maximum levels that will not affect public health.

Excessive noise can damage the inner ear. Hair cells, which transmit messages along the auditory nerve to the brain stem, are killed and replaced with scar tissue. This is known as sensineuronal or perceptive hearing loss. With exposure to excessive noise, people develop auditory fatigue, which may cause a temporary loss of hearing. Their hearing may recover after several hours away from the noise, but repeated exposure can cause permanent hearing loss. Sensineuronal hearing loss is irreversible, and it cannot be corrected.

Conductive hearing loss may develop when the eardrum or middle ear is damaged. Conductive hearing loss is usually not occupationally induced. A hearing aid that amplifies sound helps a person with a conductive hearing loss. In some cases, this type of hearing loss is reversible.

The body reacts to loud noise as it does to other types of stress. The heart receives most of the stress from loud noise; heart rate and blood pressure increase. Noise causes the body to produce adrenocorticotropic hormone (ACTH), which can cause stomach ulcers. It can also cause changes in breathing patterns, muscle tension, mobility of the GI tract, dilation of the pupils of the eyes, and secretion of saliva and gastric secretions. The immune system is also affected by excessive noise. Eosinophils and other white blood cells, and gamma globulin (a plasma protein that fights disease) become very low. Emotions are also affected by noise; people may become distressed or even angry as noise levels go up.

INDUSTRIAL NOISE

The maximum allowed daily average industrial noise is 90 dB for 8 hours a day. The Occupational Safety and Health Administration requires that for every 5 dB above 90, noise exposure must be decreased by half. Noise exposure can be controlled by reducing the noise at the source, interrupting the path between the source and receiver, and protecting the receiver, for example, with earplugs.

RECREATIONAL NOISE

Federal laws protect workers, but no laws control the amount of noise people receive when they leave the workplace. People who work in noise tend to also play in noise, and recreational noise often exceeds industrial noise. Snowmobiles, motorcycles, and power boats produce noise in the range that damages hearing. The noise in stadiums at sporting events can match that of a rock concert, where the level of the music may be as high as 200 dB. Even personal stereo headsets may reach 115 dB if the volume control is at maximum setting. For many people, hearing loss is more likely at play than at work.

NOISE IN THE HOME

The home may be besieged with noise from many sources. Loud power tools, chain saws, power lawnmowers, and snow blowers can exceed federal standards. The blender, TV, alarm clock, garbage disposal, trash compactor, vacuum cleaner, washer, dryer, dishwasher, coffee bean grinder, blow dryer, electric razor, and stereo all add to the noise level in the home. Individual appliances may produce a safe noise level, but when operated simultaneously, they can constitute a noise hazard.

HEARING PROBLEMS

Ten years ago, more than 80 million Americans had some type of hearing impairment. In this decade, the number affected is expected to increase by 28 million. While many of these people are elderly, children and adolescents are also being affected. In one study at the University of Tennessee, college freshmen had hearing losses typical of the elderly, 25% of whom report problems with their hearing.

CLEANSING, BALANCING, AND PREVENTIVE TECHNIQUES

The best prevention against hearing loss is turning down the noise. Sound is too loud if:

- you must shout to be heard above the background noise
- the person next to you can hear the music from your headset
- you cannot hear someone speaking less than 2 feet away
- speech is dulled or muffled after you leave a noisy area
- you have pain, ringing in your ears, a feeling of fullness, or pressure in your ears after noise exposure

For a do-it-yourself hearing test, hold your hand next to your shoulder as though you are taking an oath. Rub your thumb and forefinger together. If you cannot hear a distinct rubbing sound, you may have some high frequency range hearing loss. Be sure to check both ears.

Persons at risk for hearing loss should have their hearing checked once or twice a year. People with regular exposure to loud noise, newborns with a family history of hearing impairment, infants and toddlers with chronic ear infections, and people over 40 are considered at high risk. Children should visit an audiologist before starting school. People at low risk should have their hearing tested every five years.

To prevent hearing loss:

- Wear earplugs or earmuffs for dangerous noise exposure at work or at play.
- Divide noisy chores into small jobs and between the jobs give your ears a rest.
- Use sound-absorbing mats under loud appliances or machinery, and install "sound-proof" ceiling tiles in rooms where noisy activities take place.
- Purchase quiet products; do a noise level test before buying.
- Pay attention to noise-making toys. If the toy is too loud when held at arm's length, it will be much too loud for your child.

- Never use more noise to drown out background noise, such as music from your headset to drown out transportation noise.
- Stagger the use of household appliances so that they are not all running at the same time.
- Select the location of your home carefully. Try to avoid airport flight paths, high-speed freeways, and heavy truck routes. Check with the zoning board for possible future developments.

The homeopathic remedy *Arnica* can be used to help restore hearing after exposure to loud noise. *Silicea terra* may help heal damage to the ear from chronic loud noise. *Calendula* can help ruptured eardrums and deafness.

6

External Toxins: Chemicals and Metals

Chemicals

Environmental chemical pollution has been found to cause allergic sensitization. For example, people can become sensitized to low-molecular weight chemicals found in polyurethane varnish, foam, and paint. People who live in areas with high pollution have higher IgE levels (an antibody associated with allergy) than people living in areas of low pollution.

Fetuses, children, and elderly people are especially sensitive to environmental chemicals. The fetus is more sensitive to lead, mercury, and polychlorinated biphenyls than are adults. Young children have a larger body surface area in relation to their weight, a higher metabolic rate, an immature host detoxification process, an immature renal system, and an immature immune system. Elderly people have impaired host defenses, an increase in fat tissue, a loss of lean body mass, and impaired drug detoxification systems. Females are more susceptible to such environmental chemicals as lead, benzene, and alcohol.

SOLVENTS

Solvents are chemicals used to extract, dissolve, or suspend materials, such as fats and resins, that are not soluble in water. Solvents typically are organic chemicals composed of carbon and hydrogen atoms. Organic solvents can depress the central nervous system (CNS), irritate mucous membranes and tissues, and adversely affect the liver, kidneys, heart, bone marrow, and peripheral nervous system. The chemical structure of the organic solvent and the amount and length of exposure determine the effect and damage to the body.

Solvents act like general anesthetics, and they can eventually cause unconsciousness. They are lipophilic (fat-soluble), so they have an affinity for the CNS because of its high fat content. Acute organic solvent exposure can cause drowsiness, nausea, headache, dizziness, slight incoordination, rapid heartbeat, psychomotor impairment, and death from respiratory failure.

Solvents dissolved in lipid membranes are relatively protected from enzymatic breakdown and therefore they accumulate. CNS symptoms may occur after long latent periods when the accumulated solvent is released.

There is controversy over whether or not chronic low-level exposure to solvents can cause neurotoxicity. When acute solvent exposure at low levels causes symptoms, such as dizziness and slight incoordination, repeated exposure may cause permanent changes. Loss of nerve cells (neurons) can result in permanent damage because these cells do not regenerate.

All organic chemicals have irritant properties. Solvents can defat the skin due to their lipophilic properties. Exposure to large amounts of solvents can damage the skin, lungs, or eyes.

Benzene Benzene is a common solvent with a pleasant "aromatic" odor. Chemically, it is the most significant hydrocarbon, and it is used as the starting material for the manufacture of numerous products, such as phenolic and polyester resins, insecticides, and dyes.

Acute benzene exposure can cause euphoria, excitement, headache, vertigo, nausea, vomiting, dizziness, irritability, loss of consciousness, coma, irregular heartbeat, and skin rash and blisters.

Chronic exposure can cause aplastic anemia, in which the bone marrow stops producing red blood cells, or leukemia, which is cancer of the bone marrow. In the past, benzene was commonly used as an inert ingredient in pesticides.

Carbon Tetrachloride Carbon tetrachloride has the most infamous record of human toxicity because of its effect on the liver. In the past, it was used as a dry-cleaning agent, as a degreasing solvent in consumer products, and in home fire extinguishers. Exposure causes conjunctivitis, headache, dizziness, nausea, vomiting, abdominal cramps, nervousness, narcosis, and coma.

Symptoms from inhalation affect the CNS and those from ingestion affect the liver and gastrointestinal tract. Acute exposure can cause extensive kidney and liver damage in addition to cardiac sensitization. Fatalities from carbon tetrachloride are caused by kidney failure.

Ethanol Ethanol (grain alcohol) is an organic solvent that depresses the cardiovascular and central nervous systems. It is contained in perfumes and liquor, and is used in many types of industry as a solvent. It raises the pain threshold 35%, dilates blood vessels in the skin, increases gastric acid secretion, and may lead to inflammation of the stomach lining or an ulcer. Ethanol weakens all muscles, including the heart muscles, and it causes fat deposition throughout the body. It depresses cell production by the bone marrow, leading to a lack of white cells in areas of inflammation.

Ethanol causes an increased rate of infection in alcoholics, and ingesting a large amount in a short period of time can be fatal. Chronic ingestion causes cirrhosis, a scarring of the liver.

Formaldehyde Formaldehyde is used extensively in industry. The U.S. alone produces 7 to 8 billion pounds annually. Because the pure form is unstable, formaldehyde is produced in a 3% to 50% aqueous solution known as formalin. The plastics and resins industries use formaldehyde. It is also used in cosmetics, disinfectants, mouthwashes, film hardeners, wood preservatives, and biocides.

An irritant, formaldehyde affects the eyes and respiratory tract. It causes sensitization of the skin, and people can become sensitized to formaldehyde by wearing permanent press fabrics containing melamine-formaldehyde resins.

Formaldehyde is extremely toxic and at concentrations of 0.1 to 5 parts per million (ppm) can cause asthma, contact dermatitis, nausea, headache, fatigue, memory lapse, nose bleeds, and disorientation. High exposures can cause serious injury and death.

Formaldehyde is a metabolite of normal human cellular metabolism and is produced in very small amounts that the body rapidly converts to other substances.

Methanol Prolonged exposure to methanol (wood alcohol) fumes, or skin contact, can cause headache, vertigo, nausea, vomiting, abdominal cramps, mild CNS depression, sweating, weakness, delirium, metabolic acidosis, and decreased visual acuity. Methanol poisoning can be fatal because of convulsions and cessation of breathing (apnea).

When methanol is metabolized, the metabolite is more toxic than methanol itself. Ingesting 3 teaspoons of methanol has caused blindness, and 30 teaspoons has caused death. Ethanol is used as the antidote because it blocks the metabolism of methanol by the enzyme aldehyde dehydrogenase.

Methylene Chloride Methylene chloride is used in varnishes. It irritates the skin and eyes, and at high concentration it causes a drunken-like state. The body metabolizes methylene chloride to carbon monoxide.

Phenol An alcohol attached to a benzene ring, phenol denatures and precipitates proteins. Because it kills bacteria it is used in many cleaning products. It is also used in the manufacture of medications of coal tar origin, such as aspirin and sulfa drugs.

Phenol is readily absorbed by the skin, but may burn the skin with contact. It acts as a local anesthetic, and is also a CNS depressant. Phenol can cause numbness, nausea, vomiting, cold sweats, headache, irritability, and wheezing. If ingested, it severely burns the membranes of the throat, esophagus, and stomach. On a parts per million basis, phenol is as toxic by inhalation as cyanide.

Polycyclic Aromatic Hydrocarbons Polycyclic aromatic hydrocarbons (PAHs) are products of tobacco combustion, vehicular exhaust, and industrial combustion. They are lipid-soluble and are absorbed by the skin, lungs, or digestive tract, where they become concentrated in organs with high lipid content.

When PAHs are metabolized, arene oxides are formed. These are reactive, carcinogenic metabolites that attach to DNA. Antioxidants such as

selenium, vitamins A, C, E, bioflavonoids, BHA, and BHT protect against these oxides.

Tetrachlorethylene Tetrachlorethylene (PCE) is used for dry-cleaning and as a degreaser for metals. It is found in vinyl-coated, asbestos cement pipes. PCE causes eye irritation, confusion, respiratory depression, and liver damage.

Tetrachlorethylene does not evaporate or break down, so once it contaminates water, its concentration does not decrease over time. It is now classified as a potential human carcinogen. People who live next door to a dry-cleaning facility receive significant doses of PCE.

Toluene Toluene is a highly volatile chemical with a structure similar to benzene. It is now being added to gasoline to improve octane ratings. It affects the skin, irritating it and causing numbness. It also dries out the skin by defatting the surface layer. Toluene depresses the CNS. It causes fatigue, weakness, confusion, nausea, headache, and dizziness at high exposure levels.

Refineries and automobiles are common sources of toluene, as are model glue and typewriter correction fluid. Long-term toluene exposure can cause nerve damage and irregular heart rate, and has caused death. Ethanol raises blood levels of toluene by blocking its metabolism, thus causing more damage.

Trichloroethylene Trichloroethylene (TCE) decomposes to form phosgene, a highly toxic gas, and hydrogen chloride, a corrosive gas. It is used in metal degreasers, spot removers, rug cleaners, typewriter correction fluid, and disinfectants. In the past it was used as a dry-cleaning agent and fumigant.

TCE depresses the CNS and causes headaches, dizziness, and sleepiness. It irritates the eyes, nose, and respiratory tract, and causes liver and kidney damage. At high doses it causes cardiac arrest. With chronic exposure, TCE causes fatigue, memory loss, transient euphoria, and depression. It may be a carcinogen.

Vinyl Chloride Vinyl chloride is a flammable, volatile gas with a sweet odor. It irritates the skin and is a CNS depressant. In 1973, companies producing vinyl chloride began to report deaths of workers from angiosarcoma of the liver, a fatal cancer. Further investigation showed vinyl chloride exposure also causes cancer of the lungs and nervous system. Vinyl chloride is the raw material for manufacturing polyvinylchloride plastic, which is the polymer in PVC pipe, car and garden hoses, containers for margarine and oils, and plastic food wrap.

CLEANSING, BALANCING, AND PREVENTIVE TECHNIQUES

Because of their extreme toxicity, preventing exposure to solvents is of utmost importance. To minimize exposure:

- Use solvents only in a well-ventilated area.
- Wear protective clothing, such as a long-sleeved work coat and long pants.
- Use gloves, a mask, and goggles or safety glasses.
- Plan your procedure ahead of time to minimize exposure.
- Run an air cleaner if one is available.
- Take a bath or a shower immediately after you finish working with the solvent.
- Immediately wash or throw away protective clothing.
- Never store solvents inside your home.

If you have had exposure to solvents, undertake a detoxification program, preferably under the care of a physician. If a detoxification program is not available to you, take detox baths (see chapter 13) and antioxidant nutrients (see chapter 14).

Formaldehyde exposure is usually a chronic exposure from building materials, or it may be in cleaning supplies, disinfectants, and cosmetics. Read labels and avoid formaldehyde as much as possible. If you repair or build your home, select building supplies with care. Air cleaners containing sufficient activated charcoal will remove formaldehyde from the air. Wear a charcoal mask while shopping, as newly manufactured products contain high levels of formaldehyde.

Phenol is frequently encountered in cleaning supplies. Lysol contains phenol, as does PineSol. Wear gloves and a mask if you must use products containing phenol. Avoid perfumes and medications that contain phenol as a preservative.

Allergy extracts for formaldehyde, phenol, and ethanol are available. These extracts block allergic reactions to these solvents and help them to be released from the fat cells. However, because of their toxicity, many solvents cannot be diluted for testing and making extracts as can these chemicals. Homeopathic preparations can be safely used for the more toxic solvents.

Homeopathic remedies prescribed for the symptoms caused by the solvents will help to cleanse them from the body.

PESTICIDES

Rachel Carson's landmark book *Silent Spring* (1962) changed the way North Americans viewed the use of pesticides. This book led to the increased scientific study of pesticides and to improved government requirements for testing pesticides. Carson is credited with starting the environmental movement.

Pesticides are chemicals used to control weeds, insects, rodents, and other pests. They include ascaricides, rodenticides, insecticides, herbicides, and fungicides. Some chemicals currently used as pesticides were originally developed as nerve gases by Germany before World

War II. The three main categories of pesticides are carbamates, organophosphates, and organochlorines. Pesticides are toxic to humans and can cause numerous health problems.

The agriculture industry uses 90% of the pesticides in the U.S. However, pesticides also are used in paints, dentures, shampoos, disposable diapers, mattresses, paper, flea powders, hair wigs, carpets, and contact lenses. Pesticides are even used in swimming pools to control algae.

Everyone is exposed to pesticides daily. Each year, pesticides cause approximately 80,000 to 90,000 field workers to become ill and 80 to 100 to die. Pesticide residues are found in food, drinking water, air, clothing, and household furnishings. Exposure to pesticides occurs in larger amounts in schools, churches, offices, apartment buildings, and factories. The spraying of golf courses, agricultural lands, parks, and neighborhood gardens provides yet another source of pesticide exposure. Cities often have widespread spraying programs.

A single pesticide exposure may not cause problems, but combined exposures do. Many pesticides are broad spectrum and they can damage plants, birds, and humans. Pesticides may interact synergistically with each other, thus tripling or quadrupling the effect of each pesticide.

Since 1960, pesticide use has doubled in the United States. Herbicide use has increased while insecticide use has decreased. Despite this increased use of chemicals, the quantity of food production has not proportionately increased. One-third of the food crop is still lost to pests, demonstrating that there are limits to the effectiveness of pesticides.

The United States produces 1.3 billion pounds, imports 200 million pounds, and exports 400 million pounds of pesticides annually. Herbicides represent 61% and insecticides represent 21% of pesticide use.

Pesticides contain several different types of ingredients. The active ingredients are those with pesticide action against target pests. The rest of the pesticide ingredients are considered to be inert, and they are not tested for their effects. Inert ingredients include solvents, propellants, surfactants, emulsifiers, wetting agents, carriers, or diluents. While they have no pesticide action, these are not inactive ingredients. They are often biologically very active and, for humans, they may be the most toxic part of a pesticide product.

Companies may use the same active ingredient but different inert ingredients, which are considered trade secrets. The United States Federal Insecticide, Fungicide, and Rodenticide Act (FIFRA) does not require the inert ingredients to be listed. The EPA has finally examined these inert ingredients and found 50 of them to have significant toxicity for humans. Many of these 50 have now been removed from products. The EPA is now examining 65 more inert ingredients that are suspected to be toxic.

Synergists, added to the active ingredient to increase its effects, decrease the target pest's ability to detoxify the primary pesticide, frequently making the pesticide more toxic to humans. Synergism has also been noted between two chemicals in a pesticide, each of which may be of low or medium toxicity, but in combination have increased toxicity.

Pesticides have two types of action, contact and systemic. Contact pesticides act directly on the targeted pest, killing very rapidly. Systemic pesticides are applied to the soil or the leaves of the plant and may be ingested when people eat the fruits, nuts, or seeds of the plant. Systemic herbicides affect normal plant metabolism.

Organophosphate Pesticides Organophosphate pesticides were developed as chemical warfare agents. They do not persist for years in the environment, as DDT does, but they are highly toxic to humans and other mammals. More people have been poisoned by organophosphate pesticides than by any other group of pesticides. Exposure is mainly through use and application as crop-surface sprays, aerosols, baits, and fumigants. Some organophosphates include parathion, dichlorovos, diazinon, phosmet, and malathion.

Organophosphate pesticides bind to and inactivate acetylcholinesterase (AChE) within nerves. Acetylcholine, a neurotransmitter, is released from one nerve cell and binds to another nerve cell. This causes an electrical change in the second nerve cell. Acetylcholinesterase breaks down the acetylcholine so that the nerve cell is no longer excited. If AChE is inhibited, acetylcholine can continue to excite the nerve cell, leading to muscle twitching, rigid paralysis, or death.

Organophosphates are readily absorbed through the skin, lungs, and GI tract. Excessive sweating and muscle twitching result from absorption through the skin, chest tightness and excess lung secretions result from inhalation, and nausea and vomiting result from ingestion.

Most organophosphate pesticides must be metabolically converted in the liver to become biochemically active. Once activated, organophosphates are rapidly metabolized and excreted. They can easily cross the blood-brain barrier and enter the CNS, causing damage. Organophosphate pesticides have acute and chronic effects. Acutely, they can affect:

- the neuromuscular junction, causing muscular twitching, extreme weakness, and paralysis
- the respiratory muscles, causing difficulty with breathing
- the autonomic nervous system, causing increased secretions and fluid accumulation in the lungs
- the smooth muscle in the lung, causing it to go into spasm, triggering asthma
- the muscles of the GI tract and bladder, causing spasms
- the pupils of the eyes, causing constriction

Central nervous system symptoms can develop, including tremor, confusion, slurred speech, poor balance, and poor coordination. With large exposure, convulsions may result.

Chronic effects include neuropathy (pathological changes in the CNS), myopathy (any disease of a muscle), and psychological changes. The neuropathy involves the central and peripheral nervous systems and may appear up to 85 hours after the original poisoning. Peripheral nerves that control movement and sensation can be affected, but motor function changes are the most common: paralysis of the lower legs, wasted muscles, poor strength, and difficulty with movement.

Cumulative doses persist in the body, even when no exposure is occurring. Organophosphate pesticides may also block the body's detoxification mechanism, thus making related pesticides more toxic.

Exposure to organophosphates can also cause acute psychosis, loss of memory, schizophrenia, or severe depression. These symptoms can occur up to two months after an acute exposure. The psychiatric effects last at least six months and up to one year, although schizophrenia has persisted longer in some patients.

Organophosphate pesticide poisoning is treated with atropine and praladoxime. High-dose atropine counteracts the oral and gastric secretions, sweating, and autonomic nervous system effects. Another medication, metaraminol, is used to counteract the toxicity of the necessary high doses of atropine.

Carbamate Pesticides Carbamate pesticides are similar to organophosphate pesticides but they are more biodegradable and have lower dermal toxicities. The carbamates also inactivate acetylcholinesterase by binding to it, but the body rapidly reactivates it. Acetylcholinesterase levels become normal within two hours of exposure. Carbamates are considered direct inhibitors because they do not need to undergo any transformation in the body before inhibiting acetylcholinesterase.

Acute symptoms after carbamate pesticide exposure are light-headedness, nausea and vomiting, increased sweating, blurred vision, increased salivation, weakness, muscle twitching, small contracted pupils, and convulsions. Some carbamates may cause liver or kidney damage.

Carbamates are principally herbicides or fungicides. In the presence of nitrates, carbamates can be converted to nitrosamines, which are carcinogens. There is little information about the long-term toxicity or cancer-causing ability of carbamate pesticides. Treatment for carbamate pesticide poisoning is with atropine.

Organochlorine Pesticides Organochlorine pesticides are the oldest type of synthetic pesticides. They are very stable in the environment and have a high lipid solubility. Organochlorine pesticides are not as acutely toxic as the carbamates or organophosphate pesticides, but they have a greater potential for chronic toxicity.

Organochlorines are well absorbed orally and they accumulate in the fat tissue of animals, where they remain for long periods. Some organochlorines are carcinogenic and all are CNS depressants. Acute symptoms include irritability, dizziness, tremors, convulsions, and headaches. Chronic symptoms can manifest as personality changes, tremor, loss of memory, and a specific movement of the eyes called nystagmus.

In 1939, the organochlorine dichlorodiphenyltrichloroethane (DDT) was discovered to have insecticide properties. Thereafter, it was used widely for two decades. DDT has been one of the safest pesticides used in terms of acute effects. It was used directly on humans to kill lice, and it has never caused a fatal poisoning. However, DDT was banned in 1972 because of the environmental effects through its bioaccumulation.

Acutely, DDT exposure can cause numbness of the face, irritability, dizziness, poor balance, tremor, and convulsions. Subacute doses can cause the testicles to become smaller. Women who develop breast cancer tend to have higher residues of DDE, the breakdown product of DDT, in their breasts than do women free of the disease.

Chlorinated Cyclodiene Pesticides Chlorinated cyclodiene pesticides include chlordane, heptachlor, aldrin, dieldrin, endrin, and endosulfan. They are lipid-soluble and may be stored in human and animal fat for long periods of time. Many of these compounds are neuropoisons, and convulsions seem to be the first sign of toxicity. Other signs of poisoning are headaches, nausea, vomiting, dizziness, and mild chronic jerking of muscles. There may also be loss of memory and personality changes.

Chronic doses of dieldrin, heptachlor, and chlordane have caused liver cancer in mice. Aldrin, dieldrin, and endrin caused birth defects in the progeny of pregnant mice and hamsters. Aldrin and heptachlor caused death in rodent fetuses. Chlordane contains approximately 10% heptachlor. Chlordane residues remain in a home for over 30 years, causing chronic exposure and numerous symptoms in the inhabitants.

Botanical Pesticides Botanicals, which are insecticidal chemicals extracted from plants, include nicotine, rotenone, pyrethrum extracts, camphor, and turpentine. They are more expensive than the other four classes of pesticides. Pyrethroids, which are synthetic pyrethrums, are now available. They are very effective, but they are neurotoxic to humans.

HERBICIDES

Herbicides are toxic to plant enzymes and are generally thought to be nontoxic to humans, although people have died from herbicide poisoning.

Chlorophenoxy compounds are used to kill weeds next to highways and broadleaf weeds in farming. Two compounds in this group, 2,4-D and 2,4,5,-T, interfere with the growth hormone system in plants. After ingesting chlorophenoxy compounds, animals have died from ventricular fibrillation and muscle paralysis. The compound 2,4,5,-T contains a trace of dioxin, one of the most potent toxins known. It can cause skin rashes and is teratogenic (causes physical defects in developing embryos) in rats.

Dinitrophenols are another class of herbicide. Poisoning of humans causes nausea, rapid breathing, sweating, rapid heart rate, and coma. Dinitrophenols disable the mitochondria, which are the powerhouses of the cells. Chronically, these compounds can cause fatigue, sweating, thirst, and weight loss. Atropine cannot be used for acute poisoning, but ice baths and oxygen therapy have helped.

CLEANSING, BALANCING, AND PREVENTIVE TECHNIQUES

Avoiding exposure to pesticides is the preferable prevention technique. Pesticides are extremely toxic and can cause irreversible damage if the exposure is high. You can control the pesticide exposure in your home but, unfortunately, none of us can control what our neighbors use in their homes or on their yards.

Nontoxic methods of pest control can be used instead of pesticides. Remember, pesticides are more dangerous to us than the insects. It does require some effort but you can have a home with very few insects. The following measures will help control insects:

- Keep your home in good repair. Insects use any kind of crack or opening to get into your house.
- Prevent dampness next to the foundation. Moisture attracts insects both inside and outside the house.
- Keep the inside of your house clean. Vacuuming removes insects, larvae, and eggs.
- Use proper food storage, so that insects cannot feed on your food.

(For more detailed information on control of specific pests, see Recommended Books, *The Whole Way to Allergy Relief and Prevention*.)

For gardening and yard care, manually pulling the weeds will reduce the need for herbicides. Compost and manure can be used for fertilizer. Removing diseased portions of plants or even an entire tree is preferable to spraying with a pesticide. Ask your neighbors to tell you when they are going to spray their yards. Arrange to be gone for several days to several weeks while this is being done.

Hydrogen peroxide can be used on diseased trees. Spray the trees with one part food-grade hydrogen peroxide (35%) to 32 parts of water. Other plants grow better when sprayed with one ounce of 3% hydrogen peroxide per quart of water. Spray all parts of trees and other plants.

To avoid pesticide exposure:

- Wear protective clothing if you must be around pesticides. Wear long sleeves, long pants, gloves, a mask, and goggles or safety glasses.
- Launder or throw away the clothes you wore immediately.
- Shower immediately after working or being around pesticides.
- Store pesticides outside your home.

If you have had a pesticide exposure, you must do some type of detoxification program to rid your body of the pesticide residues.

Metals

Approximately 80 elements are classified as metals. Physical properties of metals include high reflectivity, electrical and thermal conductivity, and strength. In a water solution, metals can give up a negative particle, or electron, to form a positively charged ion, a cation. It is this property that determines the biological activity and toxicological characteristics of each metal.

Metals are categorized as heavy, trace, essential, nonessential, or toxic metals. Heavy metals have a specific gravity greater than 4 or 5. Trace metals, found in minute quantities in the body, are also essential metals, necessary for proper functioning of the body. However, essential metals can be toxic, depending on the dose. Copper, iron, and cobalt are all necessary in the body, but all can be toxic in high doses. Nonessential metals are not necessary for proper metabolism of the body, and they may also be toxic.

Dr. Henry Schroeder, one of the world's authorities on trace elements, noted 20 years ago that chronic toxic metal exposure is a more dangerous and insidious problem to human health than are organic substances such as pesticides.

Metals can be inhaled as fumes or dust particulates, or they can be ingested in food or water. Lung absorption depends on the particle size; particles less than 1 micron may be absorbed from the alveoli into the bloodstream. Metals may also be absorbed by the GI tract if they are sufficiently soluble. A person's age, nutrition, intake of competing metals (for example, zinc and cadmium) and the amount of food in the intestines affect the absorption of metals.

Most metals are excreted through the kidneys, but some are reabsorbed by the kidney tubules. Many metals are bound to plasma proteins and amino acids. Reabsorption is determined by the pH of the urine, the type of protein or amino acid to which the metal is attached, and whether other metals are competing for the same tubular reabsorption site.

The gastrointestinal tract also excretes metals. Lead, cadmium, and mercury are absorbed from the blood into the intestines. Metals that are attached to the cells lining the GI tract are excreted when these cells are shed.

Metals can be acutely or chronically toxic. Chronic toxicity is much more difficult to diagnose than acute. Metals are often toxic to the organs that cannot detoxify them. In chronic toxicity, a person is exposed to small doses over a long period of time. Symptoms may not develop for months to years. Acute toxicity symptoms may be different from those of chronic toxicity. Acute inorganic mercury toxicity may cause nausea, headache, diarrhea, and abdominal pain. Chronic inorganic mercury toxicity causes difficulty in swallowing, abnormal vision, hearing, taste, and smell, and poor coordination in the arms and legs.

Metals inhibit the activity of enzymes and they can bind to cofactors and vitamins. Toxic metals may displace essential metals.

ALUMINUM

Aluminum is the third most abundant element on earth and the most abundant metal. Aluminum is found in industry as a metal dust, welding fumes, aluminum soluble compounds, aluminum alkyls, and aluminum pyro powder. Coal-fired power plants, metal smelters, cement manufacturing plants, and waste incinerators are all sources of aluminum. Aluminum forms clumps or flocs with organic material, and it is often used in water-treatment plants to remove organic material.

Aluminum foil is used in cooking. Aluminum is found in soft-drink cans, antacids, paints, salt, white flour, animal and plant food, pyrotechnics, and deodorants. Some antacids contain from 35 to over 200 milligrams of aluminum per dose, and a person taking antacids could ingest 5000 milligrams of aluminum a day. (Aluminum-free antacids are available.) Buffered aspirin contains aluminum. Antidiarrheal medications, hemorrhoid medications, vaginal douches, and lipstick may contain aluminum.

Aluminum is used as a leavening agent in cake mixes, dough, and baking powders. Processed sliced cheese products often contain aluminum. Teas contain aluminum, and acidic foods in aluminum containers can leach aluminum. Acidic and alkaline foods can leach aluminum from aluminum pots. People ingest on the average from 5 to 100 milligrams of aluminum a day in the diet.

Drinking water can be contaminated with aluminum. Acid rain can leach aluminum from soil, rocks, and the sediments from the bottom of lakes. In the northeast, the amount of aluminum in surface water has increased tenfold in the past 80 years.

Aluminum enters the body through inhalation, absorption through the skin, and somewhat by GI absorption. Aluminum dust and aluminum pyro powders can be toxic to the lungs. Aluminum oxide exposure has caused pulmonary fibrosis (thickening and scarring of lung tissue) and emphysema. Aluminum builds up in the body as a person ages.

Aluminum can also cause weak bones, anemia, and abnormalities in calcium, magnesium, and phosphorous metabolism.

Aluminum interferes with the normal metabolism of nerve cells. Laboratory animals exposed to aluminum may develop neurofibrillary tangles (degenerated nerve cells) as are found in Alzheimer's disease, which is a loss of memory progressing to dementia. Patients with Alzheimer's may have normal aluminum levels in the brain, blood, and cerebrospinal fluid, but the neurofibrillary tangles will have abnormally high concentrations of aluminum. However, aluminum has not been proven to cause Alzheimer's disease.

Aluminum increases in concentration as it moves up the food chain. Meats, poultry, and dairy accumulate aluminum. Since it is not an essential metal, it is advisable to minimize your aluminum ingestion because neurological disorders are associated with cumulative doses of aluminum. Check to see if your local water contains high levels of aluminum, and avoid drinking it if it does. There has been massive fish die-off in many Scandinavian lakes because of the high aluminum concentrations.

CADMIUM

A major source of cadmium is dust from automobile tire erosion. It is also produced from burning waste. Cadmium is found in industrial effluents, plastics, fertilizers, auto exhaust, the coating on nails, rechargeable batteries, solder, coffee, soft or acidic water, and tobacco smoke. The amount of cadmium occurring in our food is increasing with these many exposures.

Cadmium is poorly absorbed from the GI tract but inhaled cadmium is absorbed readily. Once absorbed, cadmium is bound to a protein known as metallothionein, which is found in the major organs and which protects the body against cadmium's toxic effects. Cadmium accumulates primarily in the kidneys and somewhat in the liver. The half-life of cadmium is 20 years, which means that after 20 years 50% of the cadmium remains. When cadmium reaches a threshold level, damage to the kidney tubules can occur.

Structurally similar to zinc, cadmium causes damage by displacing or replacing zinc in over 200 enzymes. Cadmium is absorbed more easily when a person has a zinc deficiency.

Cadmium is toxic to the lungs. Acute exposure to cadmium dust or fumes can cause death while chronic exposure can cause emphysema. Other symptoms of chronic cadmium exposure include liver damage, anemia, high blood pressure, weak bones, bone pain, and shrinking of the testicles.

LEAD

Lead poisoning is thought to have occurred since Roman times. Because lead has a low melting point, it was one of the first metals smelted. Lead has been used extensively and has been investigated more thoroughly than any other metal.

All humans now have lead accumulations in

their bodies. We are exposed to lead from the soil, the air, and in water. Lead appears in two forms: inorganic lead and alkyl lead (used in gasoline). Exposure occurs in battery manufacturing, radiator repair, the printing industry, firing ranges, copper smelting, paint and pigment manufacturing, the plastics industry, and the rubber industry.

Until 1977 when it became regulated, lead was used in paint for pigmentation and to reduce weathering. Leaded paint can peel, flake, and chip, then be ingested by children. Children can also mouth objects contaminated with lead from dust and soil. Soil can be contaminated from lead paint as far away as ten feet from a building. Water from leaded pipes, soldered plumbing, and water cooling systems are sources of lead. Lead levels are higher in the morning when the water has been in contact with the lead plumbing all night.

The GI tract and the lungs absorb lead. The absorption of lead from the lungs depends on the particle size. Absorption from the GI tract depends on the amount of calcium, iron, fat, and protein in the diet. Infants absorb more lead than adults.

When lead is absorbed, the blood transports it to the organs of the body. The lead is then transferred into the bones, which, along with the teeth, store 90 percent of lead in the body. The rest is found in the kidneys and liver. Blood levels give an indication of recent lead exposure but do not indicate the total body burden of lead. A person can develop lead poisoning from small doses over a long period of time.

Bone storage may protect other organs from lead poisoning, but provides a source for remobilization when the body is under physiologic stress, such as pregnancy, lactation, or chronic disease. Lead is excreted by the GI tract, urine, and the shedding of skin and hair. Infants excrete more through the GI tract than adults.

Lead affects the CNS, blood, peripheral nervous system, GI tract, and kidneys. Lead poisoning causes fatigue, lethargy, insomnia, anemia, depression, irritability, headaches, tremor, and memory loss. Acute exposure can cause renal failure, severe GI symptoms, and acute brain symptoms. Chronic exposure to lead can cause mental retardation. Lead also causes subtle behavioral effects.

Lead causes a motor peripheral neuropathy, a damage to nerves that control movement. Additionally, lead poisoning causes abdominal pain, constipation, hypertension, and renal failure. Lead poisoning has caused decreased fertility, spontaneous abortion, stillbirth, and increased infant mortality. Males have had decreased sperm counts and a loss of sex drive.

Children are more sensitive to the effects of lead then are adults. Chronic lead levels have been studied by examining baby teeth that have been shed. Dr. Herbert Needleman at the University of Pittsburgh found that children with higher lead levels had lower IQ levels and more learning disabilities. When retested five years later, those children had attended more special education classes.

The lead level considered toxic has been lowered from 158 micrograms per decilitre (mcg/dl) in 1930 to 10 mcg/dl in 1990. People with blood lead levels above 25 mcg/dl require treatment.

MERCURY

Mercury occurs in three forms: metallic or elemental, inorganic, and organic. Each form has different toxicological characteristics.

Metallic or Elemental Mercury Metallic mercury is soluble in organic solvents but not in water. Metallic mercury is used in thermometers, electric switching devices, gauges, vacuum pumps, pressure-sensing devices, and in amalgams (silver fillings) used in dentistry. It is the only metal in liquid state at room temperature and it vaporizes readily.

When mercury vapor is inhaled, some is changed to inorganic mercury and some stays in the metallic or elemental form, which is more lipid-soluble. This form of mercury crosses the blood-brain barrier, where it accumulates in the brain. Mercury can damage brain cells, particularly sensation nerve cells and motor nerve cells. Elemental mercury can also accumulate in the kidneys.

Elemental mercury can produce lung damage, with inflammation of the alveoli, bronchioles, and the bronchi. Inhaling mercury fumes may cause fever, chills, shortness of breath, and a metallic taste in the mouth. This is known as metal fume fever and also occurs with the inhalation of other metals. Children younger than 30 months of age have died from pulmonary complications from inhaling mercury vapors.

Elemental mercury is poorly absorbed from the GI tract, so there is no danger for children from swallowing the mercury if a thermometer is broken in the mouth. As much as 204 grams of elemental mercury have been ingested without systemic toxicity. The danger from elemental mercury is from inhaling the fumes.

After a mercury dental filling is placed, low levels of mercury release for several years (see chapter 19, Dental Work). Chronic elemental mercury toxicity causes tremor, gingivitis (inflammation of the gums), and erethism (an abnormal state of excitement), which contributes to insomnia, shyness, memory loss, emotional lability, nervousness, and anorexia. Nineteenth-century hatters used mercury to cure beaver hides. Because of their exposure to elemental mercury, they developed neuropsychiatric symptoms and thus the term "mad as a hatter" developed.

Inorganic Mercury A portion of elemental mercury changes to inorganic mercury in the body. Inorganic mercury is a constituent of dry cells (batteries) and is used as a detonator for explosives. The compounds of mercury combined with nonmetals are known as salts. The most famous form of inorganic mercury is mercurous chloride, commonly known as calomel. Calomel was used for centuries as a primary medication. Physicians prescribed it orally to treat most major illnesses.

Approximately 10% of an oral dose of inorganic mercury is absorbed by the GI tract. Inorganic mercury salts damage the mucous membranes of the mouth, throat, esophagus, and stomach. They also cause gastroenteritis with abdominal pain, vomiting, and bloody diarrhea. Mercury salts damage the kidney, with decreased or no urination occurring about half the time. The organs of elimination of inorganic mercury are the GI tract and the kidney. Although inorganic mercury crosses the blood-brain barrier poorly, chronic toxicity causes behavioral changes.

Organic Mercury Microorganisms can convert elemental mercury and inorganic mercury into organic mercury. Organic mercury compounds are lipid-soluble and volatile.

The most significant compound is methyl mercury, which crosses the placenta and can accumulate in the fetus. Organic mercury also crosses into breast milk in toxic amounts. Up to 90% of methyl mercury is absorbed from the GI tract because of its lipid solubility. Methyl mercury moves to all body cells but concentrates in the liver, kidneys, blood, brain, hair, and skin. Hair levels correlate with blood levels, which are a good indicator of exposure.

After chronic exposure, methyl mercury toxicity develops gradually. Methyl mercury inhibits the synthesis of acetylcholine, the major neurotransmitter in the body, causing difficulty in concentration, loss of short- and long-term memory, depression, constriction of visual fields, uncoordination and an abnormal gait, numbness of the hands and feet, deafness, slurred speech, tremors of the hands, weakness, paralysis, decreased sense of smell and taste, and fatigue. The prognosis for improvement is poor. The body excretes about 1% of its organic mercury burden per day.

Organic mercury was used in the past to treat syphilis and as a diuretic. Today organic mercury is used as an antiseptic and as a preservative. Mercurochrome is an organic mercury antiseptic which, when applied to large burns, has caused death in children. Organic mercury is used as a fungicide, in embalming preparations, and in insecticide manufacturing. Until 1990, interior latex paint contained organic mercury.

Most organic mercury exposure comes from the diet and it can be concentrated in the food chain. In Minimata Bay, Japan, 25 infants were born with severe mental retardation caused by their mothers consuming fish contaminated with organic mercury from a factory discharge. Many people have been poisoned by eating grain treated with an organic mercury fungicide and intended to be used for plant seeds only, not for human consumption.

CLEANSING, BALANCING, AND PREVENTIVE TECHNIQUES

To avoid heavy metal poisoning:

- Wear protective clothing if you work in a factory or industry where there is possible exposure to heavy metals. This includes gloves, masks, suits, and safety glasses or goggles.
- If your company does not provide safety clothing or if working conditions are unsafe, in the U.S. contact the local Occupational Safety and Health Administration. In Canada, federal government employees can contact the Labour Division of Human Resources Development Canada; others can contact their provincial or territorial Department of Labour and ask for its Occupational Health and Safety division.

Cadmium Because cadmium poisoning is difficult to treat, prevention is very important. Adequate zinc helps protect against cadmium poisoning. Amino acids, calcium, copper, zinc, fiber, garlic, sulfur, iron, manganese, vitamin C, vitamin E, N-acetyl-l-cysteine, kelp, and the cabbage family decrease cadmium absorption and retention. Selenium decreases tissue cadmium and corrects hypertension.

In cadmium poisoning, the kidneys, lungs, and liver are organs of cadmium deposition and can be damaged. *Berberis vulgaris*, a homeopathic remedy, helps support the kidneys; *Kali carbonicum* is helpful for the lungs; and *Natrum sulphuricum* and *Nux vomica* are helpful for liver symptoms. *Cadmium metallicum* and *Cadmium sulfuricum* will help detoxify the cadmium from the body.

Mercury British anti-Lewisite (BAL) therapy is used to treat elemental and inorganic mercury poisoning but should not be used in organic mercury poisoning because it may cause an increase in mercury levels in the brain. Penicillamine given orally is used for less severe poisoning. DMSA (2,3-dimercaptosuccinic acid) and DMPS (2,3-dimercaptopropane-1-sulfonate) are derivatives of BAL, and have been used to treat acute and chronic mercury poisoning. DMSA is given orally. DMPS is given intravenously or intramuscularly.

Selenium, calcium, magnesium, iron, zinc, and manganese protect against organic and inorganic mercury poisoning. Vitamin C, glutathione, and cysteine may ameliorate mercury toxicity. Garlic is high in sulfur and will help chelate mercury.

Aurum metallicum, Carbo vegetabilis, Hepar sulphuris calcareum, Kali iodatum, Lachesis, Mercurius solubilis, Natrum sulphuricum, and *Sulphur lotum* are homeopathic remedies that will aid in treating mercury poisoning.

Lead Treatment for lead poisoning is with EDTA, BAL, and DMSA, all chelating agents (see chapter 15, Chelation). It takes four to five days to remove 5 milligrams (mg) of lead, when there is 50 to 100 mg of lead in the body. Zinc (60 mg daily) and vitamin C (2000 mg daily) have been used to reduce lead levels in workers in a battery factory. Copper, iron, and thiamine also have protective effects.

Alumina, Arsenicum, Platinum metallicum, Plumbum metallicum, Causticum, and *Sulphuricum acidum* are homeopathic remedies that help the body in treating lead poisoning.

Apple and garlic are herbs that help treat lead poisoning. Pectin in the diet causes lead to be excreted from the kidney.

Aluminum Avoid using baking powders made with aluminum, as well as salt that contains aluminum compounds to prevent caking. Aluminum-free antacids and buffered aspirin are available. Do not cook acidic foods (tomatoes) or alkaline foods (grains) in aluminum pots and pans. Avoid aluminum-containing antiperspirants and deodorants.

Calcium, fiber, lecithin, choline-rich foods, magnesium, vitamin C, vitamin E, and zinc prevent the absorption of aluminum or counteract its side effects. The homeopathic remedies *Plumbum metallicum, Bryonia,* and *Alumina* help cleanse the body of toxic aluminum.

7

External Toxins: Plants and Organisms

Plants

Plants can be toxic to humans in several ways. The most familiar toxic effect comes from plant pollens when they cause allergic reactions. The characteristic odors of plants are caused by aromatic chemicals called terpenes, which can also cause allergic symptoms. Some plants produce nerve poisons, internal-organ poisons, skin and eye irritants, as well as accumulating metals or minerals.

POLLENS

As part of their reproductive cycle, all seed-bearing plants produce pollen, which is analogous to human sperm. About 100 plant species produce pollen that is significant in allergic reactions and sensitivities. Problem-causing pollen must be abundant, widespread, windborne, light enough to be carried some distance, and contain specific antigens for hypersensitivity.

Trees, grasses, and weeds produce windborne pollen that causes allergic symptoms. These plants have small, unattractive flowers without nectar or scent. Plants with brightly colored, perfumed flowers are pollinated by insects and birds and generally do not affect the allergic person.

Pollen allergy symptoms include sneezing; hoarseness; increased mucus production; scratchy throat; hay fever; runny nose; itchy, red, watery eyes; and sinus symptoms of headache, pressure behind the eyeballs, tenderness over the cheekbones, pain in the frontal area, and aching teeth.

Allergic responses to pollens may also include symptoms that are not commonly thought of as pollen related. These include eczema, cold and flulike symptoms, asthma, fatigue, insomnia, depression, cramps and diarrhea, headaches, swollen lymph glands, hives, flushing, skipped heartbeats, panic attacks, and many others. During pollen season, some women may experience irregular periods, toxemia of pregnancy, or uterine hemorrhaging, especially if ragweed is pollinating.

TERPENES

Terpenes are unsaturated hydrocarbons that are widely distributed in plants. They are responsible for the taste and the odor of the plant and occur in all parts of the plant, including the pollen, but their concentration is highest in the stems, leaves, and flowers. Many sensitive people have adverse reactions to both pollen and terpenes.

These individuals develop their characteristic pollen symptoms for a given plant long before the pollen actually appears. These symptoms coincide with the rise in terpenes.

PLANT NERVE TOXINS

Plants produce chemicals that affect the human nervous system, causing a variety of symptoms. These toxins can affect the peripheral nervous system and motor coordination, and can be accompanied by delirium, stupor, and trance states. They may also cause nausea, gastrointestinal disorders, trembling, irregular or abnormally slow heartbeat, impaired respiration, dizziness, speech loss, and fatal paralysis.

Some examples of these toxins and the plants from which they come are:

- Coniine: spotted hemlock
- Nicotine: tobacco
- Pyrethrin: chrysanthemum
- Pyrollizidines: peyote
- Quinoloizidines: mescal bean
- Rotenone: legumes
- Scopolamine and atropine: deadly nightshade
- Taxol: western yew tree

Taxol is receiving attention because of its successful use in cancer chemotherapy. Nicotine and rotenone have insecticidal properties, and rotenone is safe for most mammals, except pigs. Pyrethrins are valuable as insecticides because they degrade quickly and rapidly paralyze insects.

Pyrethroids, which are synthetic pyrethrins, have been widely produced in recent years. They are more toxic to humans than the natural product, and toxic levels may cause sensations of burning or prickling of the skin, tremors, and salivation.

PLANT INTERNAL-ORGAN TOXINS

The heart, kidney, liver, and stomach may be affected by toxins from plants. Some examples of these toxins and the plants from which they come are:

- Convallatoxin: lily of the valley
- Digitoxin: foxglove
- Hypercin: St. John's wort
- Oxalates: oak tannin
- Pyrrolizidine alkaloids: fescue
- Saponins: alfalfa

Saponins cause gastric upset; hypercin and pyrrolizidine alkaloids affect the liver; digitoxin and convallatoxin affect the heart; and the oxalates obstruct the kidney tubules. However, these plant toxins can be processed so that they are beneficial rather than harmful. Digitalis, which is used in treating heart disease, is manufactured from foxglove.

SKIN AND EYE IRRITANTS

Poison ivy, poison oak, or poison sumac are well-known skin and eye irritants. The toxins in these plants are catechol compounds. Contact with the foliage of these plants causes a skin rash that may be so severe that it is disabling. In sensitive individuals, it may be very difficult to treat and healing can be very slow. Individuals exposed to smoke from the burning plants may require hospitalization to treat lung damage.

Photosensitizers are systemic plant poisons that pass unchanged through the liver and collect in the skin capillaries. When the skin is exposed to light, the capillaries leak. Phytophotodermatitis (photosensitization contact dermatitis) can occur after plants containing a chemical used as a defense against fungi and insects are crushed on the skin. When the skin is then exposed to sunlight, a blistering sunburn occurs, followed by darkened color where the plants touched the skin. Parsnips, dill, celery, figs, parsley, and mustard are some of the plants responsible for this phototoxic reaction.

MINERAL ACCUMULATORS

Some plants are toxic because they absorb inorganic materials from soil and water. Fluorides accumulate in the leaves of plants. This commonly occurs near ore smelters, refineries, and industrial plants that manufacture fertilizers, ceramics, aluminum, glass, and bricks. When animals or humans eat the leaves, symptoms may include headaches, vomiting, diarrhea, fatigue, weakness, excessive thirst, and asthma or bronchitis.

Plants growing on soil treated with nitrate fertilizers under moisture-deficient conditions accumulate nitrates. When animals consume these plants, the nitrate is metabolized to nitrite and then enters the bloodstream. The nitrite oxidizes the iron in hemoglobin so that the hemoglobin cannot transport oxygen as efficiently. This condition is called methemoglobinemia. Toxic nitrogen dioxide gas can be generated from these plants when they are stored as silage and undergo fermentation.

Volcanic activity has given Hawaii high levels of mercury in the soil, air, and water. Mercury particularly accumulates in green leafy vegetables, avocados, and papayas. People eating large amounts of these island-grown plants develop symptoms of mercury poisoning. Also, the mercury content of the water is so high that tuna weighing over 200 pounds cannot be used for food.

CLEANSING, BALANCING, AND PREVENTIVE TECHNIQUES

Pollens and Terpenes   Allergy extracts are the best protection for pollen and terpene allergies. By preventing reactions, the immune system is spared the stress and can heal. The extracts cause a release of any pollen debris or terpenes in the body. The homeopathic remedies *Allium cepa, Ambrosia, Sabadilla,* and *Wyethia* will help hay fever symptoms. *Arsenicum iodatum* will help hay fever and allergy that resembles an infection.

Washing the nose with saline nose drops helps to rinse the pollen from the nasal cavities. *BHI Allergy,* a complex homeopathic preparation, will reduce or eliminate allergic symptoms. Freeze-dried stinging nettles, quercitin, and vitamin C are also helpful.

Skin and Eye Irritants   After exposure to poison oak, poison ivy, or poison sumac, wash the affected skin with rubbing alcohol to remove the oil that causes the skin reaction. Calamine lotion helps reduce the itch and absorbs oozing from the rash. Colloidal oatmeal mixes are available, or you can make your own by finely grinding oatmeal in a blender or food processor. Use ½ cup of the ground mixture to a tub of bath water. Bathe several times a day to relieve symptoms. A charcoal poultice is useful in detoxifying poison oak or poison ivy (see chapter 17).

Several homeopathic remedies are useful in restoring balance after exposure to poison ivy or poison oak. *Rhus toxicondendron* is very effective. *Anacardium, Clematis erecta,* and *Croton tiglium* are also helpful.

Decoctions or liquid extracts of herbs can be used as a wash for poison oak or poison ivy irritations. Grindelia, gum plant, jewelweed, lobelia, mugwort, Solomon's seal, sumac, sweet fern, and witch hazel are all helpful.

Organisms

Microorganisms—bacteria, viruses, parasites, molds, yeast, and fungi—may be a source of toxins for humans. These organisms live in the soil, water, and air. Under certain conditions, they can cause health problems by generating an infection or by producing toxins.

BACTERIA

Bacteria are single-celled organisms that grow in colonies and reproduce by simple division called binary fission. They may be spheres (cocci), rods (bacilli), curved cells (vibrios), or spiral-shaped cells (spirochetes or spirilla). If the bacteria is pathogenic, and if it reaches our bodies in sufficient numbers, a bacterial infection can result.

Bacterial toxins may be divided into two classes: toxins released as the bacteria grow in the human body; and toxins produced in substances that are then ingested. (For more information, see Food, chapter 5.)

Bacteria produce several types of toxins. Exotoxins are easily separated from the bacterial cell without destroying the organism. Endotoxins are produced within a bacterial cell and are not released unless the bacteria is ruptured. Cytotoxins are a specific cell-destroying substance, and enterotoxins are exotoxins with an affinity for the cells of the small intestine.

Clostridium tetani, a common soil bacteria, enters the body through puncture wounds. The toxin that this bacteria synthesizes interferes with the neurotransmitter acetylcholine (ACC), causing tetanus or lockjaw. Because the tetanus toxin easily separates from the bacterial cell, it is considered an exotoxin.

Clostridium perfringens causes gas gangrene. The gangrene can develop in traumatic, open lesions, such as bullet wounds or compound fractures, particularly when contaminated with dirt or other foreign materials. The toxin passes along the muscle bundles, killing all cells and causing necrotic areas where the bacteria can grow. The growing bacteria produce gas in the tissues that can be heard and felt on palpation. When the bloodstream absorbs the toxin, the resulting systemic illness can be fatal unless treated.

The enterotoxin of the bacillus *Shigella dysenteriae* causes a severe form of dysentery, intestinal hemorrhaging, and gastrointestinal tract paralysis. Enterotoxin-producing *Escherichia coli* is a major cause of traveler's diarrhea.

Vibrio cholera produces a potent enterotoxin responsible for cholera. This toxin causes hypersecretion of chloride, potassium, bicarbonate, and water molecules out of the cells of the intestinal mucosa, with subsequent diarrhea. The extensive fluid loss and electrolyte imbalance can lead to dehydration and death within hours if not treated. Epidemic cholera is spread by contaminated water.

Corynebacterium diphtheriae produces an exotoxin that is responsible for the severity of diphtheria and all its pathologic systemic effects. This bacteria usually grows on epithelial tissue and causes necrosis of the cells in the area where it is growing. When the exotoxin is absorbed into the general circulation, it causes degenerative lesions in the heart, nervous system, and kidneys.

Most strains of *Pseudomonas aeruginosa* produce an exotoxin that destroys tissues. *Pseudomonas* infection is rare in healthy individuals. However, it is an opportunistic pathogen that can be devastating in immunocompromised individuals.

PARASITES

Parasites live within other organisms to obtain nourishment and shelter. This relationship may be temporary or permanent, with the parasite depending on the host organism for its existence. The parasite receives all the benefit from the association, and the host may or may not be damaged from the presence of the parasite. Medical parasites include protozoa (one-celled microscopic animals), helminths (worms), and arthropods (including bugs, flies, ticks, mites, spiders, and scorpions).

Parasites cause damage through their sheer numbers as they multiply. They obstruct vessels, destroy host cells, compete for nutrients, and their metabolic products cause inflammatory reactions. Only a few parasites release toxins that are detrimental to humans.

Protozoa *Entamoeba histolytica* causes amebic dysentery. It produces a cytotoxic enterotoxin that plays a role in tissue invasion. In virulent strains, the destruction and death of tissue cells occurs after contact.

A marine species of protozoan organisms belonging to the order *Dinoflagellata* produces toxins found in food. (For more information, see Food, chapter 5.)

Helminths Helminth comes from the Greek word meaning "worm." The term originally applied only to intestinal worms, but now includes both parasitic and free-living species of roundworms. Most helminths produce a toxic substance from secretory glands located near their mouths. These secretions are destructive to cells and are toxic to humans, enabling the worm to digest the host's tissue for food or to migrate through the tissues of the host.

Parasitic Insects and Vectors A few insects are considered parasites or act as vectors (intermediate hosts) for human disease. The louse sucks blood from humans. Their saliva is toxic to humans and causes a red, elevated papule accompanied by severe itching. The louse acts as a vector for epidemic typhus and trench fever.

Flea bites also cause a skin irritation in humans. This irritation may be only a papule, or in sensitive individuals can cause a rash. Fleas are vectors for plague and may be a mechanical vector for a number of viral and bacterial diseases.

Bedbug bites produce red itching wheals and bullae (blisters). Some individuals may have allergic symptoms with generalized urticaria (hives) and even asthma.

Ticks secrete a toxin from their salivary glands, which causes progressive paralysis. The disease has a rapid onset, and although death can occur from respiratory paralysis, most affected persons recover. Paralysis reverses quickly after removal of the tick.

Mosquitoes are distinguished from other flies by the female's elongated mouth parts, which are adapted for sucking blood, as the female cannot produce fertile eggs without a blood meal. While sucking the blood, the female mosquito injects her saliva into her victim. Antigens in the saliva may cause immediate allergic reactions as well as delayed skin reactions. A mosquito bite can cause considerable irritation with erythema (redness), itching, and swelling. Mos-

quitoes are biological and mechanical vectors for bacterial, helminthic, protozoan, and viral diseases of both humans and animals.

VENOMOUS INSECTS AND ARACHNIDS

Venomous insects cause more fatal poisonings in the United States each year than do all other venomous animals combined. These insects are from the order *Hymenoptera* and include ants, bees, hornets, wasps, and yellowjackets. They administer water-soluble, nitrogen-containing chemicals through their stinging mechanisms. Fatalities from insect stings are caused by allergic reactions in sensitized individuals. These reactions, if severe, can affect the nervous system, cardiovascular system, and respiratory function.

Scorpions inject venom into their prey through a stinger at the end of their long tails. Their venom is a toxalbumin that causes their stings to be extremely painful. Some species' stings can be fatal to humans. Scorpions are nocturnal and do not normally sting humans unless bare hands or feet come into contact with them.

Spiders all produce venom, but most do not produce sufficient quantities to harm humans. The two most important species of poisonous spiders are the black widow and brown recluse. The black widow spider can be identified by the orange hourglass-shaped spot on its abdomen. Symptoms of black widow spider poisoning include cramps, sweating, dizziness, headache, tremor, nausea, vomiting, pain, and elevated blood pressure. Death occurs rarely, and mainly in children.

The "violin" on the cephalothorax of the brown recluse spider identifies it, and it usually does not bite unless it is disturbed. The tissue and underlying muscle around the bite of this spider ulcerate and die, leaving a gaping wound. Systemic symptoms, such as anemia, nausea, vomiting, high fever, and convulsions may occur, and in rare instances, death.

VIRUSES

Viruses are organisms that are not a complete cell. They cannot replicate without host cells, and from that standpoint they can be considered a form of parasite. Viruses cause active infections, but can also remain in the body in inactive states for long periods of time. They can later reactivate to again cause acute symptoms and active infections.

Some viruses cause the destruction of cell structures that enable them to enter the cell. Others create a toxic effect by causing the body to release substances that initiate unpleasant effects. For example, many viruses increase cytokines from the immune cascade, causing the symptoms that are associated with a viral infection, such as aches, fever, and headaches.

MOLDS, YEAST, AND FUNGI

Molds, yeast, and fungi are a part of the class *Fungi imperfecti,* which contains molds and pathogenic yeast.

Molds   Molds emit mycotoxins, which can cause untoward symptoms and even death in animals and humans. However, these toxins are produced only when the molds grow on certain substances. Exposure is usually through ingesting food contaminated by mold. Although there are many of these toxins, only those affecting humans are described under Food, in chapter 5.

Molds do not have a season and, except when there is snow on the ground, are present all year. Their peak spore season is from midsummer through fall. Molds are found everywhere, both indoors and outdoors, and at all temperatures. They are particularly abundant where there is moisture and are spread by winds, insects, and humans.

Suspect a mold allergy if a person is:

- worse from 5:00 to 9:00 P.M.
- worse in damp places
- worse when working in the yard
- worse from August until frost, even after ragweed season is over
- better with snow and freezing temperatures
- worse when eating fermented products or mushrooms and other fungi
- better inside a closed house with air-conditioning or furnace on

Some symptoms and conditions caused by mold are: nasal symptoms, respiratory complaints, secretory otitis, dermatitis, urticaria, gastrointestinal distress, cerebral symptoms, depression, and allergies.

Yeast   Pathogenic yeast, such as *Candida albicans,* produce toxins that affect humans. *C. albicans* releases over 80 known toxins, many of which are produced to either kill or inhibit other competing microorganisms.

Acetaldehyde, ethanol, glycoprotein toxins, polysaccharide protein complexes, tyramine, canditoxin, mannan, and proteinase are toxic byproducts of candida metabolism. Candida toxins weaken the defense system of the body, and the presence of excessive toxins causes the mucous membranes in the gut to leak. Larger protein molecules are absorbed, stimulating antibody production. Multiple food and chemical sensitivities result.

The most important toxic substances *C. albicans* produces are acetaldehyde and ethanol. Acetaldehyde, which is chemically related to formaldehyde, disrupts cell membrane function and alters protein synthesis. It is six times more toxic to the brain than ethanol. Ethanol can cause a low-grade intoxication-like state that results in vague neurological problems. Because our metabolism cannot convert acetaldehyde or ethanol into useful materials, our body must detoxify them. If the circulating load of these toxins is too great, fatigue, poor memory, light-headedness, inability to concentrate, and depression can result.

Medical Fungi   Some fungi are pathogenic for humans. They fall into four classes:

- *Systemic or deep mycosis*: Caused by inhalation of spores and manifesting as pulmonary symptoms. If untreated can form metastatic abcesses or granulomas throughout the body.
- *Subcutaneous mycosis*: Caused by direct implantation of spores or filament fragments. Disease begins with a skin abcess or granuloma that can spread both on the skin or through the lymph system.
- *Cutaneous mycosis*: Fungi grow in the epidermis, hair, and nails. Diseases are chronic and confined to the site of the infection. Some examples of cutaneous mycosis are athlete's foot, ringworm, and fungal infections of the scalp.
- *Superficial mycosis*: Fungi are localized along hair shafts and in hardened, dead epidermal cells.

Mushrooms   Mushrooms are fleshy fungi that also produce toxins. Among these toxins are alkaloids that cause central nervous system symptoms, such as narcosis and convulsions, and in some cases hallucinations. Muscarine is an alkaloid toxin found in several species of mushrooms. Perspiration, watering eyes, and salivation are symptoms unique to muscarine poisoning. Cramps, diarrhea, headache, and blurred vision may follow.

Psilocybin and psilocin are other alkaloids. They are both hallucinogens and can produce either a good or a bad "trip," depending on several factors. The length of time the symptoms persist depends on the quantity of mushroom consumed.

Polypeptides make up another class of toxin produced by mushrooms. They are systemic poisons that attack the cells of organs, including the heart, liver, and kidneys. Death can result from eating a single cap of the *Amanita* mushroom species. Beginning symptoms include violent diarrhea, cramps, and abdominal pain. The victim may also suffer paralysis, delirium, and coma.

CLEANSING, BALANCING, AND PREVENTION TECHNIQUES

Bacteria   Homeopathy provides several remedies to detoxify and balance the body affected by bacterial toxins.

- Tetanus (lockjaw): *Hypericum, Ledum, Cicuta;* preventive for tetanus: *Arnica, Hypericum, Ledum*
- Gangrene: *Anthracinum, Arsenicum album, Kreosotum, Secale* (fingers and toes)
- Dysentery: *Aloe, Cantharis, Capsicum, China officinalis, Colchicum, Colocynthis, Ipecacuanha, Mercurius corrosivus, Mercurius solubilis, Nux vomica, Podophyllum*
- Cholera: *Camphora, Cuprum metallicum, Veratrum album;* preventive for cholera: *Veratrum album, Camphora, Cuprum metallicum*
- Diphtheria: *Lac caninum, Phytolacca, Diphtherinum, Apis*

Herbal remedies are also effective in detoxifying the body of bacterial toxins. However, some sensitive people may not tolerate herbs.

- *Dysentery*: garlic, marshmallow, prickly ash bark, slippery elm bark, bayberry, blackberry, turmeric
- *Gangrene*: garlic
- *Cholera*: garlic, goldenrod, marshmallow, prickly ash bark, slippery elm bark
- *Tetanus*: skull cap

Allergy extracts for bacteria aid in cleansing the body of both past and present infections.

Symptoms of current bacterial infections are mainly caused by allergic response to the organism. The extract reduces or eliminates these symptoms. Bacterial debris are left on the cells of the body after infections and are still allergenic. The extracts cause these debris to release, thus cleansing the body of the remains of the infection.

Parasites   The effects of toxins released during parasitic infections may be treated and the body rebalanced with homeopathic remedies.

- Hookworm and roundworm: *Chenopodium antihelminticum*
- Worms and parasites, all types: *Cina*
- Tapeworm: *Granatum, Magnesia muriatica*
- Recurrent worms: *Natrum phosphoricum*
- Worms: *Podophyllum, Ratanhia, Spigelia, Zincum metallicum*
- Amebic dysentery: *Ipecacuanha*
- Ameba: *Mercurius sulphuricus*

Herbs also help with the effects of toxins released during parasitic infections.

- *Giardia*: barberry, bayberry, echinacea, garlic, elecampane, turmeric, goldenrod
- Amebic dysentery: barberry
- Worms: pumpkin seed is an antihelmintic; garlic: roundworm, hookworm, tapeworm, and pinworms; black walnut bark: expels worms with the laxative action

Homeopathic remedies help detoxify and heal the effects of toxins released when insects bite.

- Fleas: *Ledum, Arsenicum* if glands are swollen, *Pulex*
- Bedbug: *Ledum*
- Mosquito: *Caladium;* prevents mosquito bites: *Staphysagria*
- Ticks: *Ledum*
- Lice: *Staphysagria*

The following herbs help with the toxins released with insect bites:

- Aloe vera
- Calendula
- Comfrey
- Echinacea
- Marsh tea
- Plantain
- Skullcap
- Wild hyssop
- Witch hazel

Allergy extracts for parasites help to cleanse the body of both current and past infections. These extracts also help cleanse the body after the infection by causing the release of the allergenic remains of the parasitic bodies to release from the cells.

Venomous Insects and Arachnids   Apply the following natural remedies to insect bites/stings:

- A paste made from a small amount of papain meat tenderizer and water
- Baking soda paste
- Witch hazel
- A paste of buffered vitamin C
- A cut raw onion
- Cold compresses to lessen pain and prevent the spread of toxins
- A 3% dilution of food-grade hydrogen peroxide

The following homeopathic remedies are effective treatments for insect bites.

- Bee stings: *Carbolicum acidum, Plantago, Urtica urens*
- Scorpion and spider bites: *Hypericum, Ledum, Tarentula hispanica and cubensis, Latrodectus curassavicus* (brown recluse)
- Any insect bite: *Apis, Cantharis* (bites that burn and blister), *Gunpowder, Tabacum*

Allergy extracts of insect venom help the body recover from an insect bite. In the United States, some health practitioners use a Stun Gun to treat spider bites and arrest venom damage to tissue.

This technique is particularly helpful with brown recluse spider bites, which can cause damage requiring plastic surgery.

A poultice and tea of the following herbs will help insect bites:

- Aloe
- Calendula
- Echinacea
- Mint
- Parsley
- Plantain
- Witch hazel

Viruses Effects of viral infections are helped by several nutrients. L-lysine, an amino acid, prevents viral replication. Monolaurin, a preparation of lauric acid, disintegrates the viral envelope, which prevents the virus from attaching to the cell. Coenzyme Q_{10} supports the immune system and aids with viral infections. Vitamin C taken consistently in divided doses throughout the day reduces the toxic effects of the virus.

Gelsemium is a primary homeopathic remedy for the common flu and for people who have never been well since the flu. *Arnica* is helpful in viral infections when the person feels "like he or she has been run over by a truck." *Baptisia tinctoria* is a remedy for toxic flu that came on quickly. *Pyrogenium* is also for toxic flu, but the fever is higher, accompanied by delirium. Scientific studies have shown the homeopathic preparation *Oscillococcinum* to be effective against the influenza virus. Echinacea used in herbal tincture is an important flu remedy. *Rhus toxicondendron* is a primary remedy for fever blisters and chickenpox, both of which are caused by the *Herpes* virus.

Engystol is another homeopathic preparation that is useful with viruses. This immune system stimulant can help to prevent a viral infection or shorten the course and severity of an active infection.

The following herbs are helpful for their antiviral activity:

- Balm
- Cinnamon
- Chamomile
- Echinacea
- Ginseng
- Ginger
- Goldenseal

Viral allergy extracts aid significantly in reducing the fever and malaise of viral infections. These symptoms are largely caused by an allergic response to the viral bodies. The extracts also cleanse the body of viral debris left on the cells after a viral infection.

Molds Molds cause us many types of problems. Not eating moldy foods and foods that might have mycotoxin contamination will prevent some problems.

Moisture control to prevent the growth of molds is of major importance. Keep all plumbing in good repair and be certain there is good ventilation in all parts of your house, particularly in the bathroom, laundry room, and kitchen. If you live in a humid climate, investing in a dehumidifier may be of great benefit. Air cleaners will remove mold spores.

For mold cleanup, soap and hot water, bleach, zephiran, and borax are helpful. Chemically sensitive people should avoid bleach, and some individuals may not be able to use borax. Wear a mask and gloves for mold cleanup, and wash your clothing, hair, and body afterward. Ozone generators will kill mold in hard to reach places. Ozone is a gas and will penetrate all parts of the house. However, people, plants, and animals must not be in the house while the generator is in use, or for one hour after it has been turned off. By that time, any ozone in the air will have deteriorated into oxygen.

For the mold-allergic person, allergy extracts offer the most relief. Taken regularly, they will control symptoms and help cleanse the body of any debris from molds on the cells.

Yeast Allergy extracts are extremely useful in combating the effects of ethanol and acetaldehyde produced by *Candida albicans*. Immuno-therapy with candida and T.O.E. (*Trichophyton, Oidiomycetes (Candida), Epidermophyton*) extracts also relieve symptoms associated with candida overgrowth and stimulate immune response.

China officinalis, a homeopathic remedy, is effective in combating the fermentation caused by colonization of candida in the bowel. *Natrum phosphoricum* restores acid/alkaline balance, which frequently causes symptoms to disappear.

Preparations of caprylic acid, which has fungicidal action, are very useful in treating candida infections. *Lactobacillus acidophilus* preparations restore normal gut flora. Para Microcidin, an antimicrobial, and Formula SF722 (undecylenic acid), which inhibits yeast growth, are also useful. Nystatin, Nizoral, Diflucan, and Sporonox are pharmaceuticals that reduce yeast overgrowth.

Essential fatty acids, mathake and taheebo tea, and garlic are helpful in combating candida overgrowth. Fiber decreases bowel transit time and thus reduces toxin absorption from the gut. Organic germanium increases oxygen utilization, which deters the growth of anaerobic yeast. Coenzyme Q_{10} enhances immune system function. Thyme oil and tea tree oil have antifungal properties and are helpful for skin rashes caused by yeast.

Fungi   There are many types of fungal diseases that affect people. The more serious and systemic types do require treatment by a physician.

Hydrogen peroxide will help skin or nail fungus. Dilute 35% food-grade hydrogen peroxide to a 3% or 6% solution.

3% solution: 1 ounce of 35% hydrogen peroxide in 11 ounces of distilled water

6% solution: 2 ounces of 35% hydrogen peroxide in 11 ounces of distilled water

For skin or nail fungus, or athlete's foot, soak feet nightly in a 3% or 6% solution of hydrogen peroxide. For fingernails, soak twice daily. This treatment will also work for jock itch or ringworm.

Mushrooms   Several homeopathic remedies are helpful in combating the effects of toxins consumed when eating poisonous mushrooms. *Absinthium, Arsenicum album, Belladona,* and *Camphor* will help to cleanse the symptoms of mushroom poisoning and rebalance the body.

8

External Toxins: Radiation and Electromagnetic Fields

Radiation

Radiation is the emission and propagation of waves or particles, such as light, sound, radiant heat, or particles emitted by radioactive material. The electromagnetic spectrum is composed of the following, listed from lower to higher energy and from longer to shorter wavelength: radio waves, television waves, microwaves, infrared light, visible light, ultraviolet radiation, X-rays, and gamma rays. All these energies are forms of radiation.

Radiation can be ionizing, which means it has energy high enough to ionize matter (can remove or add one or more electrons to an atom or molecule) or nonionizing, which is of lower energy. Gamma rays and X-rays are ionizing radiation, while all other members of the electromagnetic spectrum are nonionizing. Both types of radiation have biological effects.

IONIZING RADIATION

Ionizing radiation comes from natural and from manmade sources. It includes beta particles (electrons), alpha particles (two protons and two neutrons), and gamma rays (very high energy X-rays).

Natural Radiation   Natural radiation comes from cosmic radiation, isotopes in the earth's crust that decay, radon gas, carbon-14 in the atmosphere, and potassium-42 and other isotopes found in minute amounts in the body. People also receive radiation from other sources, such as diagnostic X-rays, fallout from past nuclear weapons testing, television receivers, airline travel, and therapeutic radiation.

It is estimated that 2% to 4% of the total cancer deaths in North America are caused by natural background radiation. An average radiation dose is 3.6 millisieverts per person per year. (One sievert equals 100 rems.) Dental X-rays account for an annual dose of 0.03 millisieverts (3 rems) a year, and medical X-rays account for 0.35 millisieverts a year. Airline travel accounts for 0.005 millisieverts a year from the additional cosmic radiation dose received while flying.

Isotopes   Nature is made of building blocks of matter called elements, such as oxygen, calcium, lead, and hydrogen. Elements consist of atoms, which contain protons, neutrons, and electrons. Some elements have different forms of atoms, known as isotopes, with different numbers of neutrons in the nucleus, giving the isotope a slightly different atomic weight. Elements and their isotopes have the same number of protons in the nucleus, giving them the same atomic number. Some isotopes are unstable and radioactive. When unstable isotopes change to another isotope (known as a decay product) they eject particles (alpha, beta, and gamma rays), known as radiation. This radiation can damage tissues and chromosomes.

Radioactive isotopes decay in a known pattern. The time that it takes half of the atoms to be lost is known as a half-life. Half-lives vary from less than 1 second to 4.5 billion years. When radioactive isotopes decay, they change into other elements, because protons are lost from the nucleus.

The damage that radioactive isotopes can do depends on the half-life, the type and energy of radiation emitted, the state of the isotope (gas, liquid, or solid), and the chemical interaction of the isotope with other substances. Radiation imparts energy to tissues as it passes through the body, causing damage to individual cells of the body or its genetic material, DNA.

Radon is a gas that decays to polonium, a dangerous isotope that emits alpha particles. When radon is inhaled, the high-energy alpha radiation is emitted inside the lung, and can lead to lung cancer.

Atomic bombs are made of isotopes that split apart when struck by neutrons. Two isotopes are produced from one, and these have less total mass than the original isotope. The lost mass is converted to energy, as predicted by Einstein's famous equation $E=MC^2$. This process is known as fission, and the energy emitted is radiation. Fission can cause a tremendous explosion, as in an atomic bomb, or can be controlled, as in a nuclear reactor.

The effects of radiation have been determined from the symptoms of survivors of the atomic bombs at Hiroshima and Nagasaki. Acute radiation exposure causes vomiting, malaise, fatigue, sweating, diarrhea, headache, and loss of appetite from hours to two days after irradiation. Doses above 50 Gray (Gy, an absorbed dose) cause death from injury to the central nervous system in two days. Doses between approximately 10 and 50 Gy lead to damage to the intestinal mucosa, intestinal bleeding, and death between six and nine days. Doses from one to several Gy cause suppression of the bone marrow within 48 hours.

Radiation dermatitis, hair loss, and sterility in both males and females also result from acute radiation exposure. Acute radiation affects the organs of the body that have the most rapid cell turnover—the gastrointestinal tract, the bone marrow, and the hair. These same organ systems are affected when a person receives radiation therapy. Chronic radiation exposure causes cancer in people of all ages and leukemia in children. It is now known that radiation can cause cancer at lower doses than was originally thought.

FOOD IRRADIATION   Approximately one-third of the food produced in the United States has to be discarded because of spoilage. Radiation prolongs shelf life of foods by killing insects, bacteria, fungi and viruses, and by slowing ripening. Fumigants and chemical preservatives to do not have to be used. However, when food is irradiated, unique radiolytic products (URPs) are produced. The health risk from these URPs is unknown.

Food irradiation is the only method of food preservation that the FDA considers an additive. Cesium-137 and cobalt-60 are the isotopes used to produce the gamma rays employed in food irradiation.

Radiation can bleach and change the color of the food. Some foods lose vitamins and other nutrients. Vitamin K is particularly sensitive to radiation, as are lipids and carbohydrates. Radiation destroys natural antioxidants and causes off-flavor in lipids. While radiation can affect the flavor of protein, and change the taste and texture of food, it does not make the food radioactive. Enzymes in food are radiation-resistant and require a dose five times that required by microorganisms to be inactivated. *Clostridium botulinum* is among the most radiation-resistant microorganisms.

The FDA has approved irradiation of wheat, wheat flour, pork, potatoes, spices, and whole fruits and vegetables. Only spices are currently being irradiated in significant amounts in the United States. Present laws do not require labeling of irradiated foods used in a mixture.

CLEANSING, BALANCING, AND PREVENTIVE TECHNIQUES

Radium bromatium, a homeopathic remedy, will cleanse and rebalance after radiation poisoning, and will antidote the radioactivity. *Sol* and *X-ray,* also homeopathic remedies, can be used to antidote radiation sickness. *Cadmium iodatum* will help nausea after radiation.

Soda and salt baths will cleanse radiation. For details on this type of detoxification bath, see Detoxification Baths, chapter 13.

Vitamins A, C, and B-complex and the amino acids lysine, cysteine, and methionine help to overcome any type of radioactive pollution.

NONIONIZING RADIATION

Ultraviolet, Infrared, and Visible Light
Nonionizing radiation has longer wavelengths and lower energy than ionizing radiation. Ultraviolet and infrared radiation are nonionizing radiation. The sun emits radiation from the ultraviolet range to the infrared range. Ozone in the earth's atmosphere absorbs the highest-energy ultraviolet radiation and water vapor absorbs infrared radiation.

The main source of ultraviolet radiation comes from the sun. Lesser amounts come from welding arcs, electric arc lights, and special ultraviolet lights. The amount of ultraviolet light the earth receives varies, depending on the time of day, the time of year, and the presence of clouds, snow, or water. Glass and light clothing filter out ultraviolet radiation.

Ultraviolet radiation helps to produce vitamin D in the skin, but also causes sunburn and darkens the skin. Severe sunburn blisters the skin. Chronic ultraviolet radiation exposure causes the skin to age more rapidly, increasing wrinkling and loss of skin elasticity. It can also cause skin cancer. Ultraviolet radiation can cause inflammation of the eye and the formation of cataracts.

Recent studies performed at the University of Miami, by Dr. Richard Taylor and Dr. Wayne Streileim, indicate that too much sunlight can damage the immune system. The amount of ultraviolet light that will cause a severe sunburn can damage or kill Langerhans cells in the skin. These cells are the first defense of the body against chemical toxins or infectious agents that invade the skin. This amount of ultraviolet light also decreases the circulating T-cells (white blood cells) and triggers fever blisters on the lips of people with latent *Herpes simplex* infections. One to three severe sunburns before the age of twenty doubles the chance of a person developing malignant melanoma, the most common cancer in the United States.

Infrared radiation emanates from all objects above absolute zero in temperature. For example, heat given off by a stove is infrared radiation. The sun is a major source of infrared radiation. Too much heat from the sun can adversely affect both plants and animals, causing heat exhaustion, a state of collapse brought on by depletion of plasma volume from sweating. The skin blood vessels are dilated to the extreme, but thermoregulatory centers are still functioning. The body temperature is slightly elevated.

Untreated heat exhaustion results in heat stroke. Heat gain is greater than heat loss. The body temperature becomes so high that the brain thermoregulatory centers stop functioning and the person does not sweat. As a result, the body temperature rises even higher. If the heat source is the sun, this phenomenon is known as sun stroke.

Both heat exhaustion and heat stroke may result from exposure to sources of heat other than the sun. Work situations involving the use of furnaces, boilers, or heat-producing engines are potential problems unless temperature control and protective measures are used. Some common tranquilizers interfere with neurotransmitters in the thermoregulatory centers, and people taking these drugs are very prone to heat strokes.

While too much sun can cause adverse effects, the proper amount of sunlight can have healing and cleansing effects on the body. Studies have shown that repeated short exposures to the sun lower cholesterol, triglycerides, blood pressure, and blood sugar. Fungal infections of the skin are cured or go into remission after sunlight therapy. White blood cells and antibody levels increase with treatment with ultraviolet light or sunlight in amounts that do not redden skin, and neutrophils are stimulated to engulf bacteria more rapidly. Sunlight speeds the elimination of toxic chemicals, including metals and pesticides. It also has a dramatic effect on trace minerals, making them more accessible to the body. Jaundice is reduced in both children and adults by exposure to sunlight. Many skin diseases, including acne and psoriasis, improve with exposure to sun.

Sunbathe with caution. Generally speaking, dark-skinned people can tolerate more sun than light-skinned people. Red-headed and blond people should begin with very brief exposures to the sun. Sunbathing for two minutes on each area—front, back, and sides—is the safest way to begin. Gradually increase the time by one minute each day. *Never sunburn.* Should you turn pink, do not increase the time for several days. If you still turn pink, decrease the time.

Beware of reflecting surfaces in the area where you sunbathe. Snow reflects 85% of the ultraviolet light, dry sand 17%, and grass and water around 3% to 5%. Sunbathing around snow or sand can cause you to sunburn very rapidly. Also, wet skin sunburns more easily than dry skin.

Clean skin is best for sunbathing. Fat or oil, such as those in suntan creams, oils, or lotions, when applied to the skin can stimulate the formation of cancer cells. Sunscreening agents filter out many of the therapeutic and healing effects of sunlight. Para-aminobenzoic acid (PABA), which is in many of these products, can cause genetic damage when exposed to sunlight. Many sensitive persons are allergic to PABA.

CLEANSING, BALANCING, AND PREVENTIVE TECHNIQUES

When you cannot avoid exposure to the sun, use clothing or a tolerated sunscreen to protect against ultraviolet radiation. Aloe vera gel and *Calendula* gel or ointment are very healing for cases of sunburn.

Several homeopathic remedies are helpful in restoring balance after overexposure to the sun:

- Headache from sun: *Antimonium crudum, Bryonia, Glonoinum, Lachesis, Natrum muriaticum, Natrum carbonica, Pulsatilla*
- Sunstroke or heat stroke: *Amylenum nitrosum, Glonoinum, Natrum carbonica, Sol, Staphysagria, Veratrum album*
- Sunburn: *Belladonna, Cantharis, Pulsatilla, Sol, Urtica urens*

Electromagnetic Fields

Extremely low frequency (ELF) electromagnetic fields have wavelengths of 0 to 300 hertz (hertz is a unit of frequency equal to one cycle per second) in frequency. These ELF fields are produced by alternating currents flowing along electrical lines or into electric appliances. Direct current does not produce ELF fields.

ELF electromagnetic fields are difficult to detect without special instruments. Occasionally the fields can be heard as they produce a humming noise or smelled when they produce ozone. Electricity in North America has a frequency of 60 cycles per second or 60 hertz.

Most of the rest of the world transmits electricity of 50 hertz. Microwave and radiofrequency radiation have higher frequencies.

Exposure to ELF fields occurs with the use of electric blankets, household appliances, computers, laser printers, copiers, and from electrical transmission lines. High-voltage transmission lines have very large ELF fields associated with them. The United States has regulations that set aside 100 yards of right-of-way beneath high-voltage tension lines.

Electrical currents generate magnetic fields. Household appliances have higher magnetic fields than do high-voltage transmission lines. Even so, exposure to magnetic fields from high-voltage transmission lines is usually greater than exposure to magnetic fields from home appliances due to the small amounts of time involved in the use of home appliances. When an appliance is turned off, the magnetic fields disappears. However, the electrical field remains as long as the appliance is plugged in.

Many studies have been done exposing cells and animals to ELF fields. Epidemiological studies have been done on workers in the electric industries. The results have not been consistent, but electric workers and their children have a higher risk of brain tumors. The incidence of childhood leukemia is higher in children who live near power lines that carry high voltage. Power-line exposure has also been associated with an increased incidence of suicide.

These studies support the hypothesis that ELFs act as a cancer promoter. ELF fields interact with the cell membrane and can affect hormones, calcium exchange, and tissue growth. It is postulated that the ELFs suppress the production of melatonin, a cancer inhibitor, by the pineal gland. There are now 22 studies being performed worldwide, researching the effects of ELF exposures on the risk of cancer.

Not all electromagnetic fields are harmful. Low frequency electromagnetic fields have been used to treat ulcers that expose the bare bone,

necrotic hip joints, delayed bone union, and osteoporotic bones.

The state of a person's health and the intensity of the electromagnetic exposure influences symptoms. Dizziness, confusion, hyperactivity, memory loss, sleep disturbances, mood changes, numbness, convulsions, and stress syndromes can result from repeated exposure. Some people develop frequent infections and/or allergies and sensitivities.

The following effects indicate an electromagnetic imbalance:

- symptoms that worsen before a storm and improve after it begins
- malfunction of electrical equipment when you are near
- symptoms from telephone use
- inability to find a watch that keeps time
- symptoms when near fluorescent lights
- symptoms when near transformers or high-powered electric lines
- difficulty wearing hearing aids

VIDEO DISPLAY TERMINALS

Video display terminals (VDTs) produce two types of electromagnetic fields—very low frequency and extremely low frequency. The fields from VDTs are highest at the back and side of the terminal, and drop quickly with distance. Copying machines and laser printers also emit strong electromagnetic fields, and they also drop off rapidly with distance.

The extremely low frequency fields have been associated with miscarriages, cancer, and immune dysfunction. Very low frequency fields have also been associated with pregnancy problems.

RADIOFREQUENCY AND MICROWAVE RADIATION

Radiofrequency and microwave radiation (RF-MW) are in the frequency of 3 MH (megaHertz) to 300 GH (gigaHertz). This range includes radio and television broadcasting, cellular telephone transmitters, radar, microwave ovens, medical diathermy, and hyperthermia for cancer treatment. The biological effects depend on the frequency of the radiation, the waveform, and the orientation. RF-MW have been reported to be cancer promoters and can affect the endocrine system, the blood-brain barrier, and the lens of the eye, producing cataracts.

No long-term studies have been conducted regarding the effects of low-level exposure to RF-MW radiation. Acute high exposure has caused memory loss. Biological studies have shown that pulsed radiation has more effects than continuous radiation exposure. Military personnel with RF-MW exposure have increased rates of cancer, especially of the blood and the lymphatic tissues. Exposure standards are lower in Russian and Eastern European countries than they are in the United States.

Microwave ovens should be checked yearly for leakage. If the door gasket is damaged, replace it before using the oven again. Use a well-calibrated meter to check for leakage. The dose and the time of microwave exposure that can cause problems is unknown. Do not stand in front of microwave ovens while they are in operation.

Personal radio transmitters which produce RF-MWs include cordless telephones, cellular telephones, radio-controlled toys, and business security systems. The antennas of these devices are only one to two inches away from the head and brain of the user. The brain also produces electromagnetic fields of its own. Ham radio operators have a higher incidence of leukemia than the general public.

Television sets radiate a field in all directions. The larger screens usually radiate a stronger field, which extends further out into the room. These electromagnetic fields penetrate wood and building materials, and children's beds should not be placed in an adjoining room. In animal studies, the fields from TV sets decreased

growth, affected brain function, and reduced the size of testicles in the males.

FLUORESCENT LIGHTS

Fluorescent lights operate differently than incandescent bulbs. Incandescent lights emit energy over a larger part of the visible spectrum. Fluorescent light is produced by a high-voltage discharge causing fluorescence of a chemical that coats the inside of the light. To accomplish this, a transformer raises the household current to several thousand volts. The fluorescent lights produce a much higher magnetic field than incandescent bulbs. One foot away from the fluorescent light, there is still a measurable magnetic field, and a person's head may be only a foot away from the light.

CLEANSING, BALANCING, AND PREVENTIVE TECHNIQUES

Because electromagnetic balance can be difficult to re-establish, prevention is of extreme importance. The following simple precautions can help to minimize problems.

- Choose a home that is a long distance away from transformers or high-voltage wires.
- Locate your bedroom as far away as possible from the entry of the electric current into your house.
- Keep a minimal number of electric appliances in your bedroom.
- Do not use electric blankets, heating pads, or the heater in water beds.
- Position the head of your bed to the north (best) or east (next best).
- Check your microwave for leaking, and stay at least four feet away when it is operating.
- Use a screening shield over your computer screen.
- When traveling, get out of the car periodically and walk to establish ground contact.

- Go barefooted as much as possible. Many symptoms can be relieved by standing on damp grass or in running water.
- If you have fluorescent light fixtures, use full-spectrum bulbs.

Wearing a Teslar watch is beneficial in restoring electromagnetic balance. It is a high-quality watch, containing a chip that connects the clocking mechanism and the battery into a magnetic frequency that resembles the natural field of the earth. It is weaker than the field of the earth, but because the watch is worn against the skin, its effects reach the whole body. The watch offers protection from electromagnetic pollution, eases stress and bolsters stamina. People suffering from multiple allergies frequently improve when wearing a Teslar watch. Jet lag can be significantly reduced or eliminated by wearing a Teslar watch.

In our experience, many patients with electromagnetic imbalances have improved significantly by wearing a Teslar watch. However, some patients were so imbalanced that they could wear the watch for only a few minutes each day, gradually increasing their time until they could wear it all the time. Several patients spontaneously detoxified very rapidly when they began to wear their watches. A few patients have not been able to wear Teslar watches.

Wearing diodes also helps electromagnetic imbalances. Diodes help to maintain energy levels along acupuncture meridians, to hold the body in its correct frequency, to hold energy patterns and polarity in balance, and to counteract harmful external electromagnetic energies. The number of diodes needed varies from person to person and should be checked if your health professional has the capability. Some people need to wear their diodes 24 hours a day. Others are too energized if they wear them at night.

Tachyon beads are also helpful for electromagnetic imbalances. These beads are made of special materials that emit photon (light) energy in a wavelength from 4 to 16 millimicrons. This wavelength helps maintain cellular metabolism and organize the water molecules in the body so that there is increased oxygen flow and absorption of important nutrients. Tachyon beads are available in hand and wrist bands, as well as individual beads.

Magnets can be used to cleanse electromagnetic imbalances as well as for treating many other conditions. Negative magnetic energy facilitates healing while positive magnetic energy interferes with healing. In his *Biomagnetic Handbook,* Dr. William Philpott states that negative magnetic energy:

- oxygenates tissues
- fights infections
- reduces fluid retention
- supports biological healing
- reduces inflammation
- normalizes acid-base balance
- encourages deep sleep
- relieves pain
- promotes mental acuity
- reduces or dissolves fatty deposits
- reduces fat and calcium deposits in the circulatory system

He describes treatment for many conditions, using magnets as the only modality. Most of the treatments have a cleansing and balancing effect.

Electromagnetic energy is useful for bone fractures that will not heal. Dr. Robert O. Becker of New York discovered that a flow of electrical current to the injury site is necessary for bone healing. An externally applied current facilitates healing of fractures. Magnetic therapy is also useful. Broken bones behave as two separate magnets that repel each other. Placing a magnet over the fracture site helps the fractured ends to come together smoothly. The negative magnetic energy speeds healing by pulling nutrients and oxygen into the injured tissues.

Transcutaneous Electrical Nerve Stimulation (TENS) units are very helpful in controlling chronic pain. A variety of units are available, using a variety of electrical waveforms, frequencies, pulse shapes, and current density. TENS units are also used as electrostimulators in acupuncture treatments.

Grounding techniques are very helpful in relieving electromagnetic imbalances. Allowing the bare feet to touch the earth and lying on the grass are two very simple, but effective, techniques. People who live in mobile homes should be certain they are adequately grounded. Some sensitive individuals require additional grounding over that provided by the manufacturer. This can be accomplished by driving a copper pipe two feet into the ground and attaching a copper wire to both the pipe and the metal frame or siding of the mobile home.

Electromagnetic imbalances can be relieved by a simple procedure. If performed regularly, over a period of time, electromagnetic balance will be restored. Turn clockwise (to your right), working up to 21 turns per day. Spot an object as you turn to prevent dizziness.

Geopathic Stress

Geopathic stress is an invisible pollution that can affect health. First demonstrated in 1929 by a German scientist and dowser, Gustav Freiherr van Pohl, geopathic stress is a localized geomagnetic disturbance that disrupts the homeostatic mechanisms of sensitive individuals. Pohl demonstrated a relationship between geopathic irritation zones under the beds of cancer victims and their disease, and felt geopathic stress was probably both the cause and an acceleration factor of the cancer.

Geopathic stress is caused from tectonic fissures, dislocations, faults, and underground water courses. It produces magnetic anomalies and is worse where underground streams intersect.

Since Pohl's time, the study of geopathology has continued. In 1977 the U.S. Department of Health did a study titled "Geomagnetism, Cancer, Weather, and Cosmic Radiation." This study found that cancer death rates and depth contours of the last ice age glacier correspond with horizontal geomagnetic intensity lines. Associations between cancer incidence and horizontal geomagnetic flux were demonstrated on a worldwide basis.

The study concluded that 40% to 50% of cancer may result from the effects of geopathic stress. There was also a correlation between horizontal geomagnetic flux and birth defects.

CLEANSING, BALANCING, AND PREVENTIVE TECHNIQUES

Several scientists have developed methods for detecting geopathic stress. The Bio-Physics Mersmann, Inc., has developed equipment able to identify influences of geopathic zones, locate and measure magnetic anomalies, and detect disturbed zones of an electromagnetic origin, both in the home and workplace. These measurements make preventive action possible.

Our bodies are more vulnerable when we are sleeping than they are at other times. Be certain that your bed is not over an area of geopathic stress.

Weather

Weather is considered a toxin because it can profoundly affect the human body. The effects of weather on health have been known for centuries. Paracelsus (1493–1541) stated that, "He who knows the origins of the winds, of thunder, and of the weather, also knows where diseases come from."

Biometeorology, a new multidisciplinary science, studies the effects of atmospheric phenomena on all life. Biometeorologists look at temperature, humidity, sunshine hours, wind speed, precipitation, and geomagnetic activity. According to Dr. James Rottom of the Florida International University in North Miami, about 20% of the population is weather sensitive. Other scientists feel that as much as 33% of the population is weather sensitive, which explains why people can wake up one day feeling happy and the next day depressed, even though nothing has changed in their lives.

Storms affect people adversely; many people develop symptoms each time a storm front moves through. Electromagnetic discharges from lightning travel more rapidly and much farther than the storm. These discharges are called sferics and they can cause static on car radios as far as 150 miles away. They also fill the air with positive ions. Experiments in Israel and Europe have shown that this air causes slower reaction times, more road and industrial accidents, depression, and increased surgical complications.

In contrast, the negative ions that are produced by sunlight shining through clean air, by waterfalls and heavy rain, and by running water or showers cause feelings of well-being. They have a calming, healing effect on humans. When people are exposed to negative ions, blood pressure is lowered and productivity is higher.

"Ill winds" have also been described for centuries and are called by many names, among them the mistral winds in France, chinook winds of the Rocky Mountains, and the Santa Ana winds in California. They are laden with positive ions, which decrease the production of a neurotransmitter, serotonin, in measurable amounts. Positive ions cause anxiety, aggression, irritability, physical weakness, apathy, headaches, depression, nightmares, aches and pains, nausea, and respiratory problems. These problems can begin 12 hours before the wind actually arrives.

Dr. Michel Gauquelin of the Laboratory for Cosmic and Psycho-Physiological Rhythms in Paris has correlated cold fronts with heart attacks. The incidence of heart attacks is almost double during these fronts. Post-operative complications also coincide with fronts, 60% occurring with cold fronts, and 30% with warm fronts. In Yugoslavia and Czechoslovakia surgeries are scheduled around the weather forecast because cold fronts increase blood clotting time.

Cold fronts also trigger glaucoma and asthma attacks. Angina pectoris, which is pain in the chest that may radiate down the left arm, peaks in autumn and winter. A study of 1.6 million people with circulatory problems demonstrated that these problems peak in January and February.

A chronic depression called Seasonal Affective Disorder Syndrome (SADS) occurs in winter when the days are short and gray. People develop symptoms within the same 60-day period each year. In addition to depression these people crave carbohydrates and feel better when they eat them; sleep more, but always feel tired; have no interest in sex; gain weight; feel overwhelmed by everything; have problems concentrating; avoid family and friends; have frequent infections and muscle aches.

More than 36 million North Americans suffer from this problem, and no one knows what causes SADS. Women seem more prone to this disorder than men, and it seems to run in families. Most physicians and researchers agree that this disorder is related to the changes in light that accompany the seasons. When the days become shorter and grayer, SADS begins for most people. Some researchers believe that the condition is related to a hormone called melatonin that is secreted by the pineal gland. This sleep-inducing hormone is produced in the dark. The body produces more melatonin during the winter when the days are shorter and darker.

A milder form of SADS, called Hibernation Response, causes people to feel fat, miserable, and depressed in the autumn and winter. Since the mid-1800s a reverse pattern of SADS has been known. These people have summer depression and winter mania.

Heat also causes problems for many people. Several studies point to a temperature-aggression relationship. In normally temperate areas, the incidence of murder, rape, and assault is higher in the hot, humid months of July and August. The hotter regions of the world have always had a higher incidence of aggression. Hot weather apparently stimulates the thalamus gland, which controls the human thermoregulatory system. Many of the same hormonal systems involved in heat regulation are also involved in aggression.

Heat also affects human mortality. The elderly are particularly affected by the sudden temperature change, and their death rate increases by as much as 50% during the summer.

Humidity has its effects as well. High humidity causes hot weather to feel hotter and cold weather to feel colder. In high humidity areas, mold growth is also high. (For further discussion on mold, see Organisms in chapter 7.)

Heart attacks are sometimes related to solar activity and fluctuation of the earth's magnetic field. Dr. Michael Persinger of the Neuroscience Laboratory in Sudbury, Ontario, states that weather is basically a function of the sun, referring to the connection between solar sunspot activity and the electromagnetic field of the earth. Sunspot activity increases the solar wind, which is a stream of hydrogen ions from the sun that cause magnetic storms in the earth's atmosphere. These storms decrease the strength of the earth's electromagnetic fields, which affects short-term weather and long-term climate conditions.

Changes in the geomagnetic field of the earth affect the electromagnetic field of the body and its organs. Russian scientist A. P. Dubrov has found that a short-term variation in the geomagnetic field affects the central nervous system and may trigger or affect cardiovascular function, epilepsy attacks, glaucoma, and eclampsia. These changes may also increase traffic accidents, affect blood pressure and white blood cell counts, and upset genetic homeostasis.

CLEANSING, BALANCING, AND PREVENTIVE TECHNIQUES

No matter how much we might wish it, we cannot control the weather. However, we can try to plan around it, to prevent its adverse effects on us. Some severely weather-sensitive people may require medication, but many are helped by the following nontoxic measures:

- *Negative-ion generators*: These help people who suffer from the effects of positive ions. Some air cleaners have negative-ion generators built into them, but generators that produce only negative ions are also available.
- *Natural fibers*: Some weather-sensitive people are bothered by synthetic fibers. Wearing natural fibers helps these individuals.
- *Outdoor breaks*: Many people who are bothered by positive ions generated by weather work in a closed building where numerous office machines produce high levels of positive ions. An outdoor lunch break beside a fountain will help refresh these people.
- *Showers*: Running water produces negative ions. Frequent showers will help weather-sensitive people feel better.
- *Vacations*: Weather-sensitive people should plan their vacations carefully. Waterfalls and seashores will help minimize the effects of weather.
- *Lights*: The daily use of special high-intensity lights will help controls SADS. Allowing full light to enter windows and installing a skylight will help, as will using white paint on walls.

- *Air-conditioning*: Refrigerated air-conditioning helps to reduce both heat and humidity. In dry areas, evaporative coolers will reduce the temperature, but there is a chance of mold developing in the pads of these coolers.
- *Diodes and magnets*: Wearing diodes, magnets, and tachyon beads help electromagnetically imbalanced people withstand weather changes and storms more comfortably.
- *Homeopathic remedies*: *Phosphorus* and *Sanicula aqua* help people who are worse during electrical storms and thunder- storms. *Rhododendron* helps people who are worse before and during storms, worse with barometric changes, sensitive to lightning and thunder, and who may have a weather-change headache, neuralgia, or toothache.
- *Allergy extracts*: Extracts for serotonin and/or melatonin will help people who suffer from SADS or exposure to positive ions.
- *Weather reports*: Knowing what weather is coming allows weather-sensitive people to plan ahead and to begin or have ready their particular treatments.

9

Internal Toxins

Internal Toxins

Internal toxins are those produced or stored in our bodies. They affect the body just as adversely as external toxins, but their cleansing, balancing, and prevention require different techniques from those required for external toxins.

The metabolic waste products of our cells, including carbon dioxide, dead and digested bacteria, hydrogen peroxide, and cellular debris, can sometimes be toxic. An acid/alkaline imbalance, excess lactic acid, ammonia, and free radicals produced by the body can also cause toxicity.

Microorganisms

Chemicals produced by the metabolism of microorganisms and substances released when the microorganisms are killed are internal toxins. Many symptoms of illness caused by microorganisms are caused by our allergic reaction to the organism and its metabolic products.

Microorganisms can be classified as both external and internal toxins. They are external toxins in that they enter the body from external sources, but once they are in the body, they can be considered an internal toxin. These microorganisms can include bacteria, parasites, viruses, molds, yeasts, and fungi. Regardless of the type of organism, metabolic products are released as the organism grows and multiplies in the body.

Many of these metabolic products are both toxic and allergenic to us. For more information, see Organisms in chapter 7.

Xenobiotics

Xenobiotics that have been ingested, inhaled, or absorbed through the skin and stored in the body become internal toxins. Nonpolar, fat-soluble chemicals are stored readily in the body, particularly in the lipid bilayer of cell membranes. Lipophilic chemicals are also found in fatty tissues and the brain, which has the highest fat content of any organ in the body. This accumulation of fat-soluble chemicals is called toxic bioaccumulation.

Most organs and systems of the body contain fat. When the body is stressed by heat exposure, exercise, stress, fasting, or illness, fat may be released with its toxic materials into the bloodstream. Over 300 toxins have been identified in fat. Since the body is unable to excrete these chemicals, they circulate freely, targeting various organs and body systems, and later can return to the fat. Fat is also mobilized during sleep, which may explain the severe morning symptoms of chemically sensitive individuals.

The persistence of chemicals in the body has been shown repeatedly. In Michigan in the 1970s, animal food was contaminated with polybrominated biphenyls (PBBs), which were then found in foods and cow's milk. All residents examined were found to have PBBs in their fat. When the same residents were examined five years later, the PBB levels in their bodies were unchanged. Only with a formal detoxification program were these levels decreased.

Symptoms of headaches, fatigue, irritability, memory loss, mental confusion, lack of mental acuity, "flulike" symptoms, mucous membrane irritation, skin problems, eye inflammation, and musculoskeletal pains can be caused by both endogenous and exogenous chemicals. It is important to determine which type of exposure is predominant for an individual, and to treat accordingly.

The existence of internal toxins should be considered for persons:

- who continue to have reactions and symptoms after receiving standard treatment and cleaning their environment
- with high exposure to toxic chemicals
- with higher than average toxic chemical levels in blood, serum, fat tissue, or sweat

Body Imbalances

Internal toxins can be formed when the body is under emotional stress or when the diet is unbalanced, including the intake of too much food. The intestines are the primary site affected by such an imbalance. Adjusting body chemistry by populating the intestine with different bacteria (microflora) can help to eliminate these internal toxins. If the intestines have a pH above 7, abnormal bacterial growth can flourish, interfering with the enzyme production that helps food digestion. This alkaline state has also been associated with an increased risk of colon cancer.

Lactobacilli, the normal intestinal bacterial flora, flourish at a pH of around 6.8 and produce an antibiotic that inhibits the growth of disease-causing bacteria such as *Salmonella* and *Staphylococcus.* Normal bacterial flora also prevent damage to the intestinal lining which, if damaged, may allow large molecules, more pathogens, and more antigens to cross into the bloodstream. The body may then produce antibodies or develop inflammation because of these large molecules. The large molecules, the antibodies, and the chemicals produced by inflammation must all be filtered by the liver, which is then less able to detoxify foreign chemicals. The overloaded system cannot handle incoming stimuli. Toxins accumulate and can damage regulatory enzymes and proteins. This "leaky gut" syndrome has been associated with skin inflammation, arthritis, asthma, bronchitis, and recurrent colds and earaches.

A diet that promotes the proper balance of intestinal flora contains no white flour and refined sugar, foods containing synthetic chemicals, or excessive fat. A balancing diet consists of whole grains and vegetables, which decrease the transit time—the time it takes the digested food to pass through the small and large intestines. Prolonged transit time allows intestinal waste to be reabsorbed into the blood and to be recirculated.

Natural Body Functions

BIOCHEMICAL REACTIONS

Acid-alkaline balance is essential to the proper function of the body. Biochemical reactions involving acids and alkalis control many body processes; an imbalance is toxic. Most biochemical reactions produce both energy and waste products. These waste products, lactic acid, ammonia, and urea, can be toxic if the levels become too high. Free radicals produced to an excess in the body may also be toxic.

ACID/ALKALINE BALANCE

Acids　We are all familiar with acids as substances that have a sour or sharp taste. Vinegar (acetic acid), the hydrochloric acid in the stomach, and the sulfuric acid in our car batteries are examples of common acids. In chemistry, an acid is defined as a hydrogen ion donor, an electron acceptor, or a proton donor.

Alkalis   An alkali or base is a compound that is bitter, slippery, and caustic. Household ammonia, ammonium hydroxide, is an alkali. Sodium hydroxide, sometimes called caustic soda, is a common alkali, as is potassium hydroxide, which is sometimes called caustic potash. Both compounds are also referred to as lye. In chemistry, an alkali is defined as a hydroxide ion donor, a proton acceptor, or an electron donor.

pH   A measure of whether a substance is acidic or alkaline (basic) is expressed as pH. The pH scale ranges from 0 to 14: the neutral point is 7; all values below are acidic, and those above 7 are alkaline or basic.

Acid-alkali reactions are necessary to the biochemistry of the body, and unless they occur at the proper speed and proportions, the body can develop an acid/alkali imbalance. This imbalance can be considered a toxin since the body cannot function properly and can be damaged.

For example, the pH of different parts of the body is crucial to proper digestion. For best digestive function:

- The mouth should be alkaline for the salivary enzymes to function.
- The stomach should be acid for protein processing.
- The small intestine should be alkaline for the pancreatic digestive enzymes to function.
- The large intestine should be slightly acid to maintain proper bowel flora.

Respiratory Acidosis and Alkalosis   Respiratory acidosis occurs when the lungs are unable to expel carbon dioxide as fast as it is produced. The carbonic acid level in the blood rises as a result, and arterial concentrations of carbon dioxide and hydrogen ions will be elevated. This happens when holding your breath, when there is impaired gas exchange from partial bronchial obstruction, or from a drug overdose. The body attempts to compensate by deeper, more rapid breathing.

Respiratory alkalosis occurs when carbon dioxide is eliminated faster than it is produced, as happens in hyperventilation. In respiratory alkalosis, the arterial concentrations of carbon dioxide and hydrogen ions are reduced.

Metabolic Acidosis and Alkalosis   Our blood is slightly alkaline with a normal pH range of:

- Arterial blood: 7.40 to 7.45
- Capillary blood: 7.35 to 7.40
- Venous blood: 7.30 to 7.35

If the pH of the blood rises over 7.45, metabolic alkalosis occurs. This can be caused by loss of large quantities of hydrochloric acid from the stomach, as occurs with severe vomiting. Excessive alkali therapy in treating peptic ulcers can also cause metabolic alkalosis. During metabolic alkalosis, more carbonate is deposited in the bones. At a blood pH below 7.30, metabolic acidosis occurs, as in diabetic coma when excessive acids are produced in tissue metabolism. This results from abnormal glucose combustion caused by insulin deficiency. The excessive production of lactic acid during severe exercise or hypoxia also produces metabolic acidosis. Metabolic acidosis also occurs during fasting and when excess bicarbonate is lost during diarrhea.

If metabolic acidosis continues for several hours, dissolution of bone occurs. There is a loss of carbonate from the bones, but little loss of calcium or phosphate. If the metabolic acidosis persists for several days, part of the bone will be dissolved.

When the blood becomes too acid, the respiratory center is stimulated by the brain to expel more carbon dioxide. This in turn lowers the carbonic acid levels, allowing the blood pH to return to normal range. The lungs provide a rapid mechanism for normalizing blood pH.

Buffer Systems   The pH of the blood is also maintained by buffer systems. A buffer is a chemical which, when in solution, prevents or reduces any changes that would otherwise occur when acid or alkali is added to the solution. Buffers are essential when it is necessary for the pH of the solution or system to stay relatively constant. Buffers allow the pH of the blood to stay within the normal range even though acid metabolites are constantly being formed in the tissues.

The major buffer of the body is the bicarbonate system. The bicarbonate comes from several sources. The pancreas produces bicarbonate, and carbon dioxide is converted to bicarbonate in the red blood cells. The body keeps making buffers even though the acids are stored in the connective tissue. If the body overproduces buffers in response to the acidosis, the body can become alkaline.

Hemoglobin is the next most powerful buffer in the blood and it has an affinity for the hydrogen ion. When the hemoglobin releases its oxygen, it takes up the hydrogen ion. This helps to compensate for the change in carbon dioxide concentration from venous to arterial blood.

The kidneys provide another buffering system. In metabolic acidosis, the urine is more acid. Diabetic ketosis, starvation, or severe diarrhea cause abnormally acid urine. In metabolic alkalosis, the urine is more alkaline. Severe vomiting or excess alkali therapy for peptic ulcers will cause the urine to be alkaline. The urine can also be alkaline in urinary infections when the infecting organisms split urea and release ammonia.

The urine of most people is acid because of high meat intake. If too much acid urine is produced, depleting the kidney of hydrogen ions, renal alkalosis results. This sometimes happens in severe kidney disease. Renal acidosis occurs if too much alkaline urine is produced.

CONNECTIVE TISSUE

Connective tissue, also known as mesenchymal tissue, is made up of cells designed to support, connect, and anchor the structures of the body. Connective tissue also forms a drainage system that takes up cell waste products and discharges them through the lymph system. Depending on the circumstances, it may also store these waste products.

The pH of the connective tissue and its acid/alkaline balance are essential to its proper function. When acids build up, some are flushed from the body in the urine. Other acids are locked into the connective tissues where alkalyzing reserves cannot penetrate to neutralize the acidosis. This causes the connective tissue to be too acidic, rather than going through its normal fluctuations in pH. Most people have primary mesenchymal acidosis. Consumption of meats, sugars, white flour, heat-treated oils, and antibiotics contribute to the acidosis. This acidosis affects the magnesium and potassium balance of the cells, congests the lymphatic system, and upsets calcium stores. People with high tissue acidity suffer from fatigue, headaches, and are sensitive to weather patterns.

Factors that influence the health of connective tissue include:

- the Standard American Diet of processed grains, fast foods high in fat and sugar, and few fruits and vegetables
- drugs, both prescription and recreational, do the most harm to connective tissue
- toxic chemicals, including food additives and insecticides
- stress of all kinds: environmental, emotional, or physical

- microorganisms, including viruses, bacteria, parasites, fungi, and yeast

LACTIC ACID

People who are running sprints or who have been exercising for prolonged periods of time produce excess lactic acid in their muscles. This excess lactic acid can cause muscle soreness. Anesthesia and cyanide poisoning also increase lactate levels. Ingestion of alcohol (ethanol), low blood oxygen, and severe anemia can increase lactate concentrations in the blood.

AMMONIA/AMMONIUM

Amino acids contain an ammonium group (NH_4^+). When the acids break down, these ammonium groups are used to synthesize nitrogen compounds or are converted to urea and excreted.

Ammonia is toxic to the brain. Half of the body's excess nitrogen appears as ammonia before it is converted to urea and excreted. Urea is synthesized in the liver from ammonium before the kidneys eliminate the urine. A complete block of any of the steps of the urea cycle would be fatal because the body has no other pathways to synthesize urea.

There are genetic diseases in which people have a partial block of each of the six urea cycle enzymes. These partial deficiencies cause mental retardation, lethargy, convulsions, stupor, and periodic vomiting. Ammonia toxicity can also occur in adults with liver damage. Occasionally, people with bladder infections or whose kidneys drain to the lower intestines can overproduce ammonia, which can directly enter the bloodstream, bypassing circulation through the liver.

FREE RADICALS

Free radicals contain unpaired electrons or an odd number of electrons in their outer orbitals. Oxygen sometimes forms part of free radical molecules.

Endogenous free radicals are produced in the body and our bodies cannot function properly without them. They exist in small numbers in cells, and play a role in defense against microbial invasion. They are useful in activating many enzyme reactions and are also important in hormone production.

Exogenous free radicals enter the body from external sources. Air pollution, pesticides, herbicides, cigarette smoke, ionizing radiation, toxic waste and runoff, and oxides of nitrogen produce exogenous free radicals. Excess concentrations of these free radicals and certain forms of oxygen adversely affect the body.

Free radicals can:

- be attracted to cell membranes where they can bind and cause damage
- bind to enzymes, inactivating them
- cause the breakdown of fats in cell membranes
- cause the breakdown of DNA
- cause mutations (changes in the DNA) and the death of cells
- puncture the cell membrane, allowing bacteria and viruses to enter
- exacerbate chemical sensitivity

CLEANSING, BALANCING, AND PREVENTIVE TECHNIQUES

Acid/Alkaline Balance   Dietary habits can dramatically change tissue acid/alkali balance.

- Chew food until you can feel the saliva break up the foods.
- Drink minimally with a meal and do not use liquid to wash down partially chewed foods.
- Avoid foods with high toxic residues. Animal and dairy products contain the most toxins. Fruits, vegetables, nuts, seeds, and grains contain the least.
- Eat preservative-free, high-quality foods.

- Eat foods that are produced within a 500-mile radius of your home, and eat them in their natural seasons.
- Eat a variety of foods and rotate them if you have food allergies.
- Eat in moderation. Any food or drink in excess affects the balance of the body.
- Eat only a few foods in one meal. Eating large varieties of food in the same meal taxes the enzymes needed for digestion.
- Eat fruit before noon to avoid fermentation problems.

The following diet can change the tissue acid/alkali balance as much as 85%. However, it is not for everyone. People with hyperinsulinemia will not do well on this diet. To reduce excess acidity of the tissues, eat only the following:

- *Steamed vegetables*: Any and all that you can tolerate. Do not use aluminum cookware or the microwave to prepare your vegetables. Drink the broth from the steamer seasoned with a little salt at 11 a.m. Sip slowly.
- *Grains*: One to two cups of cooked millet, brown rice, quinoa, or amaranth per day. You may also have rice crisps or Wasa crackers. Avoid oats (too acidic), corn in any form (too difficult to digest), and wheat.
- *Fish*: Poached, baked, steamed, or broiled deep-sea fish. Do not eat shellfish.
- *Chicken*: Baked, broiled, or steamed; white meat only, with the skin removed.
- *Butter*: Mix butter with equal parts of a cold-pressed oil.
- *Lemon*: In 1 quart of water daily. Sip all during the day so that you finish the quart before bedtime. Lemon will increase or decrease the body pH, depending on the need.
- *Water*: The purest tolerated water is a must for everyone, regardless of health status. The pH of the water should be between 6.7 and 7.
- *Limited herbal teas*: Consume in the evening in small sips.

Avoid the following while deacidifying the tissues:

- milk and cheese
- red meats, particularly pork; it requires six hours to get out of the stomach and is full of homotoxins
- peanuts and peanut butter
- bread and white flour
- sugars, except for very limited amounts of honey or pure maple syrup
- tea, coffee, and alcohol
- fried food of any kind
- citrus fruits, except for lemon
- raw vegetables, as they further inflame the digestive system.

Eat the following combinations:

- *Breakfast*: grains
- *Lunch*: grains and steamed vegetables
- *Dinner*: grains, steamed vegetables, and limited fish and chicken

After the tissue pH has normalized, as determined by checking the blood, urine, and saliva pH, add protein foods, such as beans and legumes. This is usually possible after 21 days. The homeopathic remedy *Natrum phosphoricum* helps with acid/alkali imbalance.

Lactic Acid   The homeopathic remedy *Lacticum acidum* helps balance lactic acid excess after exercise to reduce pain and exhaustion. An allergy extract of lactic acid will also help cleanse lactic acid/lactate excess, regardless of the cause.

Ammonia/Ammonium   Excesses of ammonia/ammonium can be cleansed from the body by an α-ketoglutaric acid supplement. Alpha-ketoglutaric acid is an amino group receptor, and it become glutamic acid after accepting the amino group.

Vitamin B$_6$, vitamin C, minerals, and increased water intake are also helpful. A low-protein diet, 1 gram per kilogram of body weight for adults and 1.5 grams per kilogram of body weight for children, will aid in reducing ammonia excess.

Free Radicals Antioxidants are compounds that protect the body against the harmful effects of free radicals. Antioxidants in the body include superoxide dismutase, catalase, glutathione peroxidase, vitamin E, vitamin A, beta-carotene, ascorbic acid, bilirubin, uric acid, selenium, and metal binding proteins. Vitamins E and A, beta-carotene, ascorbic acid, superoxide dismutase, and selenium are available as supplements.

Emotional Trauma

Both Hippocrates and Aristotle recognized the role of emotions in health and disease. Over time, however, acknowledgment of these interactions was lost. Dr. Blair Justice, the author of *Who Gets Sick,* states that "Most of medicine continues to pretend that mind and body are separated and that pathways by which attitudes and moods physically affect our organs and tissues are really imaginary . . . and that simple physical explanations will be found to account for major disorders, as if mind and brain have no physical reality."

In the early 1980s, the study of how the mind, central nervous system, hormonal system, and immune system interact began to develop. Psychoneuroimmunology was formed from the marriage of immunology, neurology, and psychology. Doctors began to acknowledge that the body did not function as separate organs, but as a complete, interdependent whole.

PSYCHONEUROIMMUNOLOGY

The brain regulates all body functions, and dysregulation of the central nervous system is now known to be a contributing factor in disease. When people lose a sense of control or become helpless, chemical changes in the body occur. Mental states, thoughts, and moods can cause changes in brain chemistry and cells.

Thus, emotions are not just in the brain; they are also in the body. Emotions affect the body physically just as physical illness affects the emotions. Researchers have found that 70% to 80% of patients who became ill had given up hope or felt helpless.

Dr. Bernie Siegel of New Haven, Connecticut notes that physical illness may be the only control some people have over life. Dr. Stewart Wolf, author of *Mind, Brain, and Medicine* states that "disease is a way of life" for some people and is how they react to the problems of life.

People who view their condition as hopeless and themselves as victims seem to conserve oxygen. They develop a slow heart rate, a lower blood pressure, and a decreased amount of hydrochloric acid secretion by the stomach.

The immune system responds adversely to stress and it is unable to identify the source of the stress, whether it is an infection, an allergic reaction, or an emotional trauma. Continued stress depresses the function and efficiency of the immune system. People can develop a flight or fight reaction on an acute level, producing high levels of adrenalin (epinephrine), noradrenalin (norepinephrine), and cortisol; elevated blood sugar; and other biochemical changes. If chemicals produced by these changes occur inappropriately and chronically, the body suffers. Disease can occur when our bodies inappropriately use mechanisms that are meant to protect us.

Emotional trauma can be a type of toxin and must be addressed, just as a chemical toxin has to be detoxified. Psychological traumas can be suppressed and forgotten by the conscious mind.

However, the subconscious and the cells remember, and their memory can adversely affect the immune, nervous, and endocrine systems and thus the health of the individual. Studies show that girls who have been sexually abused have higher than normal levels of cortisol for as long as two years after the abuse. High levels of cortisol can depress immune system function.

TRAUMA

After people experience a psychologically distressing event that is outside the range of usual human experience, they often develop post-traumatic stress disorder. In addition to fear, terror, and helplessness, symptoms include re-experiencing the traumatic event, avoidance of stimuli associated with the event, and increased adrenalin and fight/flight hormones.

Common traumas causing post-traumatic stress disorder include a serious threat to life—self, children, spouse, or friends. They may also include the sudden destruction of one's home or community, or seeing another person who has been seriously injured or killed in an accident or from physical violence. Some of these circumstances include rape, assault, airplane crashes, large fires, or bombing. The person may then have recurrent and intrusive recollections or dreams of the event.

People will avoid reminders of the traumatic event. They may feel detached from others and not interested in previously enjoyed activities. They have difficulty falling asleep or staying asleep, and show hypervigilance and an exaggerated startle effect. To be considered post-traumatic stress disorder, the disturbances must last at least one month.

The experience of an event takes place over a period of time; it does not happen all at once. The process of experiencing an event can be blocked at an early stage and remain stored in the body (brain, muscles) for years. When a person experiences an overwhelming external threat, he or she can suspend all reaction, maintaining that inhibited experience in an unassimilated form indefinitely or as long as necessary. Until the event is fully experienced, it continues to exert its effects.

ABUSE

Abuse can be emotional, psychological, physical, or sexual. Abusive behavior is intended to control and subjugate another person through the use of fear, humiliation, and verbal or physical assault. Abuse most often occurs in childhood, but it can also be inflicted on adults. Those who have been abused during childhood often enter abusive relationships when they become adults because such a situation feels familiar to them.

Emotional Abuse   Emotional abuse includes neglect, verbal abuse, and psychological abuse. It can involve constant negative comments, continual or chronic scapegoating, terrorizing, berating, and rejection. Emotional abuse is difficult to prove and in children may only come to attention through concomitant physical abuse. Abuse tends to make victims feel inadequate and helpless, and so "brainwashed" that they question the accuracy of their own memories.

Physical Abuse   Physical abuse can range in severity from bruises to death from head or internal injuries. In children under five years of age, about 10% of emergency visits are to treat injuries caused by abuse. Premature infants and stepchildren are at increased risk. Child abuse may occur more often when there is another crisis in the home. Parents who abuse their children were often abused themselves as children.

The man is the perpetrator in 95% of domestic assaults. More than 2 million women are assaulted by their male partners each year. Even though the woman is the victim, most people expect her to stop the violence, and leaving the home is usually her only option. Only the perpetrator has the ability to stop inflicting the violence. Men who batter their wives often also abuse their children.

Sexual Abuse   It is estimated that one in three women and one in four to seven men have been victims of sexual abuse as children. Sexual exploitation of children inside the family is known as incest; outside the family it is known as pedophilia. Adult forms of sexual abuse include date rape and stranger rape.

Authorities on sexual abuse estimate that about half the survivors suffer from some type of memory loss. Some survivors develop multiple personalities. Sexual abuse can cause depression, anxiety, low self-esteem, self-abusive behavior, social problems, sexual problems, and food, chemical, or sexual addictions.

STRESS

Stress has been widely blamed for making society sick today. More important than the stress is our response to it. High stress does not correlate with a high risk of illness. Stress only allows people to blame their troubles on external sources. In *Who Gets Sick,* Dr. Blair Justice discusses a number of studies on stress. In one, people who have a sense of control were shown to keep their stress chemicals from reaching damaging levels when they are under pressure.

Researchers studied a group of executives experiencing significant stress as their company was broken into a smaller company. Half the group did not become ill. Those who stayed healthy viewed change differently and considered it a chance for growth and new experience. They felt that they had a sense of control, and they were optimistic. People who had a sense of purpose and who believed in the importance and value of what they were doing had fewer symptoms of headaches, anxiety, and trouble sleeping. Control, commitment, and challenge lead to "psychological hardiness."

In other studies, people who coped poorly with stress had decreased immune responses. Anxiety and depression reduced immune system activity. People with already depressed immune systems are most prone to negative health effects from anxiety, distress, anger, or depression. Acute stress can lower the number of white cells in the immune system as well as the levels of interferon, a chemical that prevents viruses from reproducing.

Dr. Justice also reported on several studies of recently widowed people. In 1977, it was found that widows or widowers had depressed immune function after the death of their spouses. The lymphocytes, a cell of the immune system, are depressed for at least six months after the death of a loved one. In one study, the death rate of recently bereaved widows was 3 to 12 times that of married women. In another study, the death rate was 40% higher in the first six months of bereavement for a group of widowers.

TISSUE MEMORY

Emotions and memories of past experiences, both good and bad, are stored in the body. Every cell has memory and an "intelligence." Flashbacks of physical and emotional traumas can be released from the cells. Often, the memories of these traumas have been submerged or "stuffed" so that the person is not consciously aware of them.

Release of memory from the cells may be triggered by many things. Bodywork, scents, sights, sounds, words, emotional episodes, or even the administration of an allergy extract may release a memory or trigger a flashback of an event. A person usually experiences body memories first, recalling the physical pain or discomfort felt during the event. Sights and sounds follow; emotions occur last. This can set up a chain reaction as cells release other memories and chemicals.

Some psychologists doubt the validity of tissue memory, feeling that recovered memories are subconscious efforts to resolve old hurts, encouraged by current popular books and psychotherapists. While this may be true in some cases, many victims are able to find evidence that confirms the reality of their memories.

CLEANSING, BALANCING, AND PREVENTIVE TECHNIQUES

Counseling and Psychotherapy Sharing your feelings with family, friends, and church members or pastor may not be enough to help you through trauma. Professional guidance may be necessary, and counseling and psychotherapy are important cleansing tools that help reduce stress loads.

Choose a competent, licensed therapist and take particular care in this choice. In many states, anyone can work as a counselor or therapist, without proper training or license. The person you choose should be someone to whom you can easily talk, as well as someone who has had experience in dealing with the particular problems you have.

Two major fields have developed to understand human behavior: psychoanalysis and behavioral psychology. Psychoanalysis was developed by neurologist Dr. Sigmund Freud. He emphasized the interconnection between biologic and environmental influences on a person and described the mind as composed of the conscious, unconscious, and preconscious.

Behavioral psychology uses objectively measurable experimentation to study the relationship between behavior and the environment. It is felt that both adaptive and maladaptive behaviors are acquired from learning experiences, with genetic endowment also playing a role. Problem behavior is the focus. Classical conditioning is the method of treatment, which uses positive and negative reinforcement and other techniques.

Counselors and psychiatrists generally use one of these approaches in their treatment. A psychiatrist is an M.D. or a D.O. who has received medical specialty training in psychiatry beyond medical school training. A psychologist may have either a Ph.D. or an M.A. in psychol-

ogy. In most states, psychologists with a master's degree practice under the supervision of a Ph.D. Generally speaking, psychologists use less pharmaceuticals in their treatment methods, because they are not licensed to prescribe drugs. Should a prescription be necessary, psychologists enlist the help of a physician who prescribes the medication.

In addition to discussing problems and issues in counseling and analysis, other treatments help cleanse emotional trauma. These include guided imagery, gestalt therapy, art therapy, dream therapy, and dance therapy.

With any problem serious enough to affect the health of a person, professional help is both beneficial and necessary. However, there are some self-help techniques that can be done in addition to therapy.

Homeopathic Remedies There are several homeopathic remedies that help with abuse, humiliation, and physical trauma. These remedies include:

- *Aconite*: fear, rape by stranger, bruised with emotional shock
- *Anacardium*: chronic sexual abuse with humiliation and inferiority complex, possibly with multiple personalities or may hear voices with religious overtones
- *Carcinosum*: sexual abuse
- *Gelsemium*: acute shock from rape
- *Ignatia*: sciatica after grief, hysteria
- *Lycopodium*: lack of self-esteem, goes from relationship to relationship and career to career
- *Medorrhinum*: rape, incest, child abuse
- *Nux vomica*: high sex drive, promiscuity
- *Opium*: fright after rape, acute fear
- *Platina*: sexual abuse, rape, multiple personalities, hypersensitivity in vaginal area and pain with sex
- *Sepia*: rape, loss of sex drive, development of sexual aversion, then disgust

- *Staphysagria*: abuse, hurt and humiliations, acute rape remedy, recurrent bladder infections if a history of rape or incest
- *Thuja*: deep guilt from being abused, sexual identity crisis

Journaling   Journaling is an excellent self-help technique. It can involve writing in a journal either daily or at times of distress. Happy experiences can be recorded for remembering and reliving. Problems can be analyzed, often allowing a new perspective and release of misperceptions.

Journaling can also take the form of a letter that is never mailed. Sometimes burning or tearing up the letter can represent a symbolic completion or laying aside of an issue. Letters to the deceased are an excellent way of dealing with unfinished business. Anger, emotional pain, or frustration can be freely expressed with no threat of reprisal. A letter to a deceased person can also express love, pain of loss, and loneliness; this assists the grieving process with a ritual of acknowledgment and completion.

Journaling is not limited to writing. It can also be some form of artwork that unleashes emotions. Art can bypass the rigid ego and controlling intellect, allowing freedom of expression.

Journaling provides these benefits:

- feeling and experiencing the emotions of the moment rather than "stuffing" them
- venting anger in a nonviolent way
- a means to analyze problems and perceive causes and effects

Laughter and Attitude   Laughter can be a very powerful cleanser for emotional trauma and abuse. Norman Cousins, the author of *Anatomy of an Illness*, discovered in the course of his two serious illnesses that "love, hope, faith, laughter, confidence, and will to live have therapeutic value." He was able to recover by emphasizing positive emotions and laughing. Aristotle felt that laughter was a "bodily exercise precious to health." Laughing causes positive changes in brain chemistry by releasing endorphins, and it brings more oxygen into the body with the deeper inhalations. Laughter releases tension, anger, fear, guilt, and anxiety. A good laughing session can completely change your attitude.

Laugh therapy can include:

- reading comedies, cartoon books, or joke books
- watching comedies or cartoon videos
- listening to humorous tapes
- telling jokes and amusing experiences, and listening to others tell jokes or amusing experiences
- watching animals or children at play
- visiting with people you enjoy
- planning enjoyable activities for the future
- smiling as much as possible—a smile is a precursor to a laugh and increases feelings of happiness.

Our bodies have miraculous powers to heal but sometimes our own negativity shuts down this healing capacity. Positive, hopeful attitudes can be cleansing. Positive attitudes:

- give the body and mind messages to heal
- increase your confidence in your coping ability
- increase your self-esteem
- encourage concentration on "rights" rather than "wrongs"
- help you to look forward to new activities and hopes rather than dwelling in the past

Neuro Emotional Technique   Neuro Emotional Technique (NET) is a technique that has many applications. Developed by Dr. Scott Walker, a chiropractor from California, it helps release the emotions held in the body memory. It involves the use of basic muscle testing and homeopathics to achieve complete healing. It allows the removal of emotional blocks that prevent regaining health and the reestablishing of emotional balance in a nonthreatening way to the person.

Forgiveness One of the most important aspects of cleansing and balancing emotional trauma is forgiveness. A person must forgive the person who caused the trauma and in addition forgive the act itself. With time and work, this can be done. A person must also forgive himself or herself for any real or imagined wrong-doing. With total forgiveness, people can shed the burden of being victims and become victorious over the problems that made them prisoners in their own body.

Cumulative Life Experiences

We are now what we have been becoming since the day of our birth. Everything that we have encountered in life has left its mark on our personality, mentality, and body. All our life experiences, when totalled like the sum in an addition problem, can have the effect of a toxin. This cumulative toxin will be different for each person.

In a life that has been notable because of its problems, the toxin will be of considerable size and virulence. In a life that has been relatively healthy and happy, the toxic effect of the sum of life experiences will be much smaller.

Regardless of the size of the toxin from our cumulative life experiences, it must be cleansed. By cleansing and balancing each of the categories necessary for good health, the toxic effects of our experiences will be removed, one by one.

PART FOUR

How We Are Exposed to Toxins

10

Toxins in the Workplace and School

Industrial Exposures

The National Institute of Occupational Safety and Health (NIOSH) has developed a list of the ten leading work-related illnesses and injuries. The list includes: lung disease, caused by silica dust, asbestos, cotton fibers, and coal dust; occupational cancer; cardiovascular diseases; reproduction and neurotoxic disorders (brain and spinal cord problems); noise-induced hearing loss; skin diseases; and psychological disorders.

Many occupational diseases are caused by exposure to toxic substances. The long-term effects of these chemicals are unknown. Scientists have investigated only the acute effects of chemicals; they have done very few chronic studies. At least 80% of commercial chemicals have never been tested for toxicity. The synergism of chemicals (how they interact) is also not known.

INFECTIOUS DISEASES

Health care workers and laboratory workers may be exposed to hepatitis, rubella, AIDS, tuberculosis, and staphylococcal disease. Agricultural workers, veterinarians, slaughterhouse employees, hunters, trappers, forestry workers, dishwashers, cannery workers, animal handlers, ranchers, zoo attendants, and construction workers are exposed to various microorganisms, such as bacteria, fungi, protozoa, and viruses.

SKIN DISORDERS

Contact dermatitis is caused by exposure to irritating chemicals, such as solvents, cutting oils, detergents, alkalis, and acids. Chemical burns occur commonly. Some chemicals are contact sensitizers, such as epoxy resins, chromium, and plant resins. Agricultural workers frequently get contact dermatitis from exposure to plants.

Phototoxic skin reactions from tars and creosote can be seen in construction workers, roofers, road builders, and railway workers. Forestry workers and utility workers can receive phototoxic skin reactions from Queen Anne's lace and wild carrot. Agricultural workers and grocery clerks can have phototoxic skin reactions from celery, parsnips, and citrus fruits. Pharmaceutical workers can have phototoxic skin reactions from sulfonamides, and cosmetic workers from exposure to oil of bergamot.

Electronic workers, aircraft assemblers, construction workers, and painters may have contact dermatitis caused by epoxy resins. Embalmers and insulation workers can get dermatitis from formaldehyde. Tire builders, tire repairmen, and workers who wear rubber protective clothing may develop contact dermatitis from rubber accelerators. Health care workers may develop skin rashes or even anaphylactic reactions to latex gloves.

LUNG DISEASE

Workers in enzyme detergent manufacture and in western red cedar mills, animal handlers, and bakers may all develop asthma caused by sensitization to chemicals with which they are working. There are 200 agents in the workplace that can cause asthma, including grain and wood dusts. Workers who do electroplating, jewelry manufacturing, and fluorescent screen manufacturing may develop asthma because of complex salts of platinum. Textile workers who work with cotton, flax, hemp, or jute can develop chest tightness and cough because of the textile fibers they inhale. This is known as byssinosis.

Furriers, farmers, cheese washers, maple bark strippers, mushroom workers, and vineyard sprayers may develop hypersensitivity pneumonitis, in which cough, shortness of breath, fever, and chills are seen acutely. Chronic symptoms include fatigue, weight loss, and chronic lung disease.

Chronic lung disease can develop as a result of many occupations. Miners, tunnelers, quarry workers, stonecutters, sandblasters, glassblowers, and ceramic workers may develop silicosis. Coal workers, graphite workers, and workers in carbon electrode manufacture may develop pneumoconiosis. Workers who repair asbestos-containing ships, buildings, and other structures may develop asbestosis.

CARDIOVASCULAR DISEASE

Carbon disulfide exposure causes accelerated atherosclerosis. It is used in the rubber and viscose rayon industries, in the manufacture of carbon tetrachloride, and as a degreasing solvent. Chronic carbon monoxide exposure can cause heart disease. Forklift operators, foundry workers, miners, mechanics, garage attendants, and fire fighters are exposed to carbon monoxide.

Workers in the explosives manufacturing business, construction workers who do blasting, workers handling weapons in the armed forces, and workers manufacturing pharmaceutical nitrates are exposed to organic nitrates which dilate (open up) blood vessels. The body compensates by constricting (closing) blood vessels. If workers experience abrupt withdrawal, then the vasoconstriction is unopposed and they may develop angina (chest pain caused by decreased blood flow to the heart) or have heart attacks.

Dry-cleaning workers, degreasers, painters, and chemical manufacturers are exposed to solvents and propellants (freon). They may develop abnormal heart rhythms or fainting, and sudden death can occur. Agricultural workers, and organophosphate and carbamate pesticide applicators may develop rapid heart rates, high or low blood pressure, and abnormal heart rhythms.

LIVER TOXICOLOGY

Pesticide manufacturers, ceramic workers, dry cleaners, solvent manufacturers, anesthesiologists, painters, munitions workers, aircraft manufacturers, and rubber workers all have exposures to chemicals that can be toxic to the liver.

KIDNEY DISEASE

Workers welding cadmium-plated metals may develop kidney toxicity. Carbon tetrachloride, used as a solvent and in the manufacture of fluorinated hydrocarbons, can cause renal (kidney) failure. Ethylene dichloride is toxic to the kidneys, and is found in insecticides, fumigants, household cleaning fluids, and fire extinguishers. Pentachlorphenol, a renal toxicant, is used as a preservative for timber and as an insecticide, herbicide, and defoliant. Lead, cadmium, and mercury can cause renal toxicity. Beryllium is used in the manufacture of electronic tubes, ceramics, and fluorescent light bulbs, and can cause both lung and renal toxicity.

NEUROTOXICITY

Solvents used to clean electronic parts, in paint, and as degreasers are well-known causes of central nervous toxicity and peripheral neuropathy. Arsenic, carbon disulfide, carbon monoxide, lead, manganese, mercury, nitrous oxide, organophosphate pesticides, tin, toluene, trichloroethylene, and vinyl chloride are all known neurotoxicants.

REPRODUCTIVE TOXICOLOGY

Women who work with mixed organic solvents have an increased risk of congenital malformations in their offspring. Data suggest that workers with exposure to chlorprene in the rubber industry and styrene in the reinforced plastics industry, laboratory workers, and people working in the printing industry may have abnormal reproduction. Offspring of male anesthesiologists have an increase in congenital abnormalities. Female anesthesiologists have an increased risk of spontaneous abortions.

SPECIFIC CHEMICALS

- *Sulfuric acid* is used in the manufacture of phosphate fertilizers; in the production of inorganic pigments, textile fibers, pulp, and paper; and as a component of lead storage batteries. Workers in these factories have a high exposure to sulfuric acid. Other workers exposed to sulfuric acid are electroplaters, jewelers, metal cleaners, picklers, and storage battery makers. Sulfuric acid causes damage to mucous membranes and the skin. Inhaling vapors causes burning of the throat, cough, and chest tightness.
- *Acrylamide*, a known cause of peripheral neuropathy, is used to make large molecular compounds called polymers, which are used as flocculators (chemicals that cause particles to cluster together), drilling-mud additives, and surface coatings. Papermaking workers, soil stabilization workers, textile workers, and well drillers are exposed to acrylamide.
- *Aromatic amines,* used in the manufacture of textiles, paper and pulp, aqueous ink, and in the leather tanning industry,

can cause bladder cancer and methemoglobinemia.
- *Formaldehyde* exposure occurs in the production of formaldehyde resins and plastics, particleboard, paper, and in embalming. Formaldehyde has been a trigger for occupational asthma and can cause skin rashes and irritate the eyes, nose, and throat.
- *Polycyclic aromatic hydrocarbons* exposure occurs in workers in gas and coke plants, aluminum reduction plants, iron and steel foundries, coal gasification facilities, roof and pavement tarring, and application of coal-tar paints. Polycyclic aromatic hydrocarbons are known carcinogens. Workers can also suffer from skin rashes, headaches, sweating, and vomiting.
- *Styrene* is used in the manufacture of boats, wall panels, tub and shower units, and truck camper tops. Workers may experience headaches, fatigue, poor memory, and dizziness.

CLEANSING, BALANCING, AND PREVENTIVE TECHNIQUES

Preventing exposure is of paramount importance. However, sometimes prevention is difficult in an industrial setting because workers frequently have no control over their working environment. The following preventive techniques are helpful:

- *Ventilation*: Adequate ventilation will help lower levels of toxic chemicals. Properly placed exhaust fans, chemical hoods, and adequate air exchange will all increase safety in the work area.
- *Air quality*: Air cleaners may be a necessity in heavily polluted areas. Even with adequate ventilation, activated charcoal filters may be necessary to remove chemicals from the air.

- *Masks*: Wearing charcoal masks or respirators can protect workers exposed to chemicals. In heavily contaminated areas, it may be necessary to wear a mask with an air tank. When not in use, the masks should be kept in an airtight container to prevent toxic contamination inside the mask.
- *Protective clothing*: Goggles or safety glasses, gloves, jackets, coveralls, hats, and special shoes may be necessary for protection from harmful chemicals.

Office Exposures

As mentioned in chapter 5, indoor air pollution causes more problems than outdoor air pollution. Half the work force now consists of white-collar office workers who are exposed to more chemicals than in the past. Blue-collar workers continue to have industrial exposures.

The leading causes of workplace pollution are faulty ventilation, chemical contamination, biological contamination, and asbestos. The American Society of Heating, Refrigerating, and Air-conditioning Engineers (ASHRAE) publishes safety guidelines. Their 1981 guidelines defined acceptable air quality as ambient air that has no known contaminants at harmful concentrations and a majority (80%) of the workers have no complaints.

VENTILATION

One or more heating, ventilation, and air conditioning (HVAC) systems are used for buildings. Fresh outside air enters the building through intake vents. It is then combined with recirculated indoor air and passes in supply ducts through air cleaners and charcoal beds. Air cleaners filter out dust particles, and charcoal beds absorb odors. Air-tempering units regulate the temperature, and then the air is blown into rooms through room vents. Some HVAC units may have terminal units (composed of coils) that heat or cool the air.

Air exhaust fans draw the air out of the room and into a parallel system of ducts. Some exhaust air is eliminated through exhaust vents. Recirculated air passes through air filters and enters the building again. Some HVAC units also may humidify or dehumidify the air, depending on the season.

An office building should be ventilated at 15 cubic feet per minute per occupant. As a room is occupied near maximum levels, ventilation rates should increase. Local exhaust systems should be used around photocopy machines, printing equipment, or areas where solvents are used. Hoods remove the contaminated air, ducts carry it away, and air-cleaning devices purify the air. A hood must be close to the source of contamination to be effective. Fans also help to remove the contaminated air from the room and replace it with fresh air.

Poor installation or maintenance of the HVAC and local ventilation systems causes workplace pollution problems. Also, most new buildings do not permit penetration of fresh air. Faulty HVAC systems may have water leaks; poor air distribution; and inadequate cooling, heating, and dehumidification.

A common problem arises when the use of the building changes but the ventilation system is not changed to meet new needs. Sometimes intake vents are blocked, which means that the amount of air exhausted is higher than the amount of air brought in, and this causes a vacuum. Contaminated air may then be sucked into the exhaust vents and recirculated. Sometimes intake vents are directly adjacent to exhaust vents, and contaminated air is recirculated back into the building. Intake vents may be adjacent to sources of chemicals, such as car exhaust fumes that contain carbon monoxide and other toxic chemicals.

Ventilation systems are frequently shut down when no one is occupying the building. However, the building continues to outgas, and the level of contaminants builds up. If the system has been turned off, it should be restarted and run for several hours before the building is reoccupied.

Ventilation systems may be contaminated by bacteria, fungi, or animal fecal material. Molds in air conditioning systems can cause hypersensitivity pneumonia and humidifier lung. People complain most about office environments that do not have the recommended air exchanges. Floor plans and ventilation systems are designed for a certain number of people, but a building may contain 30% to 40% more people than designed levels. These buildings are always described as being "stuffy."

CHEMICALS

Indoor air pollution is the most serious chemical exposure for office workers. Our energy-efficient, airtight buildings and the increased use of synthetic materials (carpets, drapes, particleboard furniture) contribute to this problem. Other major indoor pollutants have been identified and discussed in chapters 5 and 6.

- *Ammonia* is commonly used to clean glass and other surfaces. It can burn the nose, throat, and chest and cause wheezing in asthmatics.
- *Asbestos* was used widely in buildings until the 1970s. It is now found in the air from deteriorating building materials, such as acoustical tile. The EPA states that there is no safe level of exposure to asbestos.
- *Benzene* is found in synthetic fibers, plastics, cigarette smoke, spot removers, and other solvents. Low levels can cause irritation to the liver, kidneys, and gastrointestinal tract.
- *Carbon monoxide* comes from automobile exhaust in outside air that the ventilation system brings into the building. It is also in cigarette smoke. High levels of carbon monoxide cause asphyxiation and death. Low levels cause headaches, dizziness, decreased hearing, personality changes, extra heartbeats, nausea, and vomiting.

- *Ethanol* is found in some duplicating fluids. Inhalation can cause dizziness, drowsiness, and headaches. It can also dry out the skin.
- *Fiber glass* is used for insulation in buildings. When it is inhaled into the lungs, it stays there permanently. Fiber glass also irritates the skin.
- *Formaldehyde* is used in insulation, building materials, resins, textiles, carpets, and furniture. It outgases for years from these products. With exposure, people can develop burning eyes, dizziness, coughing, breathing difficulties, and nausea. The long-term effects of formaldehyde are unknown.
- *Ozone* is used as a disinfectant and is produced in offices when oxygen molecules contact high voltages or ultraviolet light. Photocopy machines may produce ozone, but grounding them can decrease ozone emissions. Ozone promotes the formation of free radicals in the body, and when inhaled is a respiratory irritant.
- *Particulates* are particles small enough to be inhaled into the lungs. Cigarette smoke attracts other particulates in the air and allows them to be airborne for hours, when they might otherwise be removed by the exhaust system.
- *Radon gas* occurs naturally in soil and rocks. It enters buildings through soil or from contaminated groundwater and tap water. Radon has been associated with lung cancer.
- *Cigarette smoke* has been associated with lung cancer in nonsmokers who are exposed to the sidestream smoke. Sidestream smoke contains more chemicals than the mainstream smoke. Fortunately, many buildings are now being designated as nonsmoking.
- *Toluene* is used in white-out solutions. It is a skin irritant.

- *Vinyl chloride* is the building block of polyvinyl chloride, which is used in plastic products. Pipes, lighting fixtures, weather-stripping, wall coverings, electrical wires, and synthetic carpeting are examples of these products. Polyvinyl chloride can emit vinyl chloride, a carcinogen, as it deteriorates and interacts with water.

Chemicals can also irritate the skin, the largest organ of the body. Direct chemical irritants dissolve the skin or extract some essential components. Sensitizers, which include formaldehyde and duplicating fluids, cause an allergic reaction or sensitize the skin so that even a small quantity can cause a rash. Carbon paper, typing paper, typewriter ribbons, blueprint paper, and carbonless paper forms can also cause skin rashes.

CLEANSING, BALANCING, AND PREVENTIVE TECHNIQUES

Prevention of exposures in the office is preferable to dealing with adverse symptoms from these exposures. The following measures can reduce office exposure:

- *Air cleaner*: Use an air cleaner in your immediate work area. Be certain it is a model that contains activated charcoal, which removes chemicals from the air. The air cleaner should also remove particles, such as dust, dust mites, mold, pollen, bacteria, and viruses.
- *Smoking*: Do not allow anyone to smoke in your area.
- *Mask*: Wear a mask if there are chemical exposures over which you have no control. It should contain activated charcoal to help remove chemicals. Extreme exposures may require a respirator with specialized filters.
- *Protective clothing*: Wear gloves, a jacket, or a workcoat to protect your skin and your clothing. Goggles or safety glasses may also be necessary.
- *Ventilation*: Use a fan to increase ventilation and reduce chemical levels in your work area.

Make suggestions for correcting problems to your employer. If your employer does not correct the problems, in the U.S. you have the option of calling the Occupational Safety and Health Administration (OSHA), or a similar government agency that works to ensure the safety of workers. In Canada, federal government employees should contact the Labour Division of Human Resources Development Canada; other workers should contact their provincial or territorial Department of Labour and ask for its occupational health and safety division. Every employer must follow strict guidelines to ensure worker safety. If you feel that your workplace is not safe or that chemicals are not handled properly, you may need to change jobs if the working conditions and/or building are too toxic. Your health is your most valuable possession; guarding it is your most important task.

If you have health problems related to an occupational exposure see the cleansing options in part 5.

School Exposures

Toxic exposures at school can affect student behavior, academic performance, and health. Unfortunately, school exposures are rarely considered to be a cause of learning and behavioral problems. Many students in remedial programs may have unidentified sensitivities.

SCHOOL BUILDINGS

New schools can be a source of volatile organic chemicals and formaldehyde from new furniture, carpet, paint, and building materials. Many parents have noted that their children's performance deteriorated in a new school environment.

When more space is required, schools add portable classrooms because they are cheaper than adding on to a school building. The portable classrooms are typically windowless, built from inexpensive materials, usually with wood products that are high in formaldehyde. These buildings have poor ventilation, worsening indoor air pollution. Many portable buildings are placed on steel stands instead of a concrete foundation. This predisposes the space under the portable building to mold and bacterial growth, which has caused illness in both students and teachers. If the classroom has had a water leak, there may be mold in the classroom. Mold is one of the most potent and toxic allergens.

Many permanent school buildings also have mold contamination, particularly in humid climates. The HVAC units of airtight buildings can become contaminated with mold and spread it throughout the building to carpets, fabrics, and books.

Faulty or inadequate ventilation can cause poor air quality in the classroom. Lowered oxygen levels can cause drowsiness, fatigue, and poor concentration. Particulate contamination, such as dust and danders, can be spread through the classroom from dirty air ducts and vents.

TOXIC EXPOSURES

There are many toxic exposures at school:

- *Electromagnetic radiation*: Many schools are located near major transformers and high tension wires.
- *Asbestos*: Some older schools still contain asbestos tiles or asbestos fireproofing. As long as it is intact, the asbestos is not dangerous. When it becomes "friable and crumbly," asbestos becomes dangerous. Renovating can cause asbestos to become airborne.
- *Radon*: Some classrooms contain radon levels above the EPA safety level. Because radon cannot be seen, smelled, or tasted, it is important that classrooms be tested for this gas.
- *Lead*: Drinking water from water fountains can be exposed to lead in the pipes for long periods during weekends and holidays. This causes a high lead level in the water, particularly for children who drink from the fountains in the morning. Ask the school to have the lead content of the water checked.
- *Carpets*: They can harbor volatile chemicals, lead, dust, dust mites, and mold. New carpets can outgas formaldehyde.
- *Paint*: Schools tend to be painted just before school starts or while school is in session. Schools usually use enamel paint that has a slick, easy-to-clean surface. Enamel paint takes a minimum of one month to outgas at 100% ventilation and three months with less than 100% ventilation.
- *Lighting*: Most schools have fluorescent lighting. Many students are bothered by these lights, which flicker at a rate of 60 times per second. Some students have an increase in hyperactivity when they are exposed to fluorescent lights.
- *Traffic*: If schools and playgrounds are near heavily traveled highways, high concentrations of lead may be in the soil and air. Hydrocarbon levels from exhaust fumes will also be high.
- *Asphalt*: Asphalt may be encountered when schools resurface their parking lots. Sometimes this procedure takes place when school is in session, and the odors can permeate the classroom.
- *Tar*: Tar is frequently used when putting on new roofs or patching leaky roofs, work often performed during school hours. Chemically sensitive children should be kept home when either of these procedures are being done.

- *Pesticides*: Playgrounds and the interior of classrooms are treated on a regular basis with pesticides that may linger for days. Children who go out at recess can receive a high exposure to pesticides, herbicides, and chemical fertilizers from playing on grass sprayed with lawn chemicals.
- *Cleaning supplies*: Phenol and formaldehyde are frequently used as disinfectants in schools. One trip to the bathroom after these supplies have been used can mentally incapacitate a sensitive student for the rest of the day.
- *Chemicals*: Chemicals are used in biology classes (with animals preserved in formaldehyde), chemistry laboratories, or art classrooms. Even if the student is not in the classroom using the chemicals, the fumes can drift into other classrooms and make many students ill.
- *Methanol*: Methanol, and sometimes ethanol, are used in duplicating machines, often in poorly ventilated locations. Exposure causes headaches, itchy eyes, and dizziness.
- *Instructional materials*: Freshly xeroxed or mimeographed instructional materials are a toxic chemical exposure for many students. All paper is a formaldehyde exposure, including the paper in books.
- *Personal care products*: Products used by both students and teachers, including perfumes, after-shave lotions, deodorants, shampoos, hair sprays, and detergent and fabric softener scents in clothes, can cause problems for the sensitive student.
- *Animals*: Many classrooms have animals, such as guinea pigs, white mice or rats, hamsters, and rabbits. Students can react to animal dander, the bedding material in the cages, or even the urine and feces. Many people with cat allergies do not tolerate guinea pigs, hamsters, or rabbits.

CLEANSING, BALANCING, AND PREVENTIVE TECHNIQUES

The following measures are useful to protect your child from toxic exposures at school:

- *New school building*: If you have a choice of schools, do not allow your child to attend school in a new building. If there is no alternative, supply the classroom with several spider plants that remove formaldehyde from the air. Boston ferns, gerbera daisy, dwarf date palms, and bamboo palms also remove formaldehyde. An air cleaner that removes chemicals placed near your child's desk will help your child and other children in the room. Allergy extracts for chemicals will help your child to better tolerate a toxic classroom.
- *Portable buildings*: The plants and an air cleaner are also helpful in portable buildings. In addition to chemical extracts, your child may need a mold extract if the portable building contains mold.
- *Electromagnetic radiation*: Transfer your child to another school if there are high voltage powerlines nearby. Have your child wear diodes to help combat the effects of electromagnetic radiation.
- *Asbestos*: Unless the asbestos is crumbling, it should be left in place. If it needs to be removed, only persons specially trained in handling asbestos should attempt the removal.
- *Radon*: Consult professionals to treat a school radon problem. Increase ventilation, and seal all foundation or basement cracks to decrease radon levels.
- *Lead*: The use of lead in both new plumbing and plumbing repairs is now prohibited. Any school water coolers or plumbing containing lead parts should be replaced.

- *Carpets*: If your child's school has carpets find out how often they are cleaned. Donate some NeoLife Red for the school to use for cleaning the carpets.
- *Paint*: Ask to be notified when the school is going to paint. If you have an extremely sensitive child, keep him or her home on those days.
- *Fluorescent lights*: Request that your school use full-spectrum fluorescent lights.
- *Asphalt and tar*: Again, keep your child home the day these substances are being applied. A mask will help, as will an air cleaner.
- *Pesticide exposures*: Inquire about the pesticide spraying schedule and keep your child home on the days the pesticide is being applied. If lawn chemicals are applied to the playground, keep your child home on the day they are applied, and send a note to school asking that he or she not play on the grass for at least a week.
- *Cleaning supplies*: Talk to the school about the active ingredients in the cleaning supplies. If there are cleaners your child tolerates, volunteer to donate some if the school is willing to use them. Air cleaners and a mask will help. Allergy extracts for phenol, ethanol, and formaldehyde will also help with symptoms to cleaning supplies.
- *Chemical exposures*: Avoiding chemicals in science and art classes is difficult. Adequate ventilation helps, as do air cleaners. Activated charcoal masks will reduce the level of chemicals breathed. Inquire about alternative projects your child might be able to do instead of some of the more toxic lab or art projects.
- *Instructional materials*: Request that materials be prepared ahead of time and allowed to outgas before being used in the classroom.
- *Personal care products*: Having the teacher and students refrain from wearing scented products is the ideal solution for this problem. However, the chances of it happening are not high. Again, air cleaners are helpful. Allergy extracts for perfume, fabric softener, and detergent will also help.
- *Animals*: An allergy extract for animal dander will help protect your child. If the child is significantly affected, request that the animal be removed from the classroom.

11

Toxins in the Home

We spend at least one-third of our day at home. Some homes are more polluted than others. A home is sick or polluted if:

- more than one person in the same house has similar symptoms
- people who spend the most time at home have the most severe symptoms
- visitors complain of symptoms after they have been in the home
- symptoms improve or disappear when people leave the home for hours or days.
- symptoms get worse when the house is closed up for the winter
- symptoms begin after moving into a new house, after remodeling an old house, or after adding new furnishings

Sources of Home Toxins

ASBESTOS

Asbestos may be found in wall and ceiling insulation in homes built before the 1950s. Until the early 1970s it was used for insulating hot-water pipes, steampipes, furnaces and boilers, and on ceilings and walls. Asbestos was used in wallboard and spackling compound in houses built before 1977. Resilient floor tiles, refrigerators, dishwashers, ovens, and toasters may contain asbestos.

When airborne, asbestos particles can be inhaled or ingested, causing lung cancer or damage to the lungs, and cancer of the gastrointestinal tract.

FORMALDEHYDE

Formaldehyde is found in disinfectants, wooden building materials, cosmetics, molded plastics, and pesticides. Formaldehyde is also found in newsprint, paper grocery bags, carpets, draperies, permanent-press clothes, paints, shellacs, waxes, photography darkroom chemicals, and glues and adhesives.

During the 1970s, urea-formaldehyde foam insulation was pumped into walls. Many people developed burning of the eye, nose, and throat, and skin rashes. Hundreds of families had to leave their homes. The insulation is not used in homes today. Formaldehyde can also cause coughing, runny nose, sore throat, fatigue, nausea, eye and sinus irritations, and nosebleeds. Between 10% and 20% of the population is highly sensitive to formaldehyde. Monitors to test formaldehyde levels are available.

VOLATILE ORGANIC COMPOUNDS

Volatile organic compounds (vocs) are chemicals that contain carbon and hydrogen. The indoor level of vocs is two to five times that of the outdoor level. Volatile organic compounds are found in lacquers, adhesives, waxes, cleaning agents, cosmetics, paint and paint removers, inks, disinfectants, antiseptics, perfumes, mouthwashes, air fresheners, aerosol sprays, permanent-press fabrics, polyesters, synthetic fibers, drapes, dry-cleaned clothes, pesticides, and plastics.

VOCs cause eye irritations, headaches, nausea, respiratory symptoms, fatigue, and mood swings. They can also affect the reproductive system. Very little research has been done regarding the effects of VOCs, especially chronic low-level exposures.

RADON

Radon is a common indoor air pollutant that comes from uranium in rock and soil. Radon enters through cracks in a house foundation, joints in concrete slabs, around gas and water pipes, drains, and sumps. Well water is also a source of radon. In an EPA survey of 17 states, 25% of the homes tested had radon levels above the concentration for which action is recommended. The EPA estimates 20,000 lung cancer deaths each year may be due to radon exposures, although other studies have not yet been able to prove this link.

CARBON MONOXIDE

Carbon monoxide is generated from the process of combustion. Backdrafting occurs when wood stoves, fireplaces, and furnaces burn in houses that are too tightly sealed. Outdoor air should replace the indoor air that is being used in the combustion process. If it cannot, negative pressure builds up, drawing the exhaust gases back into the house.

Carbon monoxide poisoning can cause nausea and vomiting and may mimic stomach flu. Carbon monoxide poisoning causes headaches, shortness of breath, and chest pains in people with heart disease. Attached garages can be a source of carbon monoxide.

NITROGEN DIOXIDE

Nitrogen dioxide is produced when gas stoves burn. The concentration of nitrogen dioxide is two to three times higher in homes with gas stoves than in those with electric ranges. This toxin causes skin, eye, and mucous membrane irritation. It can attach to hemoglobin and interfere with hemoglobin's ability to carry oxygen. Children living in homes with gas stoves have higher rates of respiratory infections.

PARTICULATE MATTER

Particulate matter, small enough to be inhaled into the lungs, can be produced by cigarette smoke, gas stoves, wood stoves, fireplaces, kerosene space heaters, and furnaces. Particulate matter can cause eye and mucous membrane irritation. At higher doses, it causes lung disease. Particulate matter acts synergistically with other chemicals to increase the toxicity of both.

MOLDS, MICROORGANISMS, PETS, AND DUST

Molds and mildews thrive in wet areas, such as bathrooms, humidifiers, refrigerator drip pans, central air conditioning systems, heating ducts, ice machines and any area where there is a water leak. When people breathe, they release moisture into the air. Moisture is also released from washing machines, dishwashers, and houseplants. Two respiratory diseases caused by mold are humidifier fever and hypersensitivity pneumonitis.

Bacteria, viruses, fungi, pollens, pet dander, mold, and dust and dust mites can cause illness in homes. These agents can enter on people and pets or can be airborne. People have allergic reactions to pollens, molds, dust and dust mite, and animal dander. Infection can result from bacteria, viruses, and fungi.

CLEANERS AND OTHER HOME EXPOSURES

Cleaning supplies, soaps, detergents, fabric softeners, dryer sheets, waxes, bleach, perfumes, toilet articles, and room deodorizers and sprays further add to the chemical load found in the home. Hobbies and home workshops can add to home exposures. (For further discussion, see chapter 12.)

The yards around our homes become toxic if lawn chemicals, fertilizers, weed killers, or pesticides are applied to the lawn, trees, or flower beds (see chapter 6).

CLEANSING, BALANCING, AND PREVENTIVE TECHNIQUES

If your home contains any asbestos, approach it with care. People working on parts of a house may accidently dislodge asbestos particles into the air. Asbestos that is flaking can be painted over. Never try to remove asbestos; it is a job for trained professionals.

High formaldehyde levels can be reduced by sealing particleboard, plywood, chipboard, and paneling. While sealants do significantly reduce formaldehyde levels, some sensitive people are unable to tolerate them. Studies done by NASA show that spider plants and banana plants will remove formaldehyde from the air. Several plants in a room high in formaldehyde will significantly lower the levels.

Chemical cleanup of your home is the best way to remove volatile organic chemicals. Remove the following from your home:

- pesticides, paints, paint removers, lacquers, adhesives, waxes, and shellacs. Never store these products inside the house.
- scented cleaning products
- air fresheners and aerosol sprays
- dry-cleaned clothes that have not aired outside for a month

- any perfumes; after shaves; nail polish; nail polish remover; and scented soaps, lotions, and deodorants

If your home has a high radon level, seal cracks, cover exposed earth, and improve ventilation. Professional who specialize in radon control can help you solve this problem.

Mold control is very important. Monitor indoor humidity and use mold plates to determine the amount of mold contamination. Use exhaust fans in the kitchen and bathrooms to vent excess moisture to the outside. Vent the clothes dryer to the outside and repair all leaks. If the mold contamination is too great in the area surrounding the leak, the moldy materials may have to be replaced.

To avoid carbon monoxide poisoning, do not idle cars in the garage with the door closed. The wall and doorway separating the garage from the house should be airtight. If gas furnaces or stoves are used for heating, check them regularly to be certain they are functioning efficiently. Gas stoves give off both carbon monoxide and nitrogen dioxide.

Good ventilation and a properly working gas stove will decrease the indoor air pollution. Inspect furnaces yearly and clean the filters regularly. Check gas stoves, furnaces, and hot-water heaters regularly for gas leaks and carbon monoxide levels. Local gas companies have this capability. Clean and inspect chimneys yearly.

Avoid using chemicals on your lawn, trees, and shrubbery as natural fertilizers are available. Remove weeds by hand rather than using weed killers.

12

Exposure at Leisure and While Traveling

Hobbies

Hobbies often involve exposure to toxins. Paint, dyes, magic markers, oils, glues, waxes, fabrics, plastics, woods, solvents, and adhesives can contain toxic chemicals. They may also contain fungicides, pesticides, preservatives, and extenders. High doses or chronic exposures can cause skin rashes, neurological problems, respiratory diseases, lung scarring, birth defects, kidney damage, and impaired physical and mental development.

Toxic metals are found in some art and craft materials. Arsenic, cadmium, chromium, cobalt, lead, manganese, and zinc are used as pigments in paints, dyes, and ceramic glazes. Cadmium may also be in silver solders and fluxes. Lead is found in stained-glass materials.

Volatile organic chemicals are commonly found in art and craft supplies. Toluene, xylene, methylene chloride, petroleum distillate, glycol ethers, alcohols, ketones, and benzene are found in oil- and solvent-based paints, markers, finishes, glues, and coatings. Formaldehyde is used as a preservative in acrylic paints, fabric finishes, and photographic products. It is also used extensively in the manufacture of all types of paper. Hydroquinone is a chemical used in the process of developing photographs. Vapors from electric glue guns are toxic to some individuals.

Charcoal, pastels, and colored pencils create a fine dust. This dust contains sensitizing and irritating chemicals. Dust produced when cleaning ceramic greenware is a problem for some people.

Sawdust and terpene vapors from woodworking shops prohibit this medium as a hobby or an art for terpene-sensitive people.

Asbestos is sometimes a contaminant in talc and soapstone. Soapstone is often used in making jewelry. Asbestos is also used to insulate kilns. When fired, kilns produce carbon dioxide, sulfur dioxide, formaldehyde, fluorine, chlorine, lead, and cadmium.

People who do arc welding, photo printmaking, printing, and dyeline copying are exposed to ultraviolet radiation.

Professional artists, art teachers, art students, and artisans have the highest exposure to toxins in their supplies, but they tend to be more careful in the use of these materials. Children and the elderly use these products less frequently, but they may be more at risk because they are less informed of the dangers of the chemicals.

In 1988, legislation was passed that requires the U.S. Product Safety Commission to regulate the labeling of art and craft materials for health hazards. In general, products with an AP or CP seal can be used safely by small children. However, some products that bear the seal, such as metal enamels, ceramic glazes, and clays with talc, are not safe for children to use. In Canada, most consumer products containing toxic materials carry warning labels, but if you use a product frequently it would be wise to obtain a Material Safety Data Sheet from the manufacturer and follow its workplace recommendations.

CLEANSING, BALANCING, AND PREVENTIVE TECHNIQUES

Active hobbyists should work in well-ventilated areas. An exhaust fan and air cleaners are helpful. If your workroom does not have an exhaust fan, set one up by placing a square floor fan in the window. Turn the fan so that it blows to the outside. This will pull air from the room and blow it out the window, creating an exhaust.

Wearing gloves and protective clothing is helpful to keep toxins off the skin. A mask of activated charcoal will significantly reduce the inhalation of toxic fumes. You should not eat, drink, or smoke when using hazardous materials.

Use nontoxic materials whenever there is a choice. If possible, use water-based instead of solvent-based paints. Material safety data sheets are available from manufacturers for more information on many products. Ask for help to clean up a completed project. Cleanup is frequently more toxic than the actual work on a project.

Toxins from materials used with hobbies are frequently lipophilic chemicals that may be stored in the fat cells of the body. Detox baths (see chapter 13) are helpful to cleanse the body of toxins. Vitamin C, taken to bowel tolerance levels, is also beneficial.

Toxins and Travel

Travel exposes us to toxins from both the mode of transportation and the lodging facilities used on a trip.

AIR TRAVEL

Airplane travel can be dangerous for people with heart and respiratory disease. Airplane cabins are pressurized to the equivalent of 7000 to 8000 feet in altitude, which is a problem for some individuals. On international flights, attendants, passengers, and airline workers are exposed to second-hand smoke. Working as a flight attendant on smoking flights has been said to be like living with a one-pack-per-day smoker. Women who are exposed to passive smoke for three to four hours a day have an increased risk or cervical cancer.

Criteria for airplane cabin air exchange rates, environmental conditions, and air contaminants have not been established. The Federal Aviation Agency's (FAA) standard for airplane cabin carbon dioxide concentration is twice that allowed for indoor environments.

Poor air quality in commercial airlines is an increasing problem. Banning smoking on domestic flights has helped, but the problem of inadequate ventilation remains. Microorganisms, pollutants, and other materials can build up to dangerous levels. Some of the contaminants found in airplanes include:

- carbon dioxide, from breathing and dry ice
- ozone from the atmosphere
- fibers and dust
- nitrogen oxides
- volatile organic compounds from fuel and cleaning fluids
- bacteria, fungi, and viruses from food and passengers

Airplane ventilation systems draw outdoor air through the engines. The air is cooled by an air conditioner and mixed with recycled air. While on the ground, airplanes may use ground-based units, but this air is often contaminated with fumes from the ramp area. To save money, airlines use more recycled air and less fresh air.

McDonnell Douglas calculated in 1980 that cutting outdoor air intake by half would save 0.8% on fuel. Increasing ventilation twofold on a five-hour flight would increase costs by only 60 cents per passenger. The American Society of

Heating, Refrigeration, and Air-conditioning Engineers (ASHRAE) recommends a ventilation rate of 15 to 20 cubic feet per minute (cfm) per person. Economy-class passengers on a Boeing 747 flight receive less than 7 cfm. First-class has a ventilation rate of 30 to 50 cfm of fresh air per person. Related complaints from passengers and flight attendants include sore eyes, scratchy throats, nasal irritation, headaches, cough, shortness of breath, fatigue, and dizziness.

Recommended maximum carbon dioxide level is 1000 parts per million (ppm) but levels over 5000 ppm are not uncommon in airplanes. Many flights have ozone levels eight times higher than the recommended amount, causing nose, throat, and lung irritations. Adding filtration systems and using charcoal filters and disposable prefilters to take out volatile organic chemicals and ozone from the planes has been suggested.

Low humidity creates more discomfort for passengers than any other factor, causing dry eyes and respiratory and skin irritation. It is recommended that relative humidity be kept between 30% and 65%. The U.S. National Academy of Science (NAS) found that the typical relative humidity on planes was 2% to 23%. Fresh air brought inside the cabin has less than 1% relative humidity. Moisture is added to the air in cabins by passengers and flight crews breathing and perspiring. Improved ventilation would reduce the carbon monoxide, carbon dioxide, and the microorganism contamination level, but would decrease the relative humidity in the air.

Contamination with microorganisms can occur easily on airline flights. On one flight that sat on the ground for three hours in Alaska, 72% of passengers developed a strain of flu within three days. One passenger was the source of infection. Flu epidemics spread along major airline travel routes.

Air travel can also disrupt the normal body circadian rhythms, which are based on the 24-hour day. A person traveling across several time zones can become very tired and may develop gastrointestinal symptoms. This is known as jet lag. After a flight from Germany to North America, it takes three days to resynchronize psychomotor performance. It takes eight days to resynchronize if the flight direction is east.

Radiation exposure occurs during airline flights. At typical cruising altitudes of 29,000 to 39,000 feet, the radiation dose is 100 times that at sea level. Frequent flyers who log 100,000 miles a year in the air should have exposure doses monitored regularly. Pregnant women should not fly frequently because fetuses are more radiation-sensitive than adults. The International Commission on Radiation Protection recommends the maximum permissible dose for air passengers be no more than 5 millisieverts (500 millirems) a year.

Airsickness is a problem for some passengers. It is caused both by the motion of the plane and the cabin pressure. For sensitive individuals, exposure to jet fuel and the soaps, perfumes, and fabric softener on other passengers plays a role in airsickness. Other individuals may not feel well while flying because of electromagnetic disturbances. Airplane cabins frequently have a high level of positively charged ions.

On many international flights, pesticide is sprayed before passengers are allowed to deplane. The application of pesticide is a requirement of the destination country. This further adds to the toxic chemicals encountered on a flight.

Airport terminals can also be very toxic. Tobacco smoke, cleaning products, personal care products of other travelers, jet fuel and exhaust, and mold contribute to the toxicity. Many airports seem to be under perpetual construction. The building supplies used in remodeling can be a problem for many passengers.

CLEANSING, BALANCING, AND PREVENTIVE TECHNIQUES

Sensitive individuals may be helped by wearing a mask containing activated charcoal both on the plane and in the terminal building to filter toxic chemicals. Extra doses of vitamin C during the flight and in the airport will help maintain balance. Oxygen use during a flight is crucial for some sensitive individuals. Many airlines provide the service for a moderate fee, but arrangements must be made several days before the flight. Provide your own ceramic mask as the mask they will offer will be new and made of soft plastic.

Allergy extracts for chemicals will help control symptoms to the chemicals encountered in the aircraft cabins and in the airport. On international flights, an allergy extract for cigar and cigarette smoke will help with symptoms to tobacco smoke. Extracts for gas, diesel, and jet fuel will help with the chemical exposures at airports. Homeopathic pesticide extracts will help on international flights. In some cases, it may be possible to leave the plane before the pesticide is sprayed.

Magnets, diodes, or tachyon beads are excellent aids for maintaining electromagnetic balance (see chapter 8). After returning home, detox baths will help cleanse the body of toxins encountered on the trip.

If you have the tendency to be air sick, drink ginger tea and eat before you leave, avoid alcohol and carbonated beverages (except ginger ale) during the flight, and sit in the more stable seats over the wings.

Symptoms from air travel can be controlled by the balancing action of several homeopathic remedies:

- Ears that will not pop: *Kali muriaticum*
- Ear pain: *Chamomilla, Kali muriaticum*
- Airsickness: *Argentum nitricum, Cocculus indicus, Gelsemium*
- Jet lag: *Arnica, Cocculus, Gelsemium*

AUTOMOBILE/BUS/TRUCK TRAVEL

The majority of North Americans travel frequently in vehicles powered by internal combustion engines. The exhaust from these engines, whether gasoline or diesel, is a toxic exposure. Exhaust from gasoline engines contains paraffins, olefins, sulfur, sulfur dioxide, tars, ammonia, nitrogen dioxide, organic acids, zinc, metallic oxides, and unburned fuel. It also contains fragments of antioxidants, metal deactivators, anti-rust, anti-icing compounds, detergents, and lubricants. Diesel exhaust contains nitrogen dioxide, sulfur dioxide, formaldehyde, acrolein, and phenol, in addition to many hydrocarbons. For some, the toxic exposure from diesel exhaust is worse than gasoline exhaust.

Leaks from exhaust and fuel systems can find their way into older vehicles. Leaks of engine oil, antifreeze, transmission fluid, and power steering and brake fluid can cause additional chemical exposure. The exposure is worse if these leaking fluids come in contact with a hot exhaust pipe or manifold. The air conditioning/ventilation system in many vehicles draws in outside, contaminated engine air that further adds to the exposure.

Vehicle motion and exposure to exhaust fumes play a role in carsickness. Riders in the front seat are exposed to fewer exhaust fumes than passengers in the back. Many people can avoid car sickness by riding in the front seat or by driving.

CLEANSING, BALANCING, AND PREVENTIVE TECHNIQUES

Wear a charcoal mask to decrease the exposure to exhaust fumes and other chemicals encountered in a vehicle. Take less-traveled routes for both city and highway travel to avoid traffic fumes. An automobile air cleaner improves the air quality, and using a portable oxygen tank is helpful for extremely sensitive individuals.

Allergy extracts for chemicals encountered in vehicles are very helpful.

The balancing action of homeopathic remedies is also helpful for carsickness:

- Motion sickness: *Cocculus, Petroleum, and Sepia*

- Nausea: *Cocculus, Conium, Euphorbia corrolata, Nux vomica, Petroleum, Tabacum,* and *Zingibar*
- Vomiting: *Carbolicum acidum, Cocculus, Petroleum,* and *Tabacum*

BOAT TRAVEL

On powered boats, toxic exposure includes various oils and reserve fuel tanks as well as the exhaust from the engines. On passenger ships, toxic exposures are higher because of the size and complexity of the vessel. In addition to engine exhaust, cleaning supplies, carpets, drapes, heating and cooling systems, tobacco smoke, and personal care products of other passengers can be toxic exposures.

People suffering from pollen allergies, however, do well on a sea voyage because exposure to pollens is negligible.

The possibility of seasickness is common to all boats, regardless of their size. Seasickness is largely caused by the rhythmic action of the water.

CLEANSING, BALANCING, AND PREVENTIVE TECHNIQUES

Allergy extracts for chemical exposures on any size boat are helpful in maintaining balance.

On cruise ships, air cleaners will maintain air quality in the cabins. A charcoal mask will help control exposures in dining rooms, entertainment centers, and meeting rooms.

To prevent seasickness, sail on larger boats that are more stable. Stay toward the center of the boat where the rocking sensation is less. Remain on deck instead of in your cabin, and focus on the horizon and not the waves. Eat light meals of protein and carbohydrates. Avoid alcoholic beverages and drink ginger ale. Stay as still as possible if your head starts spinning, and avoid seasick passengers as nausea is "contagious."

Cocculus, Conium, Euphorbia corrolata, Nux vomica, Petroleum, Tabacum, and *Zingibar* are

homeopathic remedies that aid in clearing seasickness. Sea bands are helpful in preventing or controlling seasickness in some people. These bands fit over the wrist and have a disc that presses on an acupuncture point. Occasionally pressing the disc stimulates the acupuncture point and averts seasickness.

LODGING EXPOSURES

Hotel and motel lodging can provide an opportunity for toxic exposure. Cleaning supplies, deodorizers, carpets, drapes, and air conditioning/heating systems may outgas toxic chemicals. If smoking is allowed in the building, the toxic chemical load is even higher.

Mold can sometimes be a problem in motel and hotel rooms. It can result from a leaking roof, shower stall, or even ground contamination. Always check the room for mold as well as for chemical exposures before accepting it.

CLEANSING, BALANCING, AND PREVENTIVE TECHNIQUES

To minimize lodging exposure, ask:

- for a nonsmoking room
- that your room be aired before your arrival
- for a room not recently redecorated or sprayed with pesticides
- for a room with windows that open
- for a room away from the pool, laundry room, or heating plant
- that your room be cleaned with baking soda or not at all while you are there
- that only the beds be made and the trash emptied
- that the linens not be changed to reduce exposure to fabric softener and possible gas dryer fumes

Take an air cleaner with you and run it 24 hours a day in your room. Use your own pillow and pillowcase to minimize exposures while sleeping. Very sensitive individuals may want to supply their own linens. Do not use hotel or motel bath soaps and shampoos; bring your own.

Allergy extracts for mold and chemical toxins will help prevent problems. Take vitamin C periodically throughout the day to help cleanse the body. Wearing a charcoal mask is also helpful.

Consider traveling in the off-season to popular recreation areas. Fewer people means less exposure to personal care products and tobacco smoke. Less crowding also reduces exposure to infections.

PART FIVE

Ways of Detoxification

13

Baths, Saunas, and Hydrotherapy

Detoxification Baths

Detoxification baths are sometimes called the "poor man's sauna." Baths are very useful for people who have a toxic bioaccumulation of xenobiotics. The hot water increases blood flow and capillary action near the surface of the skin, causing faster release of toxins. The heat also increases sweating and opens pores, allowing toxin-containing perspiration to reach the skin surface more readily. Although using filtered water is preferable for these baths, city water, containing chlorine, is still effective and helpful.

Approach these baths with caution and common sense. If your chemical load is extremely high, they can make you feel very ill. Have someone in the house with you when you take your detoxification bath in case you develop symptoms and require assistance. Should you experience dizziness, headache, exhaustion, fatigue, nausea, or weakness, stop your bath. If possible, it is a good idea to have a physician supervise your detoxification program.

Your bathtub should be spotlessly clean for a detoxification bath; you are trying to rid your body of toxins, not absorb more. *Before beginning the detoxification baths take a trial series of hot, plain-water baths.*

Follow these general instructions for both the plain-water baths and the detox baths:

- Wash your body thoroughly with tolerated soap in the shower before you take your bath and scrub with a loofa sponge or a rough washcloth to remove excess body oils. Rinse thoroughly.
- Fill the tub with water as hot as you can tolerate without burning your skin. Cover the tub's overflow valve so the water level will be high enough to immerse your body up to your neck.
- Begin with a five-minute soak in hot water. Gradually build up the time by five-minute increments until you can soak for 30 minutes without experiencing symptoms. You may feel deceptively well while soaking, but it is of utmost importance that you do not overstay your time limit in the tub. Symptoms sometimes do not occur until the next day.
- Should you experience immediate intolerable symptoms, drain the tub. Sit in the tub until you feel you can safely stand and get out. If you attempt to get out of the tub while you feel weak, you might fall.
- After soaking, take a cleansing shower. Scrub thoroughly with soap and rinse well in order to remove any toxins deposited on your skin during the bath. Unremoved toxins will be reabsorbed. If you continue to perspire, repeat the shower.

- Take detox baths three times a week until your general health has improved. Then, use the baths once or twice a week.
- If you have unusual chemical exposures, increase the number and frequency of your baths.
- Some people detoxify in cycles, and detoxification baths may have to be repeated in a series. Sometimes months may pass between episodes.
- Take your tolerated dose of vitamin C before and after each bath. This will help your body to remove the toxins released into your bloodstream. If you are taking antioxidant nutritional supplements, take them before your bath.
- Drink an 8-ounce glass of water during your bath.

TYPES OF DETOXIFICATION BATHS

When you can take a plain hot-water bath for 30 minutes with no symptoms, you may begin detoxification baths. Several substances may be used in the bath to aid in detoxification. Follow the general bath instructions, adding one of the substances listed below to the bath water. Except for the Epsom salts, you may need to rotate the other substances as their effectiveness may subside quickly if some time is not allowed between use.

Epsom Salts   Epsom salts help eliminate toxins by activating fluid movement in the tissues and increasing perspiration. The salts work as a counter-irritant on the skin to increase blood supply and they also change the pH of the skin surface. The sulfur component of Epsom salts also aids to detoxifying. Sulfur springs have always been known for their medicinal and cleansing properties.

Begin with ¼ cup of Epsom salts. Gradually increase the amount with each bath until you are using 4 cups per tub of clean water. Should you experience symptoms at any level, stay at that level until you can soak 30 minutes with no symptoms.

Apple-Cider Vinegar Baths   Vinegar also works as a counter-irritant, increasing blood supply to the skin and changing the pH of the skin. Begin with ¼ cup of apple-cider vinegar in the bath water. Over a period of time gradually increase this amount to 1 cup per tub.

Clorox Baths   Use the Clorox brand of liquid bleach only, adding 2 tablespoons to a full tub of clean water. Chlorine-sensitive people cannot use Clorox.

Hydrogen Peroxide Baths   Use up to 8 ounces of food-grade 35% hydrogen peroxide in a bathtub half-full of warm water.

Soda Baths   Baking soda, or sodium bicarbonate, creates an alkalinizing bath to restore acid/alkaline balance through osmosis. They are particularly good for cleansing and drying weeping, open sores. Use eight ounces of baking soda to a tub of bath water.

Soda and sea salt baths are effective for detoxifying X-ray and radiation exposure. Use equal amounts of the soda and noniodized sea salt, building up to 1 pound of each.

Ginger Root Baths   Ginger's heating property causes sweating. It also stimulates and draws toxins to the skin surface. Cut a thumb-size ginger root into small pieces, place in a pot of water and bring to a boil. Turn off the heat and steep for 30 minutes. Strain the mixture and pour the liquid in a tub of hot, clean bath water.

Clay Baths   Clay is most frequently used in compresses or packs. However, the drawing and alkalizing action of clay baths also aids in detoxification. Use ½ cup of clay to a tub of water.

There are several types of clay on the market, all appropriate for bathing.

Burdock Root Baths   Burdock root baths help the body to excrete uric acid. They also aid in cleansing boils and clearing rashes. Simmer a level handful of burdock root in 2 quarts of water for 30 minutes. Strain into a tub of clean, hot water.

Oatstraw Baths   Oatstraw baths improve skin metabolism, which helps the body to detoxify. Simmer a heaping handful of oatstraw in 2 quarts of water for 25 minutes. Strain into a tub of clean, hot water.

Herbal Tea Baths   A number of herbal teas may be used in detox baths to aid in cleansing chemicals: catnip, yarrow, peppermint, boneset, blessed thistle, pleurisy root, chamomile, blue vervain, and horsetail. Use one cup of the brewed tea per tub of hot, clean water. Use only *one* of these teas per bath. Sensitive individuals may not tolerate the use of some of these herbs.

Saunas

TYPES OF SAUNAS

A sauna is a relatively airtight room with wooden platforms and benches. The air is kept fresh by a special ventilation system that preheats outside air before it enters the sauna. For good ventilation, the air should be exchanged six times an hour.

There are two basic types of saunas, dry and wet. No moisture is added to the sauna room for a dry sauna. Steam is used in wet saunas. The most common source of steam is a steam generator but some saunas use water poured over heated rocks for the steam source. In wet or steam saunas, the humidity is controlled to maintain 50 to 60 grams of water vapor per kilogram of air.

Electricity is the most common source of sauna heat, and infrared heat is also frequently used. The temperature should be kept between 140°–150°F for environmentally ill people and people with a heavy load of toxins.

CAUTION: Pregnant women should not sauna. The heat from the sauna may cause neural tube defects in the fetus during the first trimester of pregnancy. Since many women do not know they are pregnant during this time, women of child-bearing age should have a pregnancy test before beginning sauna treatment. Heart disease, kidney disease, and anemia are also contraindications for sauna treatment.

In modern saunas, walls and floors are often made of tile and concrete rather than wood. Cleaning is easier, which can be important in saunas that are used exclusively for detoxification regimens. The benches and platforms are best made of poplar wood to keep terpene outgasing of the wood at a minimum. In saunas where outgasing is not a consideration, they may be made of cedar, which adds its aroma (terpenes) to the air.

Sauna facilities may have cooling-off rooms in addition to shower rooms. Some sauna programs involve a gentle cooling-off, whereas others use cold showers, a dip in the lake (even through a hole in the ice), or a roll in the snow. If there are health problems, cooling off naturally or with a tepid shower is preferable.

SAUNA CLEANSING PROGRAM

The "heat stress" of a sauna is very effective in releasing fat-stored toxins from the cells. The use of a sauna is a major part of a detoxification program.

When using a sauna in a detoxification program, find a dry sauna that has been constructed to be environmentally safe with air cleaners attached to the air circulation units. Commercial saunas at health clubs tend to be too hot, have inadequate levels of oxygen, and are not environmentally well constructed.

Dry saunas are recommended because they increase sweating and so speed detoxification. A complete sauna cleansing program should include exercise, time in a dry sauna, and a cleansing shower followed by a massage. Both the exercise and sauna time should be built up gradually so that the stress to the body is minimized.

Exercise for 20 minutes, then go into the sauna. Maximum sauna time should be 30 minutes. A cleansing shower afterward washes off the toxins excreted in the sauna and prevents them from being reabsorbed. Massage stimulates, relaxes, and increases blood circulation, which aids in cleansing.

While sweating in the sauna, be sure to replace the fluids lost. Drink plenty of water, both while you are in the sauna and afterwards to help your kidneys flush toxins.

Nutritional supplements also aid in sauna cleansing, particularly the antioxidants. Oils taken orally help to bind toxins as the liver and bile remove them from the body. (See chapter 2 for more details.)

Pay attention to body odor when exercising in a detoxification program. Toxins are excreted in the sweat and can cause other people in the sauna or exercise room to react. Immediately remove towels used for the after-sauna shower; they will be impregnated with excreted toxins.

After completing a sauna, allow a period of rest. The body needs a quiet time to adjust and rebalance.

Portable saunas, sometimes called cabinet baths, are available for home use. They are available in both wet and dry models. These saunas allow the head to remain cool and the user to breathe the cleaner outside air. Take care when selecting a portable sauna because plastic parts can outgas. One- or two-person saunas constructed of wood are also available for home use. Infrared units provide the heat source for these saunas. Choose the wood for this type of sauna carefully to minimize terpene outgasing. Poplar is the best choice for sensitive people.

Hydrotherapy

Priessnitz, a Silesian peasant, founded hydrotherapy as a science in the early 1800s. He used douches (strong jets of water directed to a given area), cold purges, sweat baths, wet compresses, sitz baths, and other treatments still given today.

Hydrotherapy treatment makes use of the body's response to heat and cold. The primary reaction of the body to cold is stimulation, and its secondary reaction is invigorating, restorative, and tonic. This secondary cold effect causes smooth, soft skin, a sensation of warmth, slowed pulse, easy respirations, warmth of skin, and perspiration.

The primary effect of heat on the body is as a stimulant, and its secondary reaction is depression, sedation, and atony. The secondary heat effect causes a rapid pulse, decreased perspiration, mental tiredness, drowsiness, and muscular weakness.

Hydrotherapy increases the circulation of the blood and lymph, cleans the skin and removes impurities. It can be used to relieve pain, lower fever, decrease cramps, induce sleep, soothe the nervous system, act as a stimulant, increase physical and mental tone, and serve as a local anesthetic. It will also increase urine production and cause bowel evacuation, both of which aid in detoxification.

The duration and temperature of hydrotherapy application must be adjusted to the individual, and a health practitioner skilled in hydrotherapy should recommend the best method. The young and the old have poor heat regulation. Prolonged illness, fatigue, or anemia reduces a person's tolerance of extremes in temperature. Pressure, friction, hot drinks, and exercise can enhance reactions, but prolonged application of heat or cold can cause tissue damage and block the natural reaction.

TYPES OF HYDROTHERAPY

There are different types of hydrotherapy. Baths, including sitz, full immersion, local, and sweating baths are used. Except for the sweating bath, these baths may be hot, cold, or alternating hot and cold. Compresses are another type of hydrotherapy and may also be hot, cold, or alternating hot and cold. Full-body wet sheet packs are used cold, but blankets are used on top to make the patient sweat.

Sweat baths, vapor baths, and steam inhalations clear mucous membrane congestion. Douches are strong jets of water directed at a local or general area; showers are douches. Douches may be hot, cold, or alternating hot and cold. Cold douches to the breast bone or upper legs stimulate the kidneys; cold or alternate hot and cold compresses or douches on the abdomen stimulate the liver. Hot foot baths with ice on the back of the neck may help relieve a headache.

14

Diet and Nutrition

Fasting

We use our bodies 24 hours each day and do not often consider allowing them to rest and regenerate, other than when we sleep. We tend to take better care and pay more attention to the needs of our automobiles than we do to the condition and needs of our bodies. In an age of fast-paced technology and increased stimulation, it is important that we provide our bodies moments of rest and cleansing. Cleansing may be necessary several times throughout the year, perhaps with each change of season.

Fasting helps the body to heal and to resist diseases, infections, and toxins. It is actually an instinctual response, brought into play when the body needs all its energy to deal with disease and regeneration. Fasting frees the large amounts of energy used by the digestive organs for use elsewhere.

Sensible fasting gives the body an opportunity to return to its natural state of homeostasis. During a fast, the body produces new healthy cells to replace the discarded ones. Many people adopt a schedule of liquids-only one day each week, or liquids-only for a three-day period once each month, allowing conscious participation in an ongoing healing process rather than postponing action until a health crisis occurs.

Short-term fasting is one to three days. More than three days is considered long-term fasting.

WARNING: Do not attempt a long-term fast without medical supervision.

While true fasting requires that no food or liquid be consumed, most people drink water or unsweetened herbal teas during their fast. Total abstinence threatens the body, which adapts by lowering the metabolism and taking other measures. The toxins concentrated in our fat cells and organs are released rapidly during a true fast. They can cause problems during the fast as well as later on.

Vitamins and minerals are helpful supplements with routine eating, but do not take them while fasting because they can interfere with the cleansing process. Herbs may sometimes be used as they help to cleanse the body and regulate the glands.

FASTING MENUS

Drink at least eight glasses of liquid during the day. Use distilled water to dilute juices from fresh fruits and vegetables to prevent the digestive process from being overloaded. Either of the drinks below may be used as a fasting drink. If fresh fruits and vegetables are not available, use frozen and/or canned.

BASIC VEGETABLE
BROTH FASTING DRINK

Chop or grate the following vegetables into 1½ quarts of boiling water:

2 large red potatoes (skins included)
3 stalks celery
3 medium beets
4 carrots
Any of the following vegetables: cabbage,
    turnips, onions, turnip or beet tops.
Season with your favorite herbs. Cover and simmer 45 minutes. When slightly cool, mix in a
blender and drink warm.

"BASIC GREEN DRINK" IN A FRUIT BASE

To fresh or unsweetened pineapple juice in a
blender, add any of the following:

    celery
    radish tops
    comfrey
    burdock
    parsley
    chard
    plantain
    dandelion
    sprouts
    marshmallow
    carrot tops
    wheatgrass
    raspberry leaves

BREAKING A FAST

An important aspect of fasting is the breaking of
it. Much trauma and reversal can be eliminated
by gradually returning to solid foods over a period of three to four days. Always eat lightly and
chew foods and liquids well. Chewing stimulates the production of saliva and mixes it with
the food or liquid.

FAST BREAKING MENU

1st day: 1 fruit for breakfast
          Vegetable salad for lunch
2nd day: Add vegetable soup for dinner
          Add 1 more fruit during the day
3rd day: Add larger portions of fruit and salad
          Nuts and soured milk products
          Baked potato or squash soup
4th day: Start back on mild food

Macrobiotics

George Ohsawa coined the term macrobiotics in
California in the 1920s. Today, there are two
main schools of macrobiotics—Michio and Ave-
line Kushi in Boston and Herman and Cornellia
Aihara in Northern California. The macrobiotic
program is more than just a diet, it involves a
whole lifestyle.

The underlying principle of the macrobiotic
diet is called "the order of the universe," and relates to the way in which food can affect our mind
and body. There must be a balance between yin,
which represents expansiveness, and yang, which
represents contractiveness. Any food can be yin
or yang, depending on its properties compared to
other foods. External conditions, such as season,
and a food's size and age, also determine whether
a substance is yin or yang. By eating the proper
food, people can achieve an internal balance between yin and yang.

The macrobiotic diet stresses eating foods
grown in the same conditions as those in which
one lives, and eating as much native food as possible. For example, people who live in the northern United States and Canada should not eat
oranges, and bananas are not recommended for
anyone in Canada or the U.S. Eating non-native
foods may cause imbalances in the body, resulting in colds or flu.

The macrobiotic diet consists of 50% to 60%
whole grains, 20% to 30% locally grown vegetables, 5% to 10% beans and sea vegetables, 5% to
10% soups, and 5% condiments and other foods.
The macrobiotic diet is made of whole foods that
are cooked to preserve nutrients. Highly processed foods, sugar, commercial salt, dairy products, red meat, and poultry are avoided in the
macrobiotic diet. The macrobiotic diet is balanced and contains more vitamins, minerals,
amino acids, and essential fatty acids than the
standard American diet. On the macrobiotic diet,
the body does not have to work at balancing or
buffering foods and can spend this energy healing.

Dr. Sherry Rogers, of Syracuse, New York, has found that many people with severe chemical toxicity have healed and detoxified on a macrobiotic diet. They were able to correct vitamin and mineral deficiencies on the macrobiotic diet and gradually become more chemically tolerant. The seaweeds contain many minerals that help the body rid itself of toxic metals, such as lead and mercury. A macrobiotic diet promotes slow and gentle healing: it may take a year or more for people on a macrobiotic diet to heal totally.

On a macrobiotic diet you will have periodic discharges of old diseased cells and tissue, chemicals, drugs, and mucus that have accumulated in your body and are being eliminated.

Macrobiotic diets must be tailored precisely to each person. If you are considering starting a macrobiotic diet, you should see a macrobiotic counselor. There are also many helpful books on the macrobiotic way to prepare and cook the foods.

The macrobiotic program also includes massage, body scrubs with a hot ginger-soaked towel, deep breathing exercises with yoga and meditation, and exercise. Walking outside in bare feet, wearing cotton clothing, thinking calming thoughts, and doing meridian stretches are other parts of the program.

Nutritional Therapy

Detoxification of xenobiotics requires large amounts of energy. This energy comes from the food we eat. When we lack dietary protein, the body breaks down vital tissue protein to produce the energy it needs. This in turn decreases the concentration of Phase I and Phase II enzymes, amino acids, and peptides. With lowered enzyme concentrations, the metabolism of xenobiotics decreases.

Diets high in fat have been linked with cancer of the breast, colon, and prostate. Diets low in fat can protect the body. Many chemical building blocks of foods inhibit carcinogenesis. In studies done with mice, cruciferous vegetables (brussels sprouts, cabbage, cauliflower, and broccoli) have inhibited the induction of cancer by benzo[a]pyrene.

Vitamins and minerals, either from the diet or in nutritional supplements, are required in the chemical reactions of the detoxification process.

ANTIOXIDANTS

Antioxidants protect the body against free radicals that can damage tissues. There are two classes of antioxidants. The first consists of essential nutrients obtained from the diet and supplementation:

- Vitamin C
- Vitamin A
- Beta-carotene
- Vitamin E
- Coenzyme Q_{10}
- Cysteine/N-acetyl cysteine
- Glutathione
- Methionine

The second class is enzymes normally found in the body:

- Superoxide dismutase
- Catalase
- Glutathione peroxidase
- Glutathione S-transferase

Vitamin C Vitamin C is a carbohydrate related to glucose, the type of sugar found in the bloodstream. Humans cannot manufacture vitamin C and must obtain it from external sources. Vitamin C is essential to numerous biochemical reactions. The largest concentration of vitamin C in the body is in the adrenal glands. Lesser amounts occur in the eyes, white blood cells, pituitary gland, brain, pancreas, liver, cardiac muscle, and plasma. Vitamin C is water-soluble, so it is not stored in the body. It must be replenished frequently through diet or supplementation. Excess vitamin C is excreted within two to three hours after ingestion.

Vitamin C is contained in citrus fruits, spinach, collards, beet and turnip greens, broccoli, tomatoes, kale, potatoes, sprouts, and rose hips. However, it is difficult to obtain enough from the diet. Cooking and oxygen destroy at least half of the vitamin C in foods.

AID TO DETOXIFICATION   A deficiency in vitamin C decreases the metabolism of xenobiotics by lowering the level of cytochrome P-450. Studies have shown that vitamin C defends against reactive oxygen free radicals and lipid peroxidation.

Vitamin C is necessary for the production of the adrenal hormone, which protects the body against stress. Stress can include exposure to xenobiotics as well as other types of toxins. Vitamin C increases the therapeutic effect of different drugs, including antibiotics, so that lower doses can be taken, giving the body less to detoxify.

The diuretic effect of large doses of vitamin C stimulates urine excretion and decreases the amount of fluid in the tissues. This has a cleansing effect on the body. Chemically sensitive people lose more vitamin C from the kidneys than people who have no chemical sensitivities.

Vitamin C:

- detoxifies carbon monoxide; useful in treatment for carbon monoxide poisoning
- decreases the amount of carcinogenic nitroso compounds found in the stools of smokers
- protects against mercury toxicity
- has a detoxifying action on lead and mercury in the body
- protects against benzene exposure
- reduces the toxicity of digitalis, sulfa drugs, and aspirin
- detoxifies sulfur dioxide and carcinogens

- detoxifies bacterial toxins and poisons, such as the botulinum and diphtheria toxins

Vitamin C helps prevent and treat cancer. It is essential to the body's manufacture of interferon, decreases the spread of cancer cells, and helps control cell division. Drs. Ewan Cameron and Linus Pauling used vitamin C in terminal cancer patients and successfully lengthened their life span. Fifty terminal cancer patients, expected to die within 90 days, were given 10 grams of sodium ascorbate daily. Twenty survived for an average of 261 days. All patients showed general clinical improvement.

DOSE   A reasonable starting dose of vitamin C is 1 gram (1000 milligrams) three times daily. Add 1 gram of vitamin C daily, spreading out the doses during the day, until you get diarrhea. Then back up 1 gram; this is your bowel tolerance, and should be your daily dose. When you are under stress, are ill, or are having allergic reactions, your bowel tolerance will be higher.

Take the ascorbic acid form of vitamin C with meals and buffered vitamin C between meals. Buffered vitamin C is particularly effective for clearing allergic reactions.

During allergic reactions, 1 gram of vitamin C can be taken every 15 minutes. People with allergies and/or chemical sensitivities often tolerate large amounts, of 20 to 30 or more grams a day. If ascorbic acid powder or chewable vitamin C are taken, rinse your mouth afterward to avoid tooth enamel erosion.

Vitamin A   We can obtain vitamin A from eggs, milk fat, fish liver oils, and organ meats, especially liver. Excess vitamin A is stored in the liver and also concentrates in the eyes. Gastrointestinal disease, liver disease, or infections limit the body's ability to use vitamin A. A reduction of vitamin A levels is detrimental to the epithelial cells of the skin, glands, and mucous membranes, the lining of hollow organs, and the lining of the respiratory, alimentary tract, and genitourinary tract. Vitamin A deficiency, often accompanied by protein deficiency, causes night blindness, and itching and burning eyes. Children with vitamin A deficiency are prone to colds and respiratory symptoms, and to diseases such as measles.

Vitamin A deficiency is hard to diagnose, even from blood levels. Malabsorption, parasites, liver diseases, infectious diseases, prolonged fever, and renal disease all predispose people to vitamin A deficiency. About 40% of people in the United States are vitamin A deficient. In Canada, an autopsy of 100 subjects showed that more than 10% had no stores of vitamin A in their livers.

On the other hand, excess intake of vitamin A can cause symptoms. Bone or joint pain, fatigue, insomnia, hair loss, dryness and fissuring of the lips, poor appetite, weight loss, and enlarged liver can be caused by an excess of vitamin A.

AID TO DETOXIFICATION   Vitamin A:

- strengthens the cell wall in mucous membranes, the first site of penetration by antigens, viruses, bacteria, fungi, and chemicals and air pollutants
- is an antioxidant that protects the lipid part of the cell membrane; damage to the cell membrane may harm receptor sites for hormones and neurotransmitters

DOSE   Vitamin A can be taken in doses of 5000 to 25,000 International Units (IU) a day. Do not take large doses of vitamin A (more than 50,000 IU a day) for longer than two months. High intake of vitamin A should be closely monitored.

CAUTION: Because vitamin A and its derivatives (such as accutane) can cause fetal deformities, pregnant women should take no more than 8000 IU of vitamin A per day.

Beta-Carotene   Beta-carotene prevents damage to DNA and cell membranes. It is converted by the liver and intestines into vitamin A. People with hypothyroidism, diabetes, and people with liver disorders cannot readily transform beta-carotene into vitamin A. Nitrites from commercial fertilizers also interfere with the conversion. Beta-carotene has antioxidant properties that vitamin A does not have.

AID TO DETOXIFICATION   Beta-carotene:

- protects against singlet oxygen species (free radicals)
- is a powerful antioxidant
- protects against LDL oxidation
- protects against heart disease and cancer
- prevents damage to cellular components, especially DNA and cell membranes

DOSE   Beta-carotene can be taken in doses of 25,000 IU from one to three times a day. If the dose is excessive, the skin will become yellow, indicating that the dose should be decreased. This condition is known as carotenemia and is not dangerous.

Vitamin E   Vitamin E is found in green leafy vegetables, whole grains, milk fat, butter, margarine, vegetable oils, egg yolks, liver, and nuts. When foods are processed, cooked, or stored for long periods of time, significant amounts of vitamin E are lost.

Vitamin E is a fat-soluble vitamin. It has a great affinity for cell membranes, which contain large amounts of unsaturated fatty acids and other fats. Vitamin E prevents fats from reacting with oxygen. It is found in large amounts in the brain, pituitary gland, and adrenal glands.

AID TO DETOXIFICATION   Vitamin E:

- is the most important antioxidant found in the body
- enhances xenobiotic detoxification
- prevents oxidation of ingested fats, lipids in cell membranes, and other cell structures
- joins with lipid molecules to prevent the oxidation of vitamins A and K, and fat-soluble hormones
- helps increase oxygenation
- restores normal capillary permeability
- decreases damage to chromosomes and DNA by carcinogens and radiation
- is needed when you are exposed to smog, smoking, sun, or X-rays, which lead to cellular deterioration
- acts as an antioxidant by joining with oil-based chemicals, ozone, and nitrous oxide

Do not use polyunsaturated oils, such as margarine, because they generate more peroxides. Oils produced by high heat, chemicals, and bleaching are prone to peroxidation. The more polyunsaturated fats you consume, the more vitamin E you should take.

Vitamin E deficiency increases susceptibility to lung damage caused by ozone. Ozone is a powerful oxidant; vitamin E is a powerful antioxidant.

DOSE   Recommended doses of vitamin E are 400 to 800 IU daily, but up to 1200 IU can be taken. Always begin vitamin E supplements in small amounts.

Coenzyme Q_{10}   Coenzyme Q_{10} (CoQ_{10}) plays a critical role in energy production for the body. It is an electron carrier in the respiratory chain, which is a biochemical reaction in the body that produces molecular oxygen. Molecular oxygen is needed for the body to synthesize phosphates, such as adenosine triphosphate (ATP), which is the source of energy for all cell functions. Electrons from carbohydrates, fats, and proteins are all processed through CoQ_{10}. The body can produce CoQ_{10}, but it takes high energy to do so. It can be depleted much faster than the body can resynthesize it.

Diabetics, people with high blood pressure, people with peridontal disease, and people with heart disease have a deficiency of CoQ_{10}, and improve with oral supplementation. It is a useful treatment for congestive heart failure, angina, and cardiomyopathy, a degenerative disease of the heart muscles. Studies have shown objective improvement in heart function, decreased incidence of anginal episodes, and decreased mortality rate with CoQ_{10} supplementation.

AID TO DETOXIFICATION   Coenzyme Q_{10}:

- has antioxidant activity
- is a free radical scavenger
- seems to lower cholesterol and decrease resistance in the blood vessels
- protects normal tissue against damage caused by chemotherapy agents

DOSE   Recommended doses range from 10 milligrams (mg) once daily to 30 mg three times daily.

Cysteine   Cysteine is a water-soluble amino acid. Like all amino acids, cysteine has an amino (NH_3) group and carboxyl group (COOH), but it also has a thiol group, which is sulfur bound to hydrogen, and the most important part of the cysteine molecule.

AID TO DETOXIFICATION   Cysteine:

- acts as a reducing agent, donating hydrogen atoms to free radicals and other compounds
- prevents the oxidation of sensitive tissues that leads to aging and cancer

- helps protect against the effects of alcohol consumption
- protects (along with vitamin C) the lung cells against formaldehyde, acrolein, and acetaldehyde from tobacco smoke
- is used, along with methionine, in cases of copper poisoning
- protects (along with vitamin C) cell membranes against lipid peroxidation
- is the most potent antioxidant in the body
- detoxifies (along with vitamin C) pesticides, plastics, hydrocarbons, and other chemicals

DOSE   The recommended dietary allowance of cysteine is 25 mg per pound in adults and 55 mg per pound in children. Dr. Eric Braverman, a noted amino acid researcher from Princeton, New Jersey, recommends starting with 500 mg of cysteine daily, then building up to 3 to 4 grams daily to treat toxic exposures. People with multiple chemical sensitivities would benefit from cysteine supplementation; however, many of them do not tolerate sulfur-containing amino acids. A molybdenum supplement may increase their tolerance.

CAUTION: D-cysteine and D-cystine are toxic in humans and should not be used.

N-Acetyl Cysteine

N-acetyl cysteine (NAC), a derivative of cysteine, is thought to be an intermediate compound in cysteine metabolism, which is converted back into cysteine in the body. NAC has been studied more extensively than cysteine to determine its usefulness in cancer because, unlike cysteine, NAC is patentable.

AID TO DETOXIFICATION   N-acetyl cysteine:

- decreases the effects of a toxin produced in the intestine by *Clostridium difficile,* a bacteria related to the overuse of antibiotics
- has helped to prevent liver and heart toxicity from chemotherapy
- prevents side effects from radiation treatment, such as hair loss, skin burns, eye problems
- is used to prevent liver injury in patients who have overdosed on acetaminophen, phenacetin, and aspirin

DOSE   N-acetyl cysteine can be taken in doses of 500 mg once or twice daily but is used in much larger doses, up to 10 grams, for acute poisoning. NAC smells and tastes like rotten eggs. It is nauseating and irritating, causing some people to vomit. Cysteine does not have this smell and is better tolerated.

Glutathione

All organisms on earth contain glutathione (GSH). In humans, the liver, spleen, kidneys, and pancreas have the largest concentration of glutathione. The lens and cornea of the eye also contain a large amount. The amount of GSH in the body decreases as people age. Glutathione protects the stomach lining against hydrochloric acid.

AID TO DETOXIFICATION   Cysteine is one of three amino acids found in GSH. The others are glutamic acid and glycine. Glutathione is one of the molecules used in Phase II of detoxification. The detoxification properties of GSH come from the thiol group of cysteine. The amount of cysteine in the body determines how much GSH is produced.

Glutathione helps protect cells against the toxic effects of oxygen and its waste products. Oxidizing chemicals (often free radicals) destroy the fats in cell membranes. This is known as lipid peroxidation. Carbon tetrachloride, benzenes, plastics, dyes, and pesticides often form peroxides after Phase I metabolism. These peroxides are then reduced in Phase II metabolism by glutathione peroxidase. Selenium, magnesium, and zinc supplementation are needed for GSH synthesis and metabolism.

Glutathione has been shown to detoxify fungicides, herbicides, carbamate and organophosphate pesticides, nitrates, nitrosoamines, flavorings, plastics such as vinyl chloride, arene oxides, steroids, phenolic compounds, auto exhaust, and cigarettes. It will also detoxify epoxides produced by Phase I metabolism, toxins from *Clostridium difficile*, and many over-the-counter drugs.

Glutathione is helpful in heavy-metal poisoning. It chelates lead and cadmium from the bloodstream, and it protects against mercury toxicity.

Glutathione:

- protects the liver from developing cirrhosis from alcohol
- protects the liver and lungs from the effects of automobile exhaust
- helps protect against radiation
- prevents ulcers in people taking aspirin and other nonsteroidal drugs
- protects the integrity of red blood cells
- protects the lungs against the effects of cigarette smoke

DOSE Dr. Jeffrey Bland of HealthComm in Washington State recommends 10 to 90 mg of glutathione a day, given in three divided doses.

Methionine Methionine is an essential sulfur amino acid that must be supplied in the diet. Methionine is found in sunflower seeds, egg yolk, wheat germ, milk products, avocados, turkey, pork, beef, fish, and other meats.

L-methionine is needed for the synthesis and transport of lipids. When people are deficient in methionine, triglycerides build up in the liver and the metabolism of xenobiotics decreases. Dr. Braverman uses methionine for patients with depression, high copper levels, high cholesterol, chronic pain, allergies, and asthma.

AID TO DETOXIFICATION Methionine:

- aids in detoxifying xenobiotics
- helps remove heavy metals from the body.
- protects against the toxic effects of radiation

DOSE The recommended dietary allowance of methionine is 25 mg per pound in adults and 55 mg per pound in children. Methionine can be taken in doses of 500 mg once or twice a day.

B VITAMINS

Thiamine (Vitamin B_1) Cereal grains are good sources of thiamine, but only in the germ and outer coatings. When cereals are refined, the thiamine is lost. Enriched white flour contains 20% less thiamine than whole wheat flour. Thiamine is also found in yeast, liver, pork, fresh green vegetables, potatoes, and beans. Thiamine is destroyed by high temperatures and by soda used in foods. It is water-soluble, so it can be easily lost when the cooking water for grains and vegetables is discarded.

Thiamine is a cofactor in the oxidation process that occurs constantly in each body cell. Nerve tissue is very dependent upon carbohydrate oxidation to function properly, so nerve tissue often demonstrates the effects of thiamine deficiency first. Thiamine is needed for hydrochloric acid production in the stomach. It improves the function of the GI tract and is needed for growth.

AID TO DETOXIFICATION Thiamine:

- acts with vitamin C, antioxidants, and cysteine to counteract the effects of acetaldehyde and free radicals
- aids in the absorption and utilization of magnesium

DOSE Thiamine can be taken in doses of 25 to 50 mg daily. If it is taken for a specific deficiency, doses of 100 to 200 mg are common. Always take thiamine with B-complex, because all the B vitamins work together.

Riboflavin (Vitamin B₂)   Riboflavin is found in whole grains, yeast, liver, eggs, cheese, green leafy vegetables, peas, lima beans, and organ and muscle meats. Fruits contain very little riboflavin. As protein intake increases, the body requires more riboflavin. Riboflavin is sensitive to light and easily destroyed by cooking, antibiotics, alcohol, and oral contraceptives.

Riboflavin is needed for the metabolism of lipids, such as fatty acids. It is needed for protein synthesis and it also helps break down proteins, carbohydrates, and some fats. Riboflavin aids in growth and reproduction, and contributes to healthy nails, hair, and skin.

AID TO DETOXIFICATION   Riboflavin is converted to two coenzymes which are very active in the liver. They are necessary for the formation of oxidizing enzymes that control bodily processes. A riboflavin derivative is linked to cytochrome P-450 as a necessary component. Some tissues need riboflavin to utilize oxygen.

DOSE   Riboflavin can be taken in doses of 25 to 50 mg daily. If larger doses are taken, of 100 to 200 mg, also take a B-complex with approximately 50 mg of each B vitamin to balance all the B vitamins.

Niacin/Niacinamide (Vitamin B₃)   Niacin is found in liver, heart, kidney, beef, rabbit, turkey, chicken, ham, tuna, sunflower seeds, whole wheat, peas, peanuts, and brewer's yeast.

A B₃ deficiency causes pellagra with symptoms including diarrhea, dermatitis, and dementia. In 1915, more than 10,000 people in the U.S. died of pellagra. After ruling out microorganisms as the cause, scientists discovered that pellagra is not an infectious disease but a deficiency disease correctible through diet.

Niacin:

- helps stabilize glucose levels
- is needed for enzyme functions in the nervous system
- is necessary to epithelial cells
- is necessary to fat metabolism
- is necessary for the formation of sex hormones

AID TO DETOXIFICATION   Niacin:

- is used for electron transfer
- operates in coenzyme forms to carry hydrogen ions in all cells
- acts as a coenzyme in the energy cycle of the cell
- causes vasodilatation (opening up) of capillaries in the skin and can cause histamine release (this causes the well-known niacin flush)
- is used for detoxification regimens (see chapter 2)
- helps control cholesterol levels and is often the first medication recommended for elevated cholesterol levels

Niacin decreases fatty acid production. Three to six hours after ingestion there is a rebound, and the levels of fatty acids rise in the blood. This will mobilize toxins from the fat and allow them to be excreted.

Niacinamide, another form of niacin, plays no role in detoxification.

DOSE   Niacin can be started at a dose of 100 mg daily. It can be increased by 100 mg as tolerated, up to 2000 to 3000 mg daily. On Hubbard's program, some people are able to take 5000 mg a day. For detoxification, use short-acting niacin.

CAUTION: Liver damage can result with the long-acting form. With long term use have regular liver enzyme function tests done.

Pantothenic Acid (*Vitamin B$_5$*) Pantothenic acid is a B-complex vitamin found in organ meats—heart, liver, kidney, and brain. It is also in soy flour, sunflower seeds, buckwheat, sesame seeds, peas, peanuts, eggs, and brewer's yeast. Vegetables and fruits contain very little pantothenic acid. Breast milk is rich in pantothenic acid. Bacteria synthesize pantothenic acid in the intestines.

Pantothenic acid stimulates the production of adrenal hormones. It is essential for adrenal support and prevention of adrenal exhaustion during any type of stress. It also helps the stomach produce hydrochloric acid and aids in the synthesis of cholesterol and fatty acids. Pantothenic acid is an essential element of coenzyme A, which is needed in the utilization of nutrients and production of energy.

AID TO DETOXIFICATION Pantothenic Acid:

- helps protect against radiation injury
- counteracts the side effects and toxicity of antibiotics
- helps the intestine regain motility after intestinal operations

DOSE Pantothenic acid can be taken in doses of 25 to 100 mg daily to start, and can be increased to 1000 to 1500 mg. With larger doses, also take a balanced B-complex vitamin.

Pyridoxine (*Vitamin B$_6$*) Pyridoxine is found in brewer's yeast, sunflower seeds, whole grains, legumes, liver, lean muscle meats, fish, bananas, and nuts. Processing and cooking destroys the pyridoxine in food.

A high-protein diet, as well as cortisone and estrogen supplementation, increase the need for vitamin B$_6$. Women need extra pyridoxine while on oral contraceptives, while pregnant, and in the last two weeks of their menstrual cycle. Vitamin B$_6$ has been used to treat acne and a skin disease known as psoriasis. It is also used to treat carpal tunnel syndrome. A deficiency of B$_6$ can cause tremors, irritability, insomnia, nervousness, inability to concentrate, and a skin rash. Vitamin B$_6$ is involved in more bodily processes than any other single nutrient. When it enters the body, it is converted with the aid of B$_2$ into the coenzyme pyridoxal phosphate.

Vitamin B$_6$ is needed for the proper metabolism and use of protein, fats, carbohydrates, and hormones, such as adrenalin and insulin. It is needed for nervous system function, regulates sodium and potassium balance, and is necessary for DNA and RNA synthesis.

AID TO DETOXIFICATION Vitamin B$_6$:

- is needed for the metabolism of methionine, a sulfur-containing amino acid
- helps the transport of amino acids across cell membranes
- helps the absorption of magnesium and B$_{12}$

DOSE Vitamin B$_6$ can be taken in doses of 25 to 50 mg daily. If higher doses are taken, of 100 to 250 mg daily, also take a balanced B-complex with approximately 50 mg of each B vitamin.

CAUTION: People have developed a peripheral neuropathy from taking large doses of pyridoxine, 1200 to 2000 mg daily.

Cobalamin (*Vitamin B$_{12}$*) Vitamin B$_{12}$ is found in liver, kidney, beef, clams, oysters, sardines, crab, fish, eggs, and cheeses. Strict vegetarians and alcoholics are susceptible to a B$_{12}$ deficiency. People with B$_{12}$ deficiency may show mental apathy, memory loss, paranoia, or even psychosis before anemia develops. Studies have shown that levels of methylmalonic acid and homocysteine may be better indications of B$_{12}$ adequacy in the body than blood B$_{12}$ levels.

Vitamin B$_{12}$ deficiency causes abnormalities in the blood-forming process and nervous system. The red and white blood cell count is decreased and blood cells are enlarged and destroyed rapidly. Nervous system changes include weakness of the arms and legs, decreased sensation, problems with walking and talking (stammering), and jerking of the arms and legs. It can take five years for B_{12} deficiency symptoms to appear.

The stomach secretes a substance known as "intrinsic factor" that binds vitamin B_{12} so that it can be absorbed through the intestinal wall. About 90% of patients with pernicious anemia have antibodies against the stomach cells that produce the intrinsic factor.

Although vitamin B_{12} is a water-soluble vitamin, it can be stored by the body. Pregnancy and birth control pills can deplete vitamin B_{12}. People deficient in vitamin B_{12} and without the intrinsic factor will not be able to absorb oral vitamin B_{12}. For this reason, B_{12} is usually given as an injection. However, a recent study showed that sublingual doses of B_{12} can also be well absorbed.

Vitamin B_{12} is necessary for the maintenance of the myelin sheath (fatty covering of the nerve fibers). It plays a role in the formation of DNA and RNA in cells. Vitamin B_{12} contains cobalt and is the only vitamin that contains a mineral. It can increase energy; relieve irritability; and improve memory, concentration, and balance.

AID TO DETOXIFICATION Vitamin B_{12}:

- aids in detoxification of xenobiotics
- is active in the synthesis of the amino acid methionine

DOSE Vitamin B_{12} has been used therapeutically in doses of 30 micrograms (mcg) to 5000 mcg three times a week to once a month. Two injectable forms are available, cyanocobalamin and hydroxycobalamin. Toxicity, even of large doses, has not been noted. Nonetheless, especially with the higher doses, a balanced B-complex with 50 mg of each B vitamin is also recommended.

Folic Acid Folic acid is a member of the B-complex vitamins. It is also known as folacin and folate. It was first found in green leafy vegetables and was named after foliage. Spinach, liver, kidney, wheat bran, kale, beet greens, turnips, potatoes, broccoli, carrots, cantaloupe, Swiss chard, black-eyed peas, and lima beans are all rich in folic acid.

Folic acid can be easily depleted by stress, severe injuries, and surgery. It is needed for red blood cell formation. If folic acid is deficient, in addition to anemia, the red blood cells have a shortened life span and are shaped abnormally. People deficient in folate become weak, are fatigued, develop irritability, and may have memory problems. They may develop a sore tongue, mouth sores, poor wound healing, mental disease, inflammation of the GI tract, and decreased ability to fight infection.

Birth control pills cause folic acid deficiency. Folic acid deficiency has also been related to developmental delay, decreased resistance to infection in the child after birth, and neural tube defects, which affect the formation of the lower end of the spinal cord. The FDA has finally recognized the folic acid and neural tube defect link and allows the fortification of prenatal vitamins with more folic acid (800 mcg), though it still limits the amount of folic acid available in supplements to 400 mcg.

AID TO DETOXIFICATION Folic acid:

- is needed for the utilization of amino acids
- plays a role in methylation in Phase II detoxification

DOSE Folic acid can be taken in doses of 1 to 5 mg for specific diseases. A prescription is necessary for the larger doses. Folic acid given when B_{12} is deficient can cause neurological damage.

BIOFLAVONOIDS (VITAMIN P)

Bioflavonoids are the brightly pigmented substances found in fruit. Flavonoids are found with vitamin C in foods including citrus fruit skin and pulp, apricots, cherries, grapes, green peppers, tomatoes, papaya, and broccoli. Citrus bioflavonoids, such as tangeretin, nobiletin, and sinensetin have the greatest biological activity. Other bioflavonoids include quercetin, hesperidin, and rutin.

Bioflavonoids increase capillary wall resistance, improve varicose veins and hemorrhoids, and help prevent blood clots. Bioflavonoids have been used with vitamin C for bleeding after delivery, bleeding gums, heavy periods, hemorrhoids, nosebleeds, and skin diseases. Unfortunately, in the late 1960s, the U.S. Food and Drug Administration declared that bioflavonoids were not a vitamin and had no nutritional value.

AID TO DETOXIFICATION   Bioflavonoids:

- are antioxidants
- can chelate metals
- protect vitamin C
- decrease capillary fragility; cells depend on capillaries to bring nutrients and carry away waste material and toxins

DOSE   Although there is no standard recommended dose, most nutritionists suggest taking 100 mg of bioflavonoids for every 500 mg of vitamin C, as they work synergistically.

ORGANIC GERMANIUM

Germanium (GeOxy 132) is an organically bound trace mineral. Germanium appears to be a metal, but does not have metallic properties. Inorganic germanium is considered a metalloid and is used as a semiconductor.

AID TO DETOXIFICATION   Germanium:

- acts as a free-radical scavenger

- aids in toxic metal detoxification
- raises the level of glutathione, which is involved in Phase II detoxification
- has been used to treat mercury poisoning
- has been used to prevent radiation sickness in people who receive radiation therapy
- stimulates energy production
- increases oxygen utilization at the cell level

DOSE   Germanium can be taken in the 150 mg dose, from one to five capsules daily. A typical maintenance dose is two 150-mg capsules daily. Use only pure organic germanium. Inorganic germanium can cause renal toxicity.

L-CARNITINE

L-carnitine is an amino acid produced by the liver from the amino acids lysine and methionine. It helps convert fat into energy. If there is inadequate L-carnitine, fatty acids can build up within cells and in the blood. It reduces levels of triglyceride and cholesterol in the blood, prevents ketosis (an excess of breakdown products of fat), helps weight loss, and improves endurance. L-carnitine is found in organ meats and meats, but not in vegetables.

Genetic diseases with L-carnitine deficiencies were first discovered in 1972. Muscle diseases, including muscular dystrophy, have been helped with supplementation of L-carnitine. Dr. Ruth McGill of Texas has described an oxidative phosphorylation defect (a defect in the production of energy for the cell) in certain Gulf War veterans and in some patients with multiple chemical sensitivities who have muscular symptoms. This defect has responded to large doses of Coenzyme Q_{10} and L-carnitine.

AID TO DETOXIFICATION   L-carnitine:

- prevents buildup of plaque on artery walls
- helps metabolic liver disease

DOSE   L-carnitine can be given in divided doses of 1000 to 3000 mg a day. For genetic deficiencies, 4000 mg per day may be recommended.

ESSENTIAL FATTY ACIDS

Fatty acids are the building blocks of the fats in the human body and in plants. They are structural components of the cell membranes and of the membranes surrounding intracellular structures. Fatty acids also provide a major source of energy for the body.

There are two types of fatty acids. In saturated fatty acids, the molecules contain the maximum number of hydrogen atoms and are solid at room temperature. Saturated fats include butter and all other animal fats, coconut oil, and palm kernel oil. Unsaturated fatty acids are not fully paired with hydrogen; they are liquid at room temperature. Unsaturated fats include corn oil, soybean oil, peanut oil, cottonseed oil, linseed oil, fish oil, and marine plant oils.

Nutrients are considered essential when they have to be supplied to the body because the body cannot synthesize them. Three unsaturated fatty acids are essential: arachidonic, linolenic, and linoleic. At least a quarter of the total fats in the diet should be these essential fatty acids. Essential fatty acids take part in many biochemical reactions and biological functions.

Essential fatty acids control blood pressure and the formation of plaque in arteries. They stimulate the body's defense against cancer and infections. They enhance metabolism, bring oxygen to cells, decrease inflammation, and aid in healing. Premature aging, cardiovascular disease, obesity, and arthritis are associated with a deficiency of essential fatty acids.

Essential fatty acids are necessary for the formation of prostaglandins, hormone-like chemicals that regulate the activity of cells. They form from two types of unsaturated fats, omega-3 and omega-6. The various prostaglandins keep blood platelets from sticking together, reduce the possibility of blood clots, help remove fluid from the body, and open up blood vessels, improving circulation.

Healthy humans make sufficient prostaglandins from linolenic and linoleic acid. Should there be a block in this metabolism, evening primrose oil, which contains linoleic acid and gammalinolenic acid, and fish oils can bypass the block.

Fish oil is mainly an omega-3 fatty acid, which is more beneficial than vegetable omega-3 oils. Farm fish raised on soybean meal contain very little omega-3 oil.

Vegetable oils are excellent sources of essential fatty acids. The best sources of omega-3 fatty acids are flaxseed (linseed), rapeseed (canola), soybean, and hemp oils. Flaxseed oil is rich in linoleic acid (omega 6) and contains more linolenic acid (omega-3) than other vegetable oils. Vegetable oils must always be fresh, as rancid oils can break down to free radicals and carcinogens.

AID TO DETOXIFICATION   Fish oils:

- decrease cholesterol and triglycerides

Vegetable oils:

- speed up transit time of the stool, decreasing the buildup of toxins

Evening Primrose Oil:

- helps to relive premenstrual symptoms, improve eczema, and prevent arthritis
- helps prevent liver damage caused by alcoholism
- has been used in treatment of schizophrenia

DOSE   *Fish oil*: Take fish oil capsules with a meal, up to four to six a day. Because these omega-3 fatty acids decrease absorption of vitamin E, you should also take vitamin E supplements if you are taking fish oil capsules or eating large quantities of fish.

Vegetable oils: Take one to five tablespoons of vegetable oil per day. Borage oil, safflower oil, black currant oil, and flaxseed oil are the most helpful.

Evening Primrose Oil: One to two capsules of evening primrose oil three times a day are recommended.

MACRO AND TRACE MINERALS

Copper Copper is an essential element, but can be toxic in excess amounts. Copper is found in meats, seafood, nuts, mushrooms, chocolate, tea, dried yeast, soybeans, and some waters.

In the body, copper is found in the superoxide dismutase in the cytosol (inside the cell, but outside the nucleus), which protects against free radical damage to the mitochondria (the energy-producing portion of the cell). Copper is essential to the synthesis of thyroid-stimulating hormone produced by the pituitary gland.

In a study by Dr. Carl Pfeiffer at the Brain Bio Center in Princeton, New Jersey, only premature infants and people who were on intravenous nutrition were found to be copper deficient. Zinc deficiency accentuates copper excess, as zinc and copper are antagonistic. Zinc is lost in food processing and freezing. Copper excess is found in Wilson's disease and possibly related to post-partum psychosis, autism, heart attacks, and one type of schizophrenia.

AID TO DETOXIFICATION Copper:
- is necessary in small amounts to form hemoglobin
- activates the synthesis of several enzymes
- helps regulate essential fatty acid metabolism
- if deficient increases the toxicity of pesticides
- is a cofactor in cysteine-to-cystine production

Iron Iron is found in meats, dark green leafy vegetables, whole-grain cereals, liver and other organ meats, dried fruits, legumes, and molasses. Iron cookware is another source of iron. Women and adolescents require twice as much iron as men. Extra iron is recommended during pregnancy, for female athletes, babies up to one year old, and people who have lost a significant amount of blood through bleeding or auto-blood transfusions.

Iron combines with protein to make hemoglobin, which gives red blood cells their color and carries oxygen in the blood. Iron stores are recycled when the red blood cells are broken down.

The gene for hematochromatosis, a disease of iron overload, is quite common in the United States population. People with this disease have a mild anemia, headache, increasing fatigue, shortness of breath, dizziness, and weight loss. Iron is deposited in the tissue, including the liver, lungs, pancreas, and heart.

People who think they may be suffering from anemia should always be tested for iron deficiency or overload.

AID TO DETOXIFICATION Iron:
- decreases xenobiotic metabolism if deficient
- is in superoxide dismutase
- is found in cytochrome P-450

DOSE Iron is recommended in doses of 10 to 18 mg daily for menstruating women, and 10 mg for men. Iron-deficient patients can take 50 to 100 mg daily.

Magnesium Magnesium is found in nuts, whole grains, milk, green vegetables, and seafood. Wheat loses its magnesium in refining, and refined sugars and fats contain very little magnesium. U.S. government studies show that the average American diet supplies only 40% of the recommended daily amount of magnesium.

Dr. Mildred Seelig, a leading authority on magnesium, estimates that 80% of the population has a magnesium deficiency.

Magnesium facilitates the transport of nutrients across the cell membrane. It is needed for producing and transferring energy, contracting muscles, synthesizing protein, and exciting nerves. As a cofactor it helps enzymes catalyze many chemical reactions.

Magnesium deficiency depresses thyroid hormone levels and the microsomal lipid concentrations, which decreases xenobiotic metabolism. Magnesium is necessary for over 300 biochemical reactions in the body, so the symptoms of magnesium deficiency can vary widely. They include fatigue, depression, muscle spasms, and irritability. Muscle spasms play a role in migraine headaches, asthma, colitis, coronary artery disease, strokes, uterine hemorrhage, chronic back pain, and hypertension.

Magnesium is depleted by sweating, alcohol ingestion, fast foods, poor intestinal absorption, and diuretics. Its deficiency is rarely diagnosed. The most accurate test available today is the magnesium-loading test.

Magnesium has been used therapeutically for people with asthma, cardiac arrhythmias, and preeclampsia (a condition of pregnancy associated with high blood pressure, fluid retention, and hyperactive neurological reflexes).

AID TO DETOXIFICATION   Magnesium:

- is needed as a cofactor in ammonia detoxification
- is necessary for the synthesis of glutathione
- is a mineral activator necessary for many enzymes involved in detoxification
- is one of the most important minerals in xenobiotic detoxification

DOSE   Magnesium can be taken in a dose of 800 to 1200 mg daily. Some patients develop diarrhea with higher doses of magnesium. It is usually taken with calcium in a ratio of two calcium to one magnesium. However, if needed, magnesium can be taken in a one-to-one ratio with calcium.

Manganese   Manganese is an essential trace mineral. It is found in nuts, seeds, dried legumes, spinach, whole-grain cereals, liver, kidney, and muscle meats. Manganese is necessary for bone growth, reproduction, lipid metabolism, and the moderation of nervous irritability. It is needed for the synthesis and breakdown of protein and nucleic acids found in DNA. It is also used by the pancreas to produce insulin.

AID TO DETOXIFICATION   Manganese:

- is required in the synthesis of glutathione
- helps in the production of superoxide dismutase
- works in conjunction with molybdenum

DOSE   Manganese can be taken at a dose of 5 to 20 mg a day.

Molybdenum   Molybdenum is an essential trace mineral found in organic meats, eggs, whole grains, wheat germ, sunflower seeds, buckwheat, leafy vegetables, soybeans, lima beans, and lentils. In areas where molybdenum is low in the soil, high rates of cancer occur.

AID TO DETOXIFICATION   Molybdenum:

- helps in the synthesis and use of sulfur amino acids
- is a component of enzymes that detoxify sulfites, aldehydes, and aldehyde oxidase
- is necessary for the cells to utilize vitamin C

DOSE   No RDA has been established for molybdenum. Fifty to 500 mcg daily have been used. It is usually found in multimineral preparations and not as a separate nutrient. Some nutritionists recommend 150–500 mcg per day.

Selenium Selenium is one of the most poisonous elements known, but it is an essential trace mineral for animals and humans. Selenium is found in brewer's yeast, garlic, liver, and eggs. When foods are processed, they lose selenium.

Selenium can be toxic to humans in large doses. Too much selenium causes loss of hair, nails, and teeth; skin rashes; fatigue; and paralysis.

Men seem to have a higher need for selenium than women. Breast milk contains six times as much selenium as cow's milk and twice as much vitamin E. Cancer rates are lower where the selenium content of the soil is high. Cystic fibrosis and hypertension are more common where the selenium content of the soil is low.

AID TO DETOXIFICATION   Selenium:

- is found in glutathione peroxidase, which is necessary for the recycling of glutathione
- acts as an antioxidant, protects cell membranes, and prevents the breakdown of DNA
- enhances the function of vitamin C
- protects against the toxic effects of organic mercury
- is needed for the production of Coenzyme Q$_{10}$
- neutralizes the effects of cadmium

DOSE   The dose of selenium can be 50 to 200 mcg daily, in divided doses. Up to 400 mcg daily can be taken, but should be monitored closely. Do not take more than 400 mcg daily.

Zinc Zinc is found in meat, fish, oysters, seeds, wheat germ, onions, maple syrup, mushrooms, brewer's yeast, milk, whole grains, nuts, carrots, vegetables, herring, and liver. Vitamin A is necessary for the utilization of zinc.

Zinc is necessary for gene repair and the growth and development of reproductive organs. It can be depleted during chronic infections and inflammatory diseases. It is needed for the proper function of B vitamins and is essential to the synthesis of protein.

AID TO DETOXIFICATION   Zinc:

- is in alcohol dehydrogenase (Phase I enzyme that detoxifies aldehydes)
- is found in 90 essential enzymes
- reduces lipid peroxidation
- is a component of superoxide dismutase

DOSE   Zinc can be taken in a dose of 15 to 50 mg daily. Large doses (150 mg) suppress the immune system. Doses larger than 50 mg daily depress copper levels.

ALOE VERA

Aloe vera has been used for hundreds of years to soothe and heal cuts and burns. This succulent plant has two juices, the yellow sap in the cells beneath the thick green rind, and the gel fillet, which is the water-storage organ. The gel fillet has anti-inflammatory actions, lowers cholesterol and triglycerides, and protects the intestinal tract against ulcers. In commercial aloe vera, the fillet has been processed to contain the least possible amount of aloin from the yellow sap. Aloin is an effective, but potent laxative.

Aloe vera has been used successfully to treat allergies, anaphylaxis, chronic fatigue syndrome, colds, colic, fungal infections, genital herpes, gum infections, shingles, parasites, sprains, staph infections, stings, vaginitis, viral infections, yeast infections, stasis ulcers, warts, and frostbite.

AID TO DETOXIFICATION
- aloe vera dilates blood vessels, which increases the blood supply and thus the oxygen, and helps with detoxification

- mucopolysaccharides from the aloe vera plant form a lining through the colon to prevent toxins from reentering the body; they help in the absorption of water, electrolytes, and nutrients in the gastrointestinal tract
- acemannan (the active ingredient in the gel fillet) injects itself into the cell membrane, increasing permeability. Toxins can leave the cell more easily and nutrients can move into the cell
- aloe vera contains proteolytic enzymes, which can break down and digest dead cells, helping to cleanse the body

DOSE   Aloe vera can be taken orally in a dose of two to four tablespoons of the gel daily.

ENZYMES

Enzymes are catalysts, chemicals that accelerate reactions in the body that would otherwise be too slow. Coenzymes are proteins, contain amino acids, and have many and varied functions. They help every body reaction from nerve impulses to the regulation of hormones. Enzymes enable our bodies to renew old cells, metabolize nutrients into building blocks and energy, and remove waste products and toxins. Enzymes are essential to the function of vitamins and minerals.

Metabolic Enzymes   The most common enzymes found in the body are the metabolic enzymes. About 5000 metabolic enzymes run the body chemistry. One type of metabolic enzyme, antioxidant enzymes, converts free radicals (reactive oxygen species) into water and oxygen. This helps to detoxify the body.

Another type of metabolic enzyme is food enzymes, found only in raw foods: protease, amylase, lipase, and cellulase. They differ from the pancreatic digestive enzymes the body produces: food enzymes work in the stomach, and pancreatic enzymes work in the small intestine.

Proteases digest protein and other organisms, such as the protein coating on certain viruses, toxic debris from dead bacteria, and inflammatory chemicals produced at injury sites. Protease improves protein digestion and helps acidify the blood.

Amylase digests carbohydrates and white blood cells, such as those in pus. An abscess is a cavity filled with pus. The white cells may have killed all the bacteria, but the abscess will not resolve unless drained. Amylase can digest and pus and resolve the abscess. It can also digest viruses, including herpes, and control lymphatic swelling. Amylase and lipase can heal hives, contact dermatitis, and psoriasis. They decrease the effects of bee stings and insect bites, and help the lungs clear hardened mucus accumulations. Amylase also helps control asthma.

Lipase digests fat in food and helps to control fat metabolism. Lipase also digests the fat that surrounds viruses and it can kill some of them. Cellulase digests fiber and is not produced in the human body.

Enzyme Supplements   Enzyme deficiencies are common today. Our foods contain few if any enzymes because of cooking, processing, pasteurization, or microwaving. Heating and refining deactivate and destroy enzymes. Each enzyme requires a certain pH to function, and many diets are too acid for enzymes requiring an alkaline environment. Environmental toxins and pollutants affect our detoxification and immune systems, which require enzymes to function.

Enzyme supplementation is frequently necessary for our bodies to function optimally. Diets containing raw fruits and vegetables are also helpful. Several excellent enzyme supplements are available.

DOSE   Recommended dosages vary from brand to brand, depending on their formulation. Following is a general guide.

- as a dietary supplement, take one to two capsules or tablets with meals three times a day
- as an anti-inflammatory, take four to six capsules or tablets between meals (two hours after a meal or one hour before) three times a day. Your dosage will have to be adjusted according to symptom relief

BENEFICIAL BACTERIA

Keeping a balance between beneficial and harmful bacteria in the intestines is important to prevent harmful bacteria from taking over. Improper diet, antibiotics, other medications, alcohol, and tobacco reduce beneficial bacteria. Beneficial bacteria produce antibiotics and enhance the body's production of antibodies.

Pathological intestinal bacteria can produce toxins, which can cause hypersensitivity to the bacteria and may initiate autoimmune disease. Bacteria and tissues in the body can share antigens (substances that induce an immune reaction). A common example is the antigen shared by heart tissue and the streptococcal bacteria.

The GI tract contains a mixture of bacteria, fungi, protozoa, food particles, digestive enzymes, acids, bile, and mucins. Some pathogens of the GI tract are opportunistic organisms. If there is a minor decrease in host resistance, these pathogens colonize the GI tract and resist recolonization by the native microbes.

A change in intestinal flora can be long-lasting. People treated with antibiotics often have permanent changes in their intestinal flora. Stress also affects intestinal flora. A person who develops pathogenic bacteria flora in the intestines is under constant stress. Adrenal stress hormones decrease hydrochloric acid production in the stomach and reduce mucin production in the intestines.

Abnormal balance of bacteria in the intestines is known as dysbiosis. Dysbiosis causes impaired immune defense; intestinal wall trauma from the production of endotoxins; and production of acetic acids and hydrogen and methane gases. With intestinal wall trauma, increased intestinal permeability allows large molecules to cross the intestinal barrier and cause antibody formation. This is known as "leaky gut."

A leaky gut places an increased burden on the liver because of toxins coming in from the intestines. This increases the number of free radicals generated from the detoxification system and can lead to autoimmune diseases or inflammation of the muscles and joints.

Treat nutritional deficiencies and remove intestinal toxins as a useful first-line treatment against disease and for detoxifying the body.

Acidophilus *Lactobacilli* are one of the five major groups of intestinal bacteria. Lactobacillus refers to bacteria that produce lactic acid. *Lactobacillus acidophilus* or, as it is commonly called, acidophilus, and other organisms play an important role in the ecology of the intestines.

Lactobacillus produces at least one natural antibiotic, called acidophilin, which helps it fight off harmful bacteria. *Lactobacilli* are effective against 25 different harmful bacteria, including *Salmonella*, *Staphylococcus*, and *Streptococcus*.

Harmful bacteria in the intestine can produce a coated tongue and bad breath. They can also produce gas or bloating in the intestines. Diarrhea is often caused by an overgrowth of harmful bacteria, and acidophilus can counteract this. Acidophilus has been used to soothe sore throats and reduce cold sores. Acidophilus also produces B vitamins, which help fight stress and metabolize food.

Lactobacillus has been used for chronic illnesses in humans and animals. To be successful, a large number of *Lactobacilli* must be used and a fermentable carbohydrate source should be available for the *Lactobacilli* in the intestinal tract.

DOSE   One half teaspoon of acidophilus powder three times a day is recommended (a teaspoon equals 10 to 40 billion organisms, depending on the brand used). Capsules are also available.

Bifidobacteria   *Bifidobacteria* make up about 25% of the beneficial intestinal bacteria. *Bifidobacteria*, along with *Lactobacillus* species and *Streptococcus faecium,* produce vitamins, enzymes, and antimicrobial substances. The increased growth of *Bifidobacteria* lowers intestinal pH, lowers blood pressure, and lowers blood levels of cholesterol and triglycerides. In one study, the number of *Bifidobacteria* increased by ten times in a 14-day period when fructo-oligo-saccharide supplements were given. *Lactobacillus* growth also increased, although not as much. *Bifidobacteria* may act to detoxify carcinogens in the intestines.

Fructo-oligo-saccharides (FOS) are composed of three nondigestible carbohydrates. They occur naturally in onions, garlic, wheat, barley, and Jerusalem artichokes, but can be synthesized by reaction of sucrose with fungal enzymes. The FOS are a white powder that is approximately half as sweet as sucrose (table sugar). They are not digested by carbohydrate enzymes, but pass intact to the colon. They are used as a growth nutrient by the beneficial bacteria in the intestine, especially the Bifidobacteria. Fructo-oligo-saccharides are not used by *Salmonella, Escherichia coli*, or *Clostridium perfringens*, and are too large for candida and other yeasts to use. They may cause *klebsiella* to proliferate.

Fructo-oligo-saccharides decrease intestinal permeability and have been useful in treating musculoskeletal diseases. Because of the decreased intestinal permeability and balance of the microflora, FOS lower the toxic burden on the liver.

DOSE   Supplements of *Bifidobacteria* are available in combination with *Lactobacillus acidophilus* and fructo-oligo-saccharides (FOS).

Supplements of FOS alone or in combination with *Bifidobacteria* are taken in doses of ½ to 1 level teaspoon two to three times a day.

Taking Nutritional Supplements

All vitamins, minerals, and amino acids work together. Take a balance of all the nutrients if you are going to take supplements. It is not generally advisable to take large doses of just one nutrient. As Dr. Bland says, "Nutrients work in a symphony." Take a good-quality multivitamin and supplement extra single vitamins and minerals when needed.

Take vitamins in a form easily assimilated by the body. If a vitamin or mineral capsule/tablet passes unchanged in the stool, it was not available to the body. Vitamins that are chelated to amino acids are easily used by the body. Citrates, orotates, aspartates, picolinates, lactates, and gluconates are easily absorbed by the body.

The physical form of the vitamin is also important:

- *Powders*: More rapidly absorbed and usually contain no binders or fillers; taste may be unpleasant; can be encapsulated at home.
- *Liquids*: Absorbed well and helpful for people who have difficulty with or cannot swallow tablets or capsules; often contain sugars, flavorings, and colorings.
- *Chewables*: Helpful for children but contain sugars, flavorings, and colorings.
- *Time-release capsules or tablets*: Portions of the vitamin content are released over a period of time; many people have insufficient stomach acid to dissolve the coating to release the vitamin.

- *Tablets*: Have a longer shelf life but always contain fillers and a binder to hold the tablet together; not absorbed as well as the other forms.
- *Capsules*: Easier to swallow and absorb than tablets; contain fewer fillers and binders, but the capsule portion is usually a beef or pork exposure; some vegetable capsules are now available.

Take "clean" vitamins. Avoid brands that do not state that their product is free of common allergens, such as wheat, milk, corn, soy, egg, sugar, and yeast. Because vitamins are taken daily, they provide a constant daily exposure to these common allergens if they are present in the vitamin tablet or capsule. Avoid products that use aspartame (marketed as NutraSweet and Equal) as the sweetener.

Sensitive people may have to avoid vitamins containing herbs. Herbs are excellent for individual who tolerate them, however.

15

Allergy Extracts, Herbs, and Chelation

Allergy Extracts

Allergy extracts consist of dilutions of small amounts of antigen that are used for immunotherapy and for cleansing. They may be given either by injection or sublingually (under the tongue).

Allergy extracts are used to control allergic symptoms to the substance contained in the extract. Symptom control is desirable for the comfort of the allergic person as well as for the protection of the immune system. If the immune system is constantly stressed by adverse reactions to foods, chemicals, inhalants, or organisms, its efficiency suffers. Over a period of time, the immune system can become weak and damaged, and target organ damage can occur. If the immune cascade continues, tissue damage follows. The use of extracts protects the immune system and allows it to repair and heal. The more dilute extracts are homeopathic in nature and allow the body to release debris and toxins.

FOOD EXTRACTS

Foods to which a person is allergic can be avoided. However, some people are sensitive to many foods and their nutrition would suffer if they avoided all of them. Food extracts allow individuals to eat problem foods without symptoms and without damage to their immune systems or bodies. Food extracts can also be used to stop acute allergic reactions to foods. If there are food residues in the body, either whole food or phenolic food compounds (a naturally occurring chemical compound in foods that frequently causes allergies), the food extracts cause them to release.

CHEMICAL EXTRACTS

Exposures to chemicals are very difficult for the chemically sensitive person to avoid. We can control chemical exposures in our homes. However, when we leave our safe homes, we can be exposed to many chemicals under the control of others, such as perfume, fabric softener, hair spray, car and diesel exhaust, or pesticides.

Chemical extracts prevent and relieve reactions to chemicals. Many chemicals are fat-soluble and are stored in our bodies' fat cells. The use of dilute chemical extracts aids in the release of these chemicals.

INHALANT EXTRACTS

Inhalant extracts include extracts for pollens, molds, dust/dust mites, animal danders, feathers, and some fibers. We cannot avoid exposure to these inhalants; they are everywhere in our environment. We can choose not to have pets in order to avoid animal danders and feathers. However, we can be exposed to them on the clothes or in the homes of other people.

Inhalant extracts give relief from the allergic symptoms caused by these substances. They also stop acute allergic reactions to the inhalants.

ORGANISM EXTRACTS

The effects of an infection do not stop when the acute symptoms clear. Debris from the infectious organism remains in our cells. This debris, which may be fragments of the organism or remaining toxins produced by the organism, continues to cause allergic symptoms as long as it is in the body.

Extracts for these organisms relieve the allergic symptoms caused by these organisms and their metabolic products. The extracts also cause the debris left from the organisms to release from the cells.

Herbs

The word herb has many definitions. Some consider it a nonwoody plant that dies after it flowers. However, this definition is narrow because the bark, leaves, and berries of some trees have herbal uses. In this book, we consider an herb as any plant part that has medicinal, nutritional, or cleansing value.

The action of herbs as medicine is subtle. It is not always possible to separate the herb into specific, isolated component parts because the herb functions as a whole rather than a single active ingredient. The actual qualities possessed by herbs dictate the treatment methods. For example, a pungent, stimulating herb is used to promote warmth and to clear cold.

ACTIONS OF HERBS

The following are a few of the detoxification actions of herbs:

- *Adaptogen*: Improve body's adaptability; help the body to deal with stress; support adrenal gland and possibly the pituitary gland function; increase the resistance of glands to damage.
- *Alterative* (*depurative*) "blood cleansers": Restore proper function; are usually indicated in chronic inflammation or degeneration (skin, arthritic, autoimmune).
- *Anticatarrhal*: Remove catarrah (excess mucus) by reducing the secretion or making the secretion more fluid to flush out the infecting organism.
- *Antihelmintic*: Destroy and/or expel worms from the digestive system.
- *Antipyretic*: Prevent or reduce fevers.
- *Antiseptic*: Destroy pathogenic bacteria.
- *Aperient*: Mild laxative, promotes natural bowel movements and functions.
- *Blood purifier*: Cleanse the blood.
- *Carminative*: Expel gas from the intestine.
- *Cholagogue*: Stimulate the flow of liver bile, helping fat digestion; a natural laxative that facilitates cleansing.
- *Choleretic*: Stimulates production of bile by the liver.
- *Diaphoretic*: Promote sweating and help the skin eliminate wastes; some diuretic effects.
- *Diuretic*: Increase blood flow through the kidney and reduce water reabsorption in the kidney nephrons; some have cardioactive properties also. People with high blood pressure should not use cardioactive herbs.
- *Expectorant*: Stimulating; chemically irritate the lining of the bronchioles.
- *Hepatonic*: Tonifying action on the liver.
- *Parasiticide*: Rid the body of parasites.
- *Purgative*: Empties bowels.
- *Respiratory relaxing*: Soothe bronchial spasms and loosen mucus.
- *Rubefacient*: Cause vasodilation and a gentle increase in surface blood flow.
- *Vermifuge*: Expel intestinal worms.
- *Vulnerary*: Healing application for wounds.

ADMINISTRATION OF HERBS

Different parts of the plant are used for properties that occur at different times of the plant cycle. The carrier used for administration will partially depend on the solubility of the herb or its parts in water, alcohol, or fat (oil). Use fresh, good quality herbs, and cold pressed oils. Use glass or lead-free ceramic utensils when preparing herbs.

A few of the common carriers by which herbs may be administered are:

- *Capsule*: May be filled with herbs. The gelatin may be either of plant or animal origin.
- *Compress*: To prepare a compress, bring 1 or 2 heaping tablespoons of herbs to a boil in 1 cup of water. Dip a cotton pad or gauze into the strained liquid. Apply to body and cover if needed. Change when cool.
- *Decoction*: Prepared by soaking the herb, then boiling it in water for 5 to 20 minutes. Strain and drink the liquid hot or cold.
- *Extract*: Prepared by soaking the herbs in vinegar, alcohol, or oil for 4 to 15 days. Shake twice daily; vitamin E can be added as a preservative.
- *Infusion*: Pour 2 cups of hot liquid over ½ to 1 ounce of powdered herbs. Steep 10 to 20 minutes before drinking. Cover to prevent evaporation.
- *Ointment*: Holds herbal ingredients in a Vaseline or nonpetroleum jelly on an area for an extended time. To prepare an herbal ointment, use Vaseline or nonpetroleum jelly or oil as a base. Bring to a boil 1 or 2 heaping tablespoons of herbs in the base. Stir and strain. Allow to cool to a safe skin temperature before using.
- *Poultice*: Applies warm mashed, ground, or powdered herbs directly to the skin to draw out toxins or embedded objects from the skin, or to relieve pain and muscle spasms (see chapter 17 for specific poultices). It has to be replaced frequently to preserve the warmth. To use a poultice, clean the skin surface with an antiseptic, then oil the skin, before applying the poultice. Moisten the herbs with water, apple cider vinegar, herbal tea, liniment, or tincture. Spread to ¼- to ½-inch thick, and apply to the skin directly, or between a layer of gauze.
- *Tincture*: Used topically or in liniments, a tincture is prepared by making a solution of the herb in alcohol. (Vinegar can be used, but this makes a solution rather than a tincture.) To prepare a tincture, use 4 ounces of powdered or cut herbs. Combine with 2 cups alcohol (vodka, brandy, gin, rum, bourbon, Everclear). Shake daily, and steep for two to four weeks. Let herbs settle completely, then pour off the tincture, straining out the herbs through cheesecloth or coffee filter.

CLEANSING WITH HERBS

Herbs are primary medication for over 4 billion people—two-thirds of the world's population. While most of these people are in third-world countries, herbs are used in North America. Many lay herbalists as well as innovative physicians and health care professionals have added herbs to their therapeutic armamentarium. They are a very effective treatment for many conditions. However, some people sensitize to them very quickly, particularly people with chemical and food sensitivities. The high terpene content of herbs is partially responsible for this, and mold in improperly dried herbs also plays a role. Herbs imported from other countries are usually sprayed upon arrival, thus contaminating them with pesticides.

The focus of cleansing with herbs is to promote healing by eliminating toxins from the organs and systems of the body. This purification process begins by using aromatic and bitter herbs that initiate the purgings of the body systems. Herbalists then revitalize the systems with toning, soothing, and strengthening herbs.

Thousands of herbs have medicinal properties. However, most herbalists regularly use fewer than 25 herbs and rely on 10 to 12. The following herbs with cleansing and detoxifying properties are some of the favorites of contemporary medical herbalists:

- *Burdock root*: Increases circulation to the skin, which helps detoxify skin tissues and improves nutrition to skin cells; is a blood and liver cleanser and assists in removal of toxins through the kidneys.
- *Calendula*: Has an antibiotic effect and will cleanse the body of microorganisms.
- *Chamomile*: Used to treat headache, colds, or flu; helps to cleanse the body by improving digestion.
- *Dandelion root*: Stimulates the elimination of toxins from every cell in the body; stimulates liver secretions, breaks up stagnancy, and improves overall function; also stimulates digestion, thus improving nutrition.
- *Echinacea*: Helps prevent viral infections and will help recuperation from most illnesses; is considered a blood and lymphatic cleanser and immune system stimulant.
- *Lemon balm*: Helps reduce circulation and nervous tension; is a lymphatic cleanser
- *Licorice root*: Has antiviral and antibacterial properties and is anti-inflammatory; known as a detoxifier, especially for spleen, kidney, and liver cleansing and healing; stimulates production of interferon.

- *Siberian ginseng*: Useful for debility, exhaustion, stress, and depression; detoxifies and protects the liver from the effects of drugs.
- *Stinging nettles*: Help with arthritis, allergies and food sensitivities, gout, eczema and skin complaints, and general poor health.

Other cleansing herbs include:

- *Buckthorn, Senna, Cascara sagrada*: Increase mucus secretion and peristalsis, removing waste and killing some bacteria and parasites.
- *Garlic*: Has broad-spectrum action against bacteria, parasites, viruses, yeast, and fungus; helps to remove lead and heavy metals from tissues.
- *Goldenseal*: General cleansing; also cleans lymphatic system because of immune stimulating and antibacterial properties; stimulates bile secretion and lowers cholesterol level.
- *Cayenne*: General cleansing; particularly affects liver and blood vessels by decreasing cholesterol and increasing blood flow; also stimulates peristalsis.
- *Milk thistle*: Protects the liver against the toxic effects of pollutants, chemicals, radiation, and alcohol; is an antioxidant, stimulates the growth of new cells, assists in liver drainage.
- *Yellow dock*: Blood, lymphatic, and liver cleanser; helps kidney function, assisting in removal of toxins in the urine.
- *Ginseng*: Protects the liver from the effects of drugs and chemicals, lowers cholesterol, improves liver function, increases ability of intestines to absorb nutrients.
- *Sarsaparilla*: Binds endotoxins released by intestinal bacteria; cleans colon, liver, and blood.

- *Ginger*: Decreases cholesterol, thus cleansing blood vessels; cleansing action through bowels, kidneys, and skin.
- *Red clover*: Blood purifier.
- *Bayberry, Lobelia, Oatstraw, and Wild cherry bark*: Lymphatic cleansers.
- *Sage*: Lymphatic and blood cleanser.
- *Uva ursi*: Lymphatic and spleen cleanser, diuretic and kidney antiseptic.
- *Thyme*: Lymphatic cleanser, removes mucus from head and respiratory tract.
- *Chlorophyll*: Cleanses and mineralizes blood; cleanses colon wall by removing old waste.

As with all things in life, good quality, moderation, and balance are of prime importance. Herbs are indeed powerful medicine and should have our respect. It is our responsibility to seek information and qualified assistance before acting. Time and small doses will support our bodies to heal themselves.

Chelation

Chelation therapy is a treatment that restores blood flow in a person suffering from atherosclerosis. Commonly known as hardening of the arteries, atherosclerosis is a disease of the arterial walls that affects the whole body, slowly deteriorating the entire arterial system. Often, it is not obvious that damage has been done until a person has a stroke or heart attack or becomes senile.

Atherosclerosis is caused by several factors. Plaque, which is composed of fibrous tissue, cholesterol, and calcium, forms on the interior arterial walls. The passage becomes so narrow that the blood flow is eventually blocked. According to some sources, the most important cause of atherosclerosis is abnormal accumulations of metals. Cigarette smoking, diets high in saturated fats, high plasma cholesterol, diabetes, hypertension, and other factors are also associated with an increased incidence of this disease.

When the blood flow is reduced, vital organs become starved for oxygen and other nutrients. Cell walls lose their integrity and allow excessive calcium, sodium, and other metals to enter. When calcium accumulates in the plaque, it forms hard deposits that can be seen on X-ray. Some physicians believe that problems with calcium metabolism can also cause arterial spasms that further reduce blood flow to vital organs.

Chelation therapy is a cleansing method that removes metallic irritants and allows leaky and damaged cell walls to heal. It involves the intravenous use of a medication called ethylenediaminetetraacetic acid (EDTA). EDTA is a proteinlike molecule that binds to metal ions, making them soluble in blood. This action allows the kidneys to excrete such metals as cadmium, calcium, copper, mercury, and lead.

By removing the metallic elements, EDTA improves calcium and cholesterol metabolism, and normalizes most metallic elements in the body. This helps to prevent the formation of free radicals that most scientists now believe to be a contributing cause of atherosclerosis and other diseases. Reducing free radical proliferation allows the natural antioxidant defenses of the body to regain control.

Other conditions in which blood-flow impairment plays a role are diabetes, emphysema, macular degeneration, varicose veins, gallstones, cataracts, osteoporosis, hypertension, cancer, arthritis, Parkinson's disease, psoriasis, muscular dystrophy, and kidney diseases. All these conditions are helped with a course of chelation therapy.

While surgery is the usual treatment recommended for atherosclerosis, it offers only mechanical repair of a localized area of the arterial tree. Chelation therapy improves the flow of blood throughout the entire vascular system. Chelation can be used instead of bypass surgery or when bypass surgery has failed to give relief.

According to the American College for Advancement in Medicine (ACAM), more than 400,000 people have received over 4 million chelation treatments in the last 30 years. It is one of the safest medical procedures, yet remains a controversial treatment. This is puzzling because there has never been a death caused from chelation therapy when administered by a trained physician. Also, chelation has always been the approved treatment for lead poisoning.

As with any therapy, side effects are possible. Vein irritation, mild pain, headache, fatigue, and occasionally fever may occur. These effects tend to disappear with continued treatment. Most patients experience minimal or no side effects.

Persons receiving chelation therapy report:

- improvement in appearance, behavior, and performance
- better skin color
- more rapid wound healing
- improved memory
- increased energy
- increased capacity to exercise
- improved kidney function
- disappearance of angina pain
- amelioration of cardiac symptoms
- improved vision
- disappearance of senility
- disappearance of leg cramps
- healing of gangrenous limbs
- normalization of blood pressure
- disappearance of impotence
- increased blood flow that warms a previously cold limb

Objective evidence of effectiveness can be provided by comparison of pre- and post-therapy diagnostic tests.

When intravenous chelation is used, benefits occur rapidly. Oral chelating agents are available and do help, but more slowly. Dr. Richard Passwater of Maryland first began using the term oral chelation to refer to nutritional supplements and specific foods that help cleanse blood vessels and improve blood flow. Vitamin E, vitamin C, B-complex vitamins, and bioflavonoids all have chelating properties. Aspartic acid, L-aspartate, orotic acid, and orotate salts of calcium, magnesium, and zinc are all excellent oral chelating agents. The trace minerals selenium, manganese, zinc, vanadium, chromium, potassium, and silicon have chelating effects. Chelating amino acids are glutathione, cysteine, glutamic acid, and glycine.

Other food supplements that function as oral chelating agents are lactic acid, acetic acid, citric acid, lecithin, B-15, and germanium. Fiber, garlic, the enzymes bromelain and papain, bee pollen, thymus and adrenal glandular supplements are also helpful.

Formulations are available that contain balanced amounts of the oral chelating agents. These formulations may be used as supplementation to intravenous chelation therapy or alone.

Crataegus oxyacantha berries (English hawthorn), as an herbal tincture, is a very effective oral chelating agent in helping heart problems. *Crataegus* acts on the heart muscle as well as on plaque in the arteries. It lowers and regulates pulse, strengthens a thready pulse, and reduces chest pain. When combined with cayenne, the mixture slowly reduces cholesterol deposits and provides relief from high blood pressure.

16

Exercise and Bodywork

Exercise

Exercise? But I can't because:
    I'm too tired!
    My back/head/feet hurt!
    I'm too old to start!
    I look bad!
    I don't have time!
    It won't help!
    I don't feel like it!
    I get enough exercise at work!
    It's too hot/cold!

Do any of these excuses sound familiar? We have all used one or more of them to avoid exercise. Some of us may have used all of them!

EFFECTS OF EXERCISE

Exercise plays an important role in cleansing our bodies. However, exercise should not be used just when there is a problem, but should be a lifelong habit and an activity that you enjoy. Lack of exercise allows toxins to build up in our bodies, destroying the balance. Calcium leaches from the bones and is excreted in the urine, further contributing to the imbalance.

Physical activity stimulates the development and maintenance of bone tissue, muscle mass, strength, and endurance. It helps to excrete toxins and restore balance in many body systems. Exercise is a powerful tool that can be used to detoxify the body and to improve and maintain good health.

Studies show that exercise:

- speeds up removal of toxins and waste materials from the cells
- increases blood flow that carries nutrients and oxygen to every cell
- increases lymph circulation
- can shorten the duration of an allergic inflammatory cascade
- increases levels of high-density lipoprotein (HDL) cholesterol
- helps lower blood pressure
- helps prevent heart attacks
- helps maintain appropriate blood-sugar levels
- increases body temperature
- prevents formations of gallstones by increasing the solubility of cholesterol in bile
- restores lung power, endurance, and strength
- increases muscle flexibility and strength
- improves bone structure and support for the body
- can reverse adult-onset diabetes
- aids in weight reduction programs

It has also been demonstrated that exercise can improve mental health. Exercise:

- decreases anger/hostility, fatigue/inertia, and tenseness/anxiety
- reduces the perception of stress
- elevates mood with release of endorphins
- improves mental abilities, learning potential, memory, and cognitive skills with increased oxygen levels
- improves self-image and self-confidence

TYPES OF EXERCISE

For any type of exercise:

- Wear clothes and shoes that fit and support your body.
- Use equipment that fits your body.
- Shower immediately after any type of exercise and wash your clothes to remove the toxins in your sweat so you do not reabsorb them.

Aerobic Exercise Aerobic exercise is the best type of exercise and should be done at least three times a week. To be aerobic, the exercise must raise your heartbeat to the proper range. However, you should always be able to carry on a conversation while you exercise. If you cannot, you are exercising too hard. Monitor your heart rate to be certain that you achieve your proper heartbeat range determined by the pulse.

The general formula for determining your proper pulse rate is:

- Ideal Exercise Heartbeat Rate Per Minute = 220 minus your age. This figure multiplied by 0.6 gives the low number for your pulse range. Multiply by 0.85 to get the high number for your pulse range.

Any pulse between those two numbers is within your target heart rate zone. Moderate aerobic exercise for a longer period of time is more effective than strenuous exercise in short bursts.

Aerobic exercise will:

- rapidly cleanse chemical toxins from the blood
- increase oxygen utilization and the function of oxygen-dependent metabolic pathways
- allow your heart and blood vessels to function more efficiently
- enhance endocrine function
- stimulate the production of endorphins, which help to mask pain and bring about a feeling of euphoria
- cause a lower resting pulse rate
- increase your endurance

WALKING Brisk walking is the very best exercise. The heart works at a safe "exercising" rate and promotes cardiovascular fitness. A regular walking program will promote cleansing by:

- increasing oxygen uptake
- improving circulation and muscle tone
- improving resting and active pulses
- promoting weight loss
- building endurance
- releasing toxins in the sweat and breath

In addition to the physical benefits, walking also helps emotional cleansing. It can reduce anxiety and tension, and even alleviate depression.

If you choose walking for exercise, find a safe place to walk. Pollen-sensitive patients may have difficulty walking in heavily vegetated areas during pollen season. Chemically sensitive patients should find an area away from traffic. If you walk after dark, walk in a well-lighted area, both for protection and so you can see obstacles in your path. Wear reflective tape on your shoes and shirt or jacket to make you more visible to motorists.

RUNNING Running is a popular method of exercise in North America. Estimates place the numbers of joggers at just over 33 million. Running:

- increases elimination of toxins
- increases oxygenation to cells
- improves blood transport
- improves lung capacity
- reduces body fat
- increases muscle
- strengthens legs, muscles, and bones

If you follow a sensible program, running can be good for you. Even though it is a high-impact exercise, if done properly it can entail very little risk. You should warm up before you run to prevent strains and sprains. Warming up causes muscles and tendons to become more flexible and to elongate to accommodate the longer range of motion required for running.

Watch for warning signs of injury. Pain in the knee, hip, and ankle are indicators that serious injuries are possible unless care is taken. Burning pain in muscles while exercising and extended cramping after exercising are also indications that the exercise is too strenuous. Take additional nutritional supplements, wait a few days, then run more slowly. Pain that persists for more than 48 hours should be checked by a physician.

SWIMMING Regular long-distance swimming produces the same benefits as running, cycling, or cross-country skiing. It causes you to become fit very rapidly. You can get into good shape by swimming twice a week for 15 minutes.

The water makes exercise easier, especially for those who are overweight. If you stand in water up to your neck, you become 90% lighter. The water pressure improves your circulation by 25%, and painful joints move more easily in water.

Exercise in the pool may be in the form of swimming laps, running, walking, jumping, or using a kickboard. The water acts as a giant cushion for these activities. It absorbs the shock from jumping and provides low-impact exercise. Because water has more resistance than air, walking or running in water makes your leg muscles, heart, and lungs work hard even though your speed for these activities will be slower. Water exercise sessions are available at some public pools. When you use the pool for exercise, there are a few precautions to consider. Either begin your activities slowly in the water, or do warm-up activities before you get in the water. If the pool water is chlorinated, wear padded goggles to help protect your eyes. Some swimmers are more comfortable using a nose clip to prevent water from entering the nose. If you are allergic to chlorine, take a chlorine extract before and after swimming, and shower immediately after the swimming session.

CYCLING Bicycle riding is an aerobic exercise and has the added benefit of also being useful for transportation. It is not a weight-bearing activity and therefore is less stressful to your joints. Bicycling provides as much benefit as jogging. It will increase your circulation, improve blood transport, increase oxygenation to cells, and increase elimination of toxins.

Stationary bicycles offer more environmental control than outdoor bicycles. You can ride and breathe the air in your safe home. The best stationary bicycles have fan blades in the wheel and handlebars that move. The fan circulates the air, and the handlebars exercise your upper body. This type of bicycle offers you the options of exercising various areas of your body separately. There are not pauses in pedaling as there are when you ride on the street. If you exercise at the proper level, sweating will help your body excrete toxins.

CROSS-COUNTRY SKIING Cross-country skiing is considered to be one of the best, if not the best, form of exercise. Unlike downhill skiing, anyone can cross-country ski, as the techniques are simple. You use both your arms and legs and get twice the workout you would walking or running at the same speed. It is good for the heart and lungs, and there is not the shock and stress to the feet and ankles that there is in running. Cross-country skiing also burns calories, up to 1000 calories an hour for a good skier.

There are exercise machines that allow the same movements as cross-country skiing. These machines can be used indoors all year long.

Exercise for the Environmentally Ill For those who are acutely ill with environmental illness, a limited amount of gentle to moderate exercise will help to alleviate the inflammatory processes of reactions. A limit is necessary to prevent placing an added burden on the adrenal glands that are already stressed from the allergic state. A five-minute brisk walk or a few minutes on an exercise bicycle is enough to clear an individual from an allergic reaction and provide some cleansing. If you are home-bound, you can walk briskly about a safe room, flail your arms vigorously, do bicycle exercises, or yoga.

The advantage of exercise for the sensitive patient are:

- increased oxygen uptake and utilization
- increased blood transport to carry nutrients and oxygen to the cells and waste products and toxins away from the cells
- Increased stimulation of endorphins

Martial Arts Martial arts are traditional disciplines of Far Eastern countries, such as Japan, China, and Korea. They are also a form of exercise, and they emphasize balance, agility, and coordination. While there are several forms of martial arts, the two that are helpful for body balancing and health are Chi Kung and Tai Chi.

CHI KUNG (QIGONG) Chi Kung (pronounced Cheekung) is a Chinese term applied to the many different forms of exercise that work with the chi (breath). Chi, in addition to an association with respiration, facilitates adaptation to our environment, supplies energy for our ongoing regeneration, and provides resistance to disease.

Kung means discipline, one who spends time practicing. Chi Kung can be interpreted to mean to practice breathing in order to increase chi pressure. With practice, this internal power can be felt flowing through and out of the body. The discipline required to build this internal power also favorably affects the mental abilities of all styles of Chi Kung practitioners.

With any form of Chi Kung, one is able to increase the flow of hormones produced by the endocrine glands. This builds up the immune system and increases available vital force. The organ exercises cause a flushing of the toxins, waste materials, and sediment from the organs. They convert the fat stored in the layers or sheaths of connective tissue (fascia) into chi energy. This energy is then stored within the fascia and is available to protect the soft organs and support them in their healthy functioning. Both Heller bodywork and Rolfing massage techniques (see Bodywork, below) work with the fascia from the outside in. Chi Kung works with this same fascia from the inside out, to allow for free-flowing energy in the body.

It is believed that fascia, the most pervasive tissue within the body, is the means by which the chi is distributed along acupuncture routes. Research has demonstrated that the flow of bioelectric energy in the body encounters the least resistance between the fascial sheaths. These routes have also been found to correspond to the well-documented classical acupuncture meridians. These meridians often run parallel with the cardiovascular system.

Two-thirds of the blood supply for the liver, kidneys, stomach, and spleen passes through the abdominal area. When chi is stored and subsequently released on command, the abdomen acts like a very efficient heart, thus saving the heart muscle.

The body needs active motion. Chi Kung-type exercises provide active motion to enhance and strengthen the body as a whole rather than stressing a congested, weakened out-of-balance body. The meditative aspects of Chi Kung can increase circulation and the production of lymphocytes without affecting blood pressure the way running and aerobic exercises do. The Chinese use Chi Kung for treating chronic diseases. Three basic therapeutic principles support the effectiveness of Chi Kung.

- Restoring vitality: The depleted energy reserves of the body are replenished through rest and recuperation of the physical systems. Internal control quiets overexcited and fatigued parts of the brain. The environment within the central nervous system is then conducive to restoring vitality.
- Storing physical energy: Deep relaxation or sleep reduces oxygen consumption by around 30% and decreases the metabolic rate by about 20%. Attaining and retaining this state during a waking period stops energy loss, facilitates energy storage, and assists in conditions of weakness or debilitation such as chronic fatigue syndrome.
- Massaging the organs in the abdominal cavity: The range of movement in the diaphragm is three to four times greater during abdominal breathing than it is during regular breathing. The abdominal organs are rhythmically massaged, thus stimulating the stomach and intestines, improving digestion and absorption, and reducing blood congestion in the lower abdomen. Improvement in these functions alleviates chronic constipation.

TAI CHI Tai Chi is part of Chinese medicine and philosophy that, in turn, is part of Taoism. Tai Chi is a series of continuous, slow, fluid, smooth and graceful movements. These move-ments are performed in a relaxed manner, but with knees slightly bent and a straight and upright posture. The Tai Chi exercise is a series of consecutive moves and has been described as "meditation in motion," because concentration is focused on the moves.

When correctly performed, Tai Chi exercises the cardiopulmonary system, stimulates blood circulation, relaxes the joints, and encourages mental relaxation. It involves much time to learn and as much dedication to perfect as a martial art. Most people view it as a mild exercise. Should you decide to try Tai Chi, you will be surprised by how easy it is to begin, as well as the resulting feeling of well-being.

In Tai Chi emphasis is on the movement and coordination of breath, the internal environment rather the external manifestation. A breath guides the physical form. Tai Chi uses the attention of the mind, combined with the feeling and the movement of the body. The muscles, tendons, and bones are brought into a different rhythm, providing a new vitality. This, in turn, feeds back information to the mind and feelings.

TREATMENT OF INJURIES FROM EXERCISE

Homeopathy offers healing and balancing remedies for injuries and other problems from exercising.

- *Arnica*: for trauma, sore bruised feeling, muscle fatigue
- *Bellas perenis*: for tennis elbow, sore muscles
- *Bryonia*: an important first-aid remedy, for injury or trauma worse with motion
- *Lacticum acidum*: for pain and/or exhaustion after exercise
- *Magnesia phosphorica*: for sore muscles after exercise
- *Rhus toxicodendron*: for pain better with movement, trauma to joints, back pain

- *Ruta grav*: for tennis elbow, frozen shoulder, trick knees, and overuse of joints
- *Strontium carbonium*: for bone pain and injury to the ankle

Two homeopathic ointments are helpful for exercise injuries:

- *Arnica gel*: for temporary relief of bruises; minor muscle and joint aches and pains; swelling from minor falls, blows, sprains, and strains; simple headache; sports injury; and overexercising.
- *Traumeel*: for minor sports injuries, sprains, bruises, and inflammation

Aloe vera decreases inflammation associated with athletic injuries, such as joint sprains, tendonitis, and blisters.

Bodywork

Bodywork can be seen as sensorimotor education, where the bodyworker is a facilitator. The body responds externally and internally to friction on the skin, pressure on deeper tissues, and sensory input around the joints. Bodywork can change habitual neuromuscular responses as well as guide in the creation of new and more appropriate responses. Parts of the body that have become desensitized can relearn how to provide the brain with the information necessary to the tissue's normal, healthy function.

Most physicians and practitioners agree that most of the body's processes rely on movement of fluids, and that bodywork is an effective means of promoting fluid circulation. To survive and function every cell must continuously receive nutrients, oxygen, hormones, antibodies, immune modulators, and water, while toxic wastes are taken away from the cell. This cycle of receiving and expelling involves movement.

Muscle activity is involved in all movement. Stimulation of the nerves activates muscles. The ease of the movement depends on the coordination and function of both the central and peripheral nervous systems at the time of stimulation. Movement, then, results from the unifying activity of the mind and the body.

Bodywork improves movement: lazy muscles are encouraged to work, and connective tissue is softened and stretched. It also increases circulation, which facilitates cleansing and the removal of waste material.

The cleansing action of bodywork:

- promotes elimination of toxic waste
- relieves congestion
- improves blood and lymph circulation
- increases the oxygen supply to cells
- increases the availability of nutrients to the cells, muscles, and bones
- acts as a mechanical cleanser, pushing out wastes
- improves liver function
- eliminates excess fluid in the tissues
- eliminates waste fluid from muscles
- balances the nervous system, which affects all body systems

Bodywork can heal and cleanse on all levels. Touching the body also touches the mind, the emotions, and the spirit.

All bodywork can help us to understand that our bodies are:

- living, growing systems that continually change
- functioning, interwoven, dynamic processes
- interacting with our environment, both physical and metaphysical

THE ROLE OF STRESS

Stress of all types also affects the body and its movements. The way we react to stress reflects the way we have learned to react to potential problems. Stress can help us identify our weak points and focus on strengthening them.

Three important factors help us cope with stress:

- accurate anticipation
- effective control
- positive feedback for coping responses

Bodywork helps us learn and develop appropriate responses in these areas. Comforting a child or an adult with soothing touch alleviates the shock and fear of trauma. The pathways carrying the sense of touch to the brain are thicker, faster, and more numerous than the pathways carrying pain. Distraction from the pain allows the body to receive relaxation (alpha) impulses. With less pain, the person is able to re-evaluate the stressful situation. When anxiety levels decrease, the response to pain changes. As relaxation continues, muscle contractions begin to release. Bodywork increases circulation and the resulting oxygenation aids in restoring comfort and mobility, initiating a positive internal feedback loop.

Bodywork gives physical, emotional, and mental benefits:

- Physical: strengthened immune system, improved muscle tone, reduced blood pressure, reduced physical stress, increased flexibility and movement, and increased relaxation
- Emotional: reduced emotional stress and anxiety, and improved self-image
- Mental: increased ability to concentrate, reduced mental stress, and enhanced stress management

TYPES OF BODYWORK

Any type of bodywork directly affects the nerves, organs, and circulation, and indirectly affects the body as a whole. All bodywork techniques have one thing in common: By contact with the skin they stimulate specific receptors, resulting in a specific reaction. The exact receptors that are stimulated and the resulting effect depends on the manner of skin contact.

Cautions   Some physical conditions preclude vigorous, stimulating, and/or deep bodywork. Before requesting bodywork, weigh any extreme condition or extraordinary circumstance. If you are under a physician's care, always request an evaluation before getting bodywork.

As a general rule, do not seek stimulating, vigorous, or deep bodywork if you:

- have a fever
- have an external injury to the skin
- have a concussion, sprain, or an incompletely knit broken bone
- are in poor health or extremely weak physical condition
- have inflammation
- suffer from high blood pressure
- have recently consumed alcohol or smoked
- have either a completely empty or an extremely full stomach
- have an unidentified severe pain

You must communicate with your bodywork practitioner or therapist; both of you must be aware of your general physical, mental, and emotional condition. Your practitioner also needs to know what medications you are taking or have taken recently. Common sense dictates the appropriate type of therapy. If you are in doubt, be sure to ask questions.

If bodywork is entered into too enthusiastically, it is not uncommon for a person to feel nauseated or headachy. Shorter, more frequent sessions may be necessary in order to avoid rapid detoxification.

Because of overlapping in techniques, bodywork is difficult to categorize. A few basic types of bodywork discussed here are:

- soft tissue

- connective tissue–fascia
- meridians
- energy and healing touch

Soft-Tissue Bodywork   Soft-tissue massage may range from gentle, nurturing stroking to more vigorous classic Swedish massage.

SWEDISH MASSAGE   Swedish massage is the most familiar style of soft-tissue bodywork. It involves treatment of the entire external body, except the reproductive organs and body orifices. The person is always draped and may undress to a personally comfortable degree. Oil, powder, or alcohol are mediums often used to help the therapist's hands glide over the skin surface. Swedish massage has a set pattern of stretching the limbs and an active stimulation of skin and soft tissue.

Strokes are rhythmic, follow muscle groups, and always end stroking toward the heart. A few of the basic strokes are:

- Effleurage: Glides across the skin with no attempt to move deep muscles.
- Petrissage: Gently lifts muscle mass and gently wrings or squeezes it.
- Friction: Small circular movements that move the tissues under the skin.
- Tapotement: Gentle tapping that provides contrast and tension release.

MANUAL LYMPHATIC DRAINAGE
CAUTION: *This technique must only be practiced by a completely trained professional.*

Developed in the 1930s by Emil Vodder of Denmark, manual lymphatic drainage (MLD) can be regarded as one of the large-surface massage methods. It involves manual techniques that are not used in any other classical form of massage.

In MLD, the skin is always kneaded, never stroked. The technique consists of a combina-

tion of round or oval, small or large, and deep or shallow circular movements, all of which knead the skin. The length of treatment of a particular body part, the use of certain pressure, and the speed of the movements can be explained, but not taught. The sensitivity and intuition of the practitioner are vital to this type of massage.

Because the effect of MLD is largely derived from mechanically displacing fluids and the substances they carry, the techniques developed and taught by Vodder must be executed precisely. Experience shows that the more exact the technique, the better the results. The amount of pressure used depends on the state of the tissue to be treated; the softer the tissue, the softer the massage.

The basic principles of manual lymphatic drainage are:

- The proximal area (area closer to the center of the body) is treated before the distal (area farther from the center of the body) so that the proximal area is emptied to make room for the fluid flowing in from the distal end.
- The techniques and variations are repeated rhythmically, usually five to seven times, either at the same location in stationary circles or in expanding spirals.
- As a rule, no reddening of the skin should appear.
- MLD should *not* elicit pain.

Connective Tissue–Fascia Bodywork   In addition to the skeletal system, the other supportive structure in the body is connective tissue, or fascia. It fastens muscles to bones and bones into joints, surrounds every nerve and vessel, holds all internal structures in place, and envelops the body as a whole.

Connective tissue has many different shapes and properties. It is made up of fluid, cellular, fibrous, and crystalline constituents. It can be quite diffuse and watery, or it can form a tough, flexible meshwork. Tendons and ligaments have extraordinary tensile strength, superior to steel wire.

Connective tissue has limits on its ability to regenerate and maintain resilient properties. Poor nutrition and sedentary habits weaken all the connective tissues of the body, stiffen them, and can shorten their effectiveness, even in a young adult. Over time, connective tissue eventually dries and stiffens.

Over the centuries, many deep-tissue techniques for manipulating the connective tissue framework have been developed and used with success. Direct pressure and stretching are among the most effective means for increasing energy levels and pliability in all forms of connective tissue. This increase happens in several ways:

- Warmth from the practitioner's hands contributes some thermal energy.
- Temperature and viscosity far beneath the skin surface are affected by deep manipulation, pressure, motion, and friction.
- Squeezing, stretching, and contorting the connective tissues causes flushing and assists with cleansing.
- Large amounts of toxins and wastes can be moved out of the intercellular fluids and into the bloodstream where they can be eliminated.

ROLFING   One recent and popular connective tissue massage is rolfing, developed by Ida Rolf who established the Rolfing Institute in Boulder, Colorado, in 1972. Rolfers use fingers, knuckles, forearms, elbows, and sometimes even tools to exert pressure or stretching forces on the connective tissues in an effort to energize and reshape it.

This pressure and stretching, carefully applied at specific points and in specific directions, softens and lengthens the connective tissues to make them more malleable. The release of thickened and strained areas proceeds systematically, session by session, area by area. The rate of metabolism of the entire system improves.

Rolfing also addresses the structural properties of connective tissue. Lack of use, misuse, poor postural habits, and chronic strains may cause asymmetries and imbalances. Some connective tissues may thicken and shorten; others weaken and lengthen. Muscle sacs develop excess fiber, and ligaments overextend and cannot support the joints. Sheets of fascia bunch up and become glued to themselves or to their neighbors with hydrogen bonds.

When these various related problems become widespread, a deep-tissue practitioner is needed to rearrange and actually "sculpt" these deformed and glued structures. A more efficient distribution of weight and a broader range of motion are then possible.

Meridian Bodywork   All living things have a vital energy. The Chinese call it *chi*, the Japanese call it *ki*, the East Indians call it *prana*, and the Tibetans call it *rlun*. Wilhelm Reich, an Austrian psychoanalyst (1878–1957), called it *orgone*, and later scientists are calling it bioplasma. It has been described as an electromagnetic energy that influences both the body and the psyche.

Meridians are the pathways along which this vital energy flows; however, scientific research has not yet identified a physical phenomenon demonstrating this pathway. With slight curves, or brief horizontal jags, meridians move along a vertical plane. The meridians are bilateral, duplicating themselves on each side of the body.

Of the 59 meridians, the 12 organ meridians and two of the extra meridians are most commonly used in treatment. The organ meridians are: lung, large intestine, stomach, spleen, heart, small intestine, urinary bladder, kidney, pericardium (cardiovascular system), triple warmer (endocrine system), gall bladder, and liver. The two extra meridians are the governing vessel and the conception vessel.

The organ meridians are named for the organ affected or controlled by the energy flow along that particular meridian. In addition, meridians are classified as either yin, where the energy mainly flows upward, or yang, where the energy mainly flows downward. The terms and concept of yin and yang are from Chinese medicine. Yin is the more passive and receiving; yang is active, aggressive, and outgoing.

Although these meridians have no physical trace in the human body, both the vital energy and the circulatory systems of blood and lymph flow through them. It has been observed that many of the meridian pathways run closely parallel to the pathways of one or more main nerve branches.

The circulation of energy and nutrients starts at the first regular meridian, the lung, and over a 24-hour period moves through all the meridians. This cycle repeats continuously throughout life. Each meridian has a two-hour interval in which a maximum of vital energy is reached. Each cycle also has a sequential directional flow, moving from a yin meridian to a yang meridian.

ACUPUNCTURE   To balance the energy in the body, slim needles are applied to specific points along meridians. By both the placement and the manipulation of the needles (twirling, vibrating, heating, and electric current), the therapist can sedate, stimulate, or tonify (tone). Acupuncture points can be located with electrical measuring devices. The electrical resistance of the skin is consistently lower at acupuncture points.

Pulses are available at the skin level all along the meridians. However, the practitioner usually takes the organ pulses at the wrist, to diagnose the condition of the energy flow in the body. Treatment is based on the findings from reading the pulses.

In addition to its role as an anesthetic for surgery in China, acupuncture has been used successfully for centuries as a preventive form of medicine and to facilitate the body's repair of diseased conditions. For example, in cases of paralysis, acupuncture assists nerves in the affected area to recover their ability to transmit impulses. In organ congestion, stimulation along various points of the meridian allows the organ to receive energy and dispel blockage, helping the body return the organ to full functioning capability.

MOXIBUSTION   Moxibustion is most often used in conjunction with an acupuncture treatment, but it can be used alone. Moxibustion is used to stimulate the flow of energy between yin and yang points of the physical body, and to bring warmth to a cold and/or congested area. The technique allows the heat generated to penetrate the skin and deeper muscle layers.

Moxa is the name given to the smoldering tinder of mugwort leaves and/or root (*Artemesia vulgaris*). The moxa is prepared, then shaped into either a cone or stick form before use. The cone is usually placed on top of a thin slice of ginger or garlic root, on a thin layer of salt, or on the top of an acupuncture needle. The stick is held above the skin. The moxa is lit and allowed to smolder until the patient feels the heat to a comfortable level. Pain is *not* a part of the process. The practitioner always monitors the moxibustion process and removes the moxa before the skin starts to blister.

SHIATSU   Although the roots of Shiatsu can be traced to China 3000 years ago, Tokujiro Namikoshi of Japan revived this technique in 1930. Shiatsu is a form of acupressure and has been described as a dance over and along the meridians of the body. The practitioner maintains the attitude of observer. The practitioner's body weight rather than muscle strength is used to allow the hand/fingers to penetrate into the meridian.

Pressure is applied rhythmically and perpendicularly. The practitioner uses the balls of the fingers and thumbs as well as the base of the thumb. The pressure is varied according to the body part and the condition being addressed. Eleven positions of the hands and fingers can be used. Eight types of pressure can be applied: steady, sustained, graded, concentrated, suction, slowing, vibrational, and palm stimulation.

Giving attention to specific points along a meridian affects various muscles and joints directly. Muscle tension caused by contracted tendons and muscle fibers can be released by stimulating a point along the meridian that is related to the particular muscle/joint. In addition, specific complaints, such as migraine headache, tension headache, nausea, vertigo, stiff neck, sciatica, and many other complains can be addressed by stimulating associated meridian points.

REFLEXOLOGY In the early 1900s, William H. Fitzgerald, an American physician, rediscovered the centuries-old Chinese method of foot massage, which he called zone therapy. The points used are nerve endings on the feet that reflex the entire body. This same map of points is on the head, ears, eyes, and palms of the hands.

The zones run longitudinally along the foot, with the head, eyes, and ears being mapped on the tip of the big toe, across the tips of the toes to the little toe. Each foot represents one half of the body. The inside of each foot reflexes the spinal column. The soles, upper parts of the foot, and around the heel and ankle all have reflex points to the organs and skeletal structure. The lymphatic system is also included in the reflex mapping.

Treatment consists of using the thumbs to apply firm pressure. Gentle holding and gentle squeezing of the feet before treatment will familiarize the recipient with the touch, as well as warm the tissue that will be massaged.

When the tissue, tendons, and fluids have been warmed, massage is more comfortable and effective. Tender areas will indicate where concentration of time and energy is needed. Pressure should be firm, but *not* painful. Areas of tightness, swelling, or congestion should be gently massaged to relax the muscle, disperse excess fluid, and/or break up congestion. Because reflexology is very easy to overdo, the usual treatment is only twenty minutes.

Working the reflexes can cleanse the body. Reflexology can relieve headaches, clear congested sinuses, reduce the pain of menstrual cramps, ease a backache, and reduce swelling in a "trick" knee.

Energy and Healing Touch Healing touch is what the name implies—touch that heals. The practitioner touches the patient to reconnect him or her with healing energy that affects the mind, body, and spirit.

REIKI Reiki is a hands-on system of healing that restores and balances the life force energy within the body. It is thought that Reiki originated in Tibet centuries ago, but Dr. Mikao Usui of Japan rediscovered the basic system in the mid- to late 1800s.

Reiki balances and strengthens the body's energy, promoting its ability to heal itself. This healing system touches a person on all levels: body, mind, and spirit. Treatment involves a practitioner placing hands on a patient's body in a passive way with the intent to transfer energy and bring the person back into balance. Treatments are carried out in a quiet environment and last about an hour. Although Reiki is a complete treatment, it maximizes the results from other treatments such as massage, chiropractic, physiotherapy, and acupuncture.

THERAPEUTIC TOUCH Dolores Krieger, a professor of nursing at New York University, demonstrated in controlled studies in 1972 that touch has positive physiologic effects. In placing hands on a patient, the uniquely human aspect of concern for the individual is communicated.

The practitioner must be settled and calm before laying on hands. The idea is to communicate love, support, and caring while either touching, holding, or lightly stroking the patient in a nonthreatening manner. This is done while respecting the person's sense of privacy and private body space. The practitioner acts as a support system, providing a healthy energy field for the repatterning of the patient's weak and imbalanced energy flow.

Therapeutic touch interaction can provide relaxation, reduction of pain, acceleration of healing, and alleviation of illness.

17

Other Ways of Detoxification

Compresses, Poultices, and Packs

When used for cleansing the body, compresses, poultices, and packs stimulate circulation, cause sweating that excretes toxins, and draw out impurities. They are noninvasive treatments that can help to rid the body of many different toxins and even infections. If a rash should develop after a treatment, do not use again.

COMPRESSES

A compress is a soft pad of gauze or cloth applied to a body part with varying pressure to control hemorrhage. Compresses may also be moistened with water or medication to reduce pain or prevent infection, and applied with little or no pressure. They may be applied warm or hot to stimulate circulation of blood or lymph and to heat cold joints. When applied cold they soothe pain and reduce swelling.

Some common compresses and conditions they may be used to treat are:

- *Epsom salts*: Dissolve Epsom salts in hot water and apply as a compress to draw out boils or any type of infection. Epsom salts can also be dissolved in hot water for soaking infected fingers, hands, toes, and feet.
- *Ice or cold*: Ice or cold compresses can be used for bursitis, strains, sprains, sore throats, arthritis, inflammation, fever, headaches, hemorrhoids, and swelling.
- *Heat*: Heat compresses can be used to relieve the pain of earaches, cystitis, diverticulitis, flatulence, and headache.
- *Alternating hot and cold*: Alternating hot and cold compresses applied over the affected area will help flush fluids in the area, pushing out waste products with the cold (contractive) phase, and bringing in fresh fluid (blood and nutrients) with the hot (expansive) phase. This treatment will help many conditions, including inflamed ovaries, nephritis, hepatitis, hemorrhoids, glaucoma, and sinusitis.
- *Herbal*: Specific herbal compresses can be used for bruises, swelling, hematomas, and pain. See Administration of Herbs in chapter 15 for instructions for making an herbal compress.

POULTICES

Poultices are used to relieve pain and congestion, reduce inflammation, promote absorption or resolution of an abscess, diminish tissue swelling and tension, soften crusted lesions, encourage muscle relaxation, stimulate healthy granulation, and deodorize or disinfect.

Clay can be used in poultices, either as a clay-water paste or in a clay-glycerine mixture. Sterilize the clay in a 350°F oven until heated through before mixing with the water or glycerine. Apply the paste to the skin and cover; keep moist. Clay poultices may be left on for 6 to 10 hours.

A charcoal poultice is helpful for skin ulcers. Mix equal parts of charcoal powder and olive oil and apply to the ulcer. A poultice of cornstarch and fresh lemon juice, or cornstarch and witch hazel, alleviates the itching of mosquito bites.

Herbal poultices are made from crushed herbs or a paste of herbs, moistened and applied directly to the body or between a layer of gauze. The poultice should be ¼ to ½ inch thick. Hold it in place with tape or an elastic bandage, and leave it on at least three hours. A poultice can be left on all night. Most poultices are applied warm and should not be reheated. When the first one cools, use a second poultice. (See Herbs in chapter 15 for information on preparing herbal poultices.)

Many different conditions can be helped with an herbal poultice:

- Arthritis: cabbage or comfrey leaf
- Boils: flaxseed
- Bruises: comfrey or hyssop
- Bursitis: green cabbage leaf or comfrey leaf
- Inflammation: elderberry
- Insect bite: honey, plantain, or lobelia
- Neuritis or neuralgia: mullein or mustard
- Phlebitis: papaya, mullein tea, or comfrey
- Varicose veins: mullein
- Warts: comfrey root or leaf, or chickweed
- Superficial wounds: aloe vera juice and/or comfrey

PACKS

Castor oil packs have a drawing power as deep as 4 inches into the body. Use undyed cotton cloth or wool flannel; wool flannel is preferable. Soak the flannel in cold-pressed castor oil.

Wring the cloth so it is wet, but not dripping. Apply the cloth to the affected area of the body and cover with plastic. Cover the plastic with a towel and place a heating pad over the towel. The heating pad should be as warm as can be tolerated. Leave the pack on for 1 to 1½ hours. Wash off remaining oil with a water and baking soda mixture.

Some health care practitioners feel that the flannel cloth can be stored in a covered pan or Ziploc bag and reused numerous times before it is washed. Others feel that one or two uses before washing and reusing are appropriate. The number of safe uses can be partially determined by the toxicity of the area being treated.

Clay packs may be used to reduce edema and to resolve boils. Clay has good drawing power and will draw toxins and excess fluid out of the body through the skin. There are many clays that make good packs, such as Green Clay, Indian Healing Clay, and Bentonite Clay.

To make a clay pack, mix the clay until it is soft and has no lumps. It should be the consistency of a heavy ointment or cream cheese. Apply to the affected area to a ¼-inch thickness. Leave on for one-half to one hour.

Various types of packs may be used to help many conditions:

- Celiac disease: castor oil pack over abdomen
- Cystitis: hot trunk pack
- Diabetes: castor oil pack from lower ribs to pubis
- Diverticulitis: castor oil pack or cold trunk pack
- Fever: cold trunk pack
- Tendonitis: hot castor oil pack on affected tendons
- Tonsillitis: cold throat pack
- Liver pain: hot castor oil pack over the liver
- Immune depression: hot castor oil pack over the thymus

Charcoal Therapy

Charcoal is a supreme cleanser of the body. Because it is very porous, charcoal has a large surface area to adsorb (attract and hold) toxins. For example, 1 pound of charcoal can adsorb 80 quarts of ammonia gas. Charcoal will adsorb chemicals, drugs, gases, body wastes, and foreign proteins.

Activated charcoal is the best for detoxification or cleansing purposes. Activated charcoal is made by the controlled burning of the source material, then subjecting it to steam or air at elevated temperatures. This causes a network of internal pores that greatly increases its surface area and adsorptive capabilities. Common source materials for charcoal include coal, sawdust, bone, peat, wood char, and papermill wastes. Charcoal made from coconut or black walnut shells has high adsorptive powers.

Finely pulverized charcoal has the most effective cleansing power. Charcoal capsules and tablets help, but their efficiency is below that of powdered charcoal. While it is possible to make your own charcoal, in terms of purity and effectiveness it is better to purchase it at a health food store or drug store.

Charcoal can be used as a deodorizer for air and water, as well as a chemical filter in masks and air cleaners. If placed in an open container in a room, it will remove odors, including the odor of cigarette smoke. Charcoal powder will also remove odors from skin ulcers if it is placed on the ulcer or in a dressing.

Taken orally, charcoal removes the odor from intestinal gas. In most cases the effectiveness of charcoal is determined by the dosage and by how quickly it is given after a toxic exposure. The first dosage is eight to ten times the estimated weight of the toxin. Food and bile interfere with charcoal's effectiveness, yet adsorption is still rapid. Charcoal forms a stable complex with toxins and does not subsequently release them for reabsorption into the bloodstream.

Charcoal works better in an acid than an alkaline medium. It adsorbs mineral acids, alkalis, and salts poorly; for this reason, it does not adsorb nutrients. Charcoal adsorbs a large number of toxins extremely well, including acetaminophen, alcohol, amphetamines, aspirin, chlordane, cocaine, cyanide, gasoline, iodine, kerosene, Malathion, morphine, narcotics, nicotine, pesticides, phenol, and radioactive substances.

Charcoal has cleansing capabilities in several different forms:

- *Slurry*: Charcoal stirred into water forms a slurry, which is more effective than induced vomiting or stomach lavage (pumping the stomach) to remove poison. It is totally safe to use in acute poisonings; no contraindications are known. For caustic agents such as lye, use large amounts of charcoal. Larger amounts of charcoal must also be used to adsorb gasoline, lighter fluid, kerosene, and cleaning fluids. Use charcoal equal to twice the weight of the poison consumed.

- *Poultice*: Charcoal combined with water and ground flaxseed (as a thickening agent) makes a poultice that can be used almost anywhere on the body's surface. Use 3 tablespoons ground flaxseed combined with 1 to 3 tablespoons charcoal and 1 cup of water. Let set for 20 minutes or heat gently to thicken. Spread approximately ¼-inch thick over a square of white paper towel. Cover with another paper towel. Apply to the affected area and cover with plastic, then a towel, and leave the poultice in place for six to ten hours. After removing the poultice, rub the skin with a cold, wet cloth. Poultices are extremely effective for venomous bites, such as spider bites and bee stings.

- *Mini-poultices*: Apply charcoal to a Band-Aid. Either rub a charcoal tablet on damp Band-Aid gauze until it is black, or dip the damp gauze into charcoal powder. Place the Band-Aid over the insect bite. Mini-poultices are effective for ant, mosquito, and chigger bites. They will also detoxify poison ivy eruptions.

- *Tablets and capsules*: Intestinal gas and bloating can be treated with four capsules or eight tablets of charcoal taken three to four times per day. This treatment also helps with malodorous stools and bad breath originating both from the mouth and gastrointestinal tract.
- *Powder*: Charcoal powder can be placed directly on the skin to reduce swelling by absorbing excess fluid and the products of inflammation. It will also adsorb toxins, bacteria, carcinogens, products of allergies, and wound secretions.

A variety of conditions can be treated with charcoal:

- *Acetaminophen (Tylenol) poisoning*: Can be treated with oral charcoal.
- *Aspirin poisoning*: Fatalities can be prevented by giving charcoal. It is more effective when given at the first signs of poisoning from allergy or overdose.
- *Theophylline overdoses*: This respiratory tract medication has a narrow therapeutic range and overdoses are a common occurrence. People taking this drug should keep charcoal on hand to treat these overdoses.
- *Cancer*: Controls pain when applied with poultices, which also adsorb the toxins produced by the cancer and chemotherapy.
- *Mushroom poisoning*: Can be treated with charcoal powder capsules or tablets even as long as 24 hours after consuming the mushroom.
- *Wound dressings*: Disinfects and deodorizes wounds and is quite effective when added to dressings.

Oxygen Therapy

Oxygen is an odorless, tasteless, colorless gas found in elemental form in the atmosphere. The oxygen in the atmosphere comes from the metabolism of green plants. It is found in almost all plant and animal substances. Oxygen is essential for maintaining life in all organisms on earth, with the exception of anaerobic bacteria.

Oxygen is to our bodies what gasoline is to our cars. Oxygen is necessary to all biochemical processes in the body. Almost all oxygen consumption occurs on the cell membranes. Two-thirds of the body's oxygen consumption is used to burn fuels in the production of adenosine triphosphate (ATP), which is the primary molecule that accepts energy from the breakdown of these fuels. The ATP donates this energy to the cells of the body once it has been broken down to adenosine diphosphate and a phosphate group. This process is the body's main energy-producing reaction.

Oxygen also aids in altering compounds for structural purposes. It is consumed in both the processes of oxygenation and of dehydrogenation of existing compounds, changing their composition to be more useful to the body. In addition, oxygen is consumed to alter compounds for protective purposes. White blood cells use oxygen to kill the bacteria they have ingested. Toxic compounds are converted to harmless derivatives through oxidation reactions.

With an abundance of oxygen, our bodies can function properly, fighting off disease and eliminating chemical toxins. We can live without food, water, and sleep for several days, but we can live without oxygen for only a few minutes. Irreparable brain damage occurs after that time. Our cells stop producing sufficient ATP, and they become disorganized, unable to function.

Oxygen is supplied by air inhaled into the lungs. Red blood cells carry oxygen from the lungs to all parts of the body. After releasing the oxygen, they pick up carbon dioxide from the blood plasma and return it to the lungs where it is expelled from the body.

Oxygen deficiency, or oxygen starvation at the cellular level, can lead to disease. Poor diet, abuse of alcohol, air pollution, drugs, and lack of exercise all greatly reduce the amount of oxygen available to the cells. This can have adverse effects on the immune system. When the cells receive insufficient oxygen, they turn to sugar fermentation as another source of energy. Cellular metabolism becomes dysfunctional, causing the cells to become unhealthy and weak. They lose their immunity and become vulnerable to infection.

Without sufficient oxygen, digestion is affected. Production of gastric secretions requires calcium, water, and oxygen. Low or dilute gastric secretions and the resultant poor food assimilation lead to overeating in an attempt to obtain enough nutrition.

Without sufficient oxygen, the body is unable to cleanse or repair itself. Vitamin C is not assimilated properly, causing the breakdown of collagen. This permits veins and arteries to harden. Hardening of the arteries in older people leads to strokes and degeneration of the brain. The liver, the major organ of cleansing and detoxification, cannot repair its cells without sufficient oxygen.

The use of oxygen is an important aid in cleansing the body. Added oxygen is used by the body to oxidize or burn up toxins. If oxygen therapy is given consistently and for long enough, the body can cleanse itself of all toxins. Anaerobic microorganisms will be unable to live in the oxygen-rich environment.

There are several methods of administering oxygen for cleansing:

- Inhalation therapy
- Hyperbaric oxygen therapy
- Hydrogen peroxide therapy
- Ozone therapy
- Stabilized oxygen therapy

INHALATION THERAPY

Oxygen is given as an inhalant to treat such respiratory problems as asthma, bronchitis, emphysema, and pneumonia, in which lung function is impaired, and the body is not receiving sufficient oxygen. In this type of therapy, oxygen eases the labored breathing caused by these disease processes. The concentration of oxygen available to the lungs is increased, thus increasing the amount of oxygen available to the body and helping to compensate for the impaired lung function.

Oxygen will also help destroy any harmful anaerobic microbes that might be present, without harming helpful aerobic microorganisms. Anaerobic microbes may be viral, bacterial, or fungal.

Oxygen plays a very important cleansing role when used as an inhalant to clear allergic reactions. It helps to stop any allergic reaction, regardless of the symptoms. There does not have to be difficulty in breathing for oxygen to be of benefit, as it has a biochemical effect, reversing the allergic and inflammatory cascade.

In reactive or inflammatory processes, hemoglobin (the oxygen-carrying protein in red blood cells) releases more oxygen to the cells fighting the reaction or foreign substance. Providing more oxygen to these active cells also allows an increase in ATP release, which accelerates the process of detoxification.

If a mask is used, oxygen should be administered at the rate of 5 to 6 liters per minute. If a cannula (nasal tube) is used, the rate should be 2 to 3 liters per minute. Use the oxygen for 15 to 30 minutes to clear the reaction. If the reaction has not stopped, extend the time another 15 to 30 minutes. Do not use the oxygen continuously for more than 5 hours.

Ceramic masks and special tubing are available for people who do not tolerate plastic masks and tubing. An oxygen tank and oxygen for emergency use can be obtained by prescription from a physician familiar with your condition.

HYPERBARIC OXYGEN THERAPY

In hyperbaric oxygen therapy, oxygen is administered under pressures greater than atmospheric pressure (barometric pressure) at sea level. Very little oxygen is dissolved in the blood at normal barometric pressure. Under increased pressure, enough oxygen dissolves to meet the average requirements of the body. The body then uses the oxygen dissolved in the blood rather than that bound to hemoglobin, which is less readily available.

Hyperbaric oxygen results in:

- decreased cardiac output
- increased blood-brain barrier permeability
- improved red cell elasticity, thus improving micro-circulation
- reduced fatigue and increased physical endurance
- suppressed respiratory reactivity to carbon dioxide

Hyperbaric oxygen treatments are carried out in chambers in which the pressure can be raised to several atmospheres higher than sea level. The chambers may be large enough to hold several people or may hold just one patient. There are now mobile hyperbaric oxygen chambers that can be moved to locations where they are needed.

The person receiving treatment remains in the chamber for a prescribed amount of time, depending on the condition being treated. The most common condition treated with hyperbaric oxygen is decompression sickness, commonly known as the "bends." The bends are caused by a rapid reduction of environmental pressure that allows inert gases in the body tissues to form bubbles. Divers may suffer from the bends if they return to the surface too quickly.

Other conditions that have been successfully treated with hyperbaric oxygen therapy include:

- Carbon monoxide and smoke poisoning. Cyanide, hydrogen sulfide, and carbon tetrachloride poisonings have been successfully treated with hyperbaric oxygen therapy.
- Crush syndrome, compartment syndrome, and other acute traumatic ischemia (mechanical obstruction of blood supply). Crush injuries to limbs involving injury to muscle, bone, skin, connective tissue, and nerves respond well to hyperbaric oxygen therapy. Most of the benefit is obtained from counteracting the effects of anoxia and ischemia occurring in these injuries.
- Infections. Oxygen is a broad-spectrum antibiotic, cleansing the body of microorganisms, both anaerobic and aerobic. However, the pressure must be above 1.3 atmospheres for aerobic organisms to be affected. Soft tissue infections, osteomyelitis, and gas gangrene have all been effectively treated with hyperbaric oxygen therapy. Treatment of other infections would also be effective with this technique.
- Skin transplantation. Skin transplants or skin flaps with marginal survival possibilities because of circulatory or nutritional disturbances have been saved with hyperbaric oxygen therapy. It is of particular value in burn cases or cases requiring extensive plastic surgery or skin grafting.

Hyperbaric oxygen has also been successfully used in cases of fat embolism, air embolism during surgery or catheterization, coronary artery occlusion and myocardial infarction, and management of serious neurological disturbances resulting in coma.

HYDROGEN PEROXIDE THERAPY

One of the simplest sources of healing oxygen can be found in food-grade hydrogen peroxide

(H_2O_2), which comes in a 35% solution. The more familiar 3% hydrogen peroxide found in pharmacies has been altered by the addition of various stabilizers and toxic metals. Ozone bubbled through water becomes hydrogen peroxide. Nascent oxygen is then released from the hydrogen peroxide.

Hydrogen peroxide occurs naturally from atmospheric ozone, in rain and snow, and in the running water of mountain streams, where the continuously moving water is naturally aerated. Raw vegetables and fruits contain natural hydrogen peroxide. The body's immune system combines free oxygen with some of the body's water to create hydrogen peroxide as part of its defense against invading pathogens. It is released from human blood platelets and white cells when they are disturbed by particulate matter irritating their membranes.

In the body, the increased oxygen provided by hydrogen peroxide helps digestion, aids liver function and repair, slows collagen breakdown, relieves hypoxia, and helps prevent wound infection.

Hydrogen peroxide also reduces the stress and pain of chronic infection and disease. It has been used to treat heart and blood vessel diseases, pulmonary diseases, infectious diseases, immune disorders, Parkinson's and Alzheimer's diseases, migraine headaches, cancer pain, and blood and lymph node cancers.

Ingestion of Hydrogen Peroxide Use only diluted 35% pure food-grade hydrogen peroxide and always keep it refrigerated.

Dilute 35% pure food-grade hydrogen peroxide as follows:

- Use 5 ounces of distilled water, fruit juice, or milk to dilute the amount of hydrogen peroxide recommended below.
- Alternatives are to drink the peroxide in orange juice and eat a bite of orange or banana to remove the aftertaste.

- *Do not mix* with carrot juice, carbonated juice, or alcoholic drinks.
- Take it on an empty stomach, one hour before or after a meal or medicine.
- Stir the drops into the diluting substance and take according to the following schedule.

    Day 1: 1 drop
    Day 2: 2 drops
    Day 3: 3 drops
    Day 4: 4 drops

    Take it once, twice, or three times a day.
- Continue, if you choose, adding a drop per day until day 16. Many people choose to stop at ten drops.
- If your stomach becomes upset, stay at that level or go back a level.

There is a limit to how much the body can eliminate in a 24-hour period. If undesirable cleansing symptoms occur, go off the program for a few days to give the body a chance to catch up with elimination. Then begin where you left off or at a lower level.

If Candida overgrowth or ulcers are a problem, begin the program very slowly. One drop a day for the first week may be your tolerance level. For very serious complaints, it is possible to ingest as much as 25 drops three times a day for one to three weeks. Then reduce intake to twice a day until the problems are gone. This treatment may take six months or longer to complete. After your problems have been eliminated, a good maintenance program is 5 to 15 drops per week, depending on the amount of cooked or processed foods in the diet.

CAUTION: Always follow hydrogen peroxide treatment with *acidophilus* replacement. For discussion of acidophilus therapy, see Beneficial Bacteria in chapter 14.

Since this is a cleansing process, you will likely have both ups and downs as your body gradually releases toxins long stored in the organs. Because the body tries to maintain homeostasis, these reactions will be temporary, usually lasting three days. If your energy level is already low, you might be uncomfortable for as long as a week. Reactions might include skin eruptions, nausea, diarrhea, headache, unusual fatigue, a cold, sinus flare-up, ear infections, or flu.

Intravenous Administration   Hydrogen peroxide in a diluted solution can be administered intravenously for a rapid response in more serious infections. It helps to reoxygenate the cells and stimulate the immune system. Viral infections respond more rapidly than bacterial infections.

Other Uses for Hydrogen Peroxide   To make your own safe 3% solution, add 1 ounce of 35% food-grade hydrogen peroxide to 11 ounces of distilled water.

CAUTION: 35% hydrogen peroxide is flammable and can be harmful. It should always be diluted and handled with care. Rinse immediately and thoroughly with water if it gets on the skin. People with organ transplants CANNOT use hydrogen peroxide. The immune system will be strengthened and will reject the transplant as a foreign body. However, it is safe to use if you have plastic or metal implants.

- *Body spray*: After a shower or bath, dry off. Spray your body with a 3% dilution of hydrogen peroxide and let dry. This restores the acid mantle that soap removes.
- *Mouth rinse*: Use a 3% dilution of hydrogen peroxide as a mouth wash to fight tartar and plaque.
- *Gum disease*: Add enough 3% diluted hydrogen peroxide to baking soda to form a paste. Apply to gums.
- *Facial freshener and acne control*: Apply a 3% dilution of hydrogen peroxide on a cotton ball to the skin after washing your face. WARNING: Be careful to avoid eyes.

- *Nasal spray*: Use 1 part 3% dilution of hydrogen peroxide to 1 part distilled water.
- *Food purifier* (meat, fish or vegetables): Mix 1 ounce of 35% hydrogen peroxide with 1 gallon of water. Pass the food through this bath. It is not necessary to soak the food or to rinse it afterward.
- *Wound cleanser* (also prevents infection): Pour a 3% dilution of hydrogen peroxide over the wound. Capful amounts are usually sufficient unless the area is quite large. Thick foaming indicates that infectious material is being killed. Repeat the hydrogen peroxide flow over the wound. Be aware that the damaged tissue will be sensitive; do not repeat more than three consecutive times. If necessary, you may repeat the treatment several hours later.

OZONE THERAPY

Ozone is triatomic oxygen, a molecule containing three atoms of oxygen instead of the usual two. It is created in nature by solar radiation ionizing oxygen at higher altitudes. Electric discharge also produces ozone, causing the fresh smell accompanying lightning and rain. Copy machines, some appliances, and electric trains have high-voltage discharges that cause ozone to form. Ozone is also produced when nitrous oxides and hydrocarbons react in the presence of sunlight. Refineries, factories, automobiles, and chemical manufacturing plants produce ozone in this way.

Ozone is unstable and cannot be stored. It has to be produced as it is needed for treatment. Ozone is usually produced when air or oxygen passes through a high-energy field. An ozone-producing apparatus is called an ozone generator. Ozone generators can be used to detoxify homes and workplaces of molds and chemicals. Ozone kills mold and oxidizes chemicals so that they are less harmful.

An important cleansing agent, ozone has disinfectant properties and is antibacterial, antiviral, antifungal, and antiparasitic. Ozone can be used to purify drinking water, for disinfecting utensils, and for sanitizing air. Ozone can be used to treat municipal water supplies and swimming pools. Ozone treatment of industrial waste water, lakes, ponds, and fisheries is of both economic and environmental importance. Pesticides are difficult to remove from water by reverse osmosis and distillation, but they are reduced by ozone treatment.

In microdoses, ozone has important medical uses. In such small doses, it can be used both topically and internally. Topically, it is used to treat skin disorders. It is used rectally or vaginally, and an ozone bath can provide as much benefit as a hyperbaric oxygen treatment with much less cost and equipment. In high concentrations, ozone is toxic to the epithelium (lining) of the lungs and is therefore not administered medically in nebulizers.

Bacteria and viruses can be cleansed from the blood with ozone. A pint of blood is drawn from the person and placed in a special infusion bottle. Ozone is forced into the bottle and thoroughly mixed with the blood. The ozone molecules give up their third oxygen atom, in a process that inactivates the microorganisms. The treated blood is then given back to the patient. Some practitioners use direct intravascular injections of pure oxygen/ozone mixtures.

Ozone also has antitumor properties. It is believed that the special peroxides formed by ozone in the blood seek out and destroy diseased cells. These diseased or infected cells have lower levels of protective enzyme activity and are less stable. The hydroxyperoxides react with the cell membrane lipids, invading the cell and destroying disease. The hydroxyperoxides have no effect on healthy cells except for oxygenating their environment and enhancing circulation.

Cleansing effects of ozone include:

- activation of enzymes involved in oxygen radical or peroxide scavenging
- acceleration of glycolysis (breakdown of glucose) in red blood cells
- activation of the citric acid cycle (the energy-producing cycle of the body)
- increase of blood oxygen, blood fluidity, and red blood cell pliability
- increase of bactericidal, viricidal, and fungicidal properties

STABILIZED OXYGEN THERAPY

Stabilized oxygen is a liquid oxygen supplement that contains stabilized electrolytes of oxygen. Several companies make stabilized oxygen, and most of them use sodium chlorite in solution. When taken orally, the chlorine-oxygen molecule enters the bloodstream intact. In the bloodstream, the oxygen molecule has a greater affinity for hemoglobin and leaves the chlorine, which is then excreted through the kidneys. The oxygen-enriched blood stimulates the functions of white blood cells and reduces the clumping of red blood cells.

Sodium chlorite and the chlorite ion are a rich source of oxygen and are anti-inflammatory, bactericidal, and fungicidal. The oxygen they release is also effective in combating viruses. These substances and chlorine dioxide (a reaction product) can reduce the severity and duration of diarrhea and stomach flu. Although chlorine oxides are unstable, the manufacturing process has stabilized them. Their half-life in the body is approximately 12 hours, and they do not initiate free radical activity in the body.

Stabilized oxygen can be used to purify water. It is effective against coliform bacteria, streptococcus, staphylococcus, fungus, and *Giardia lamblia*. It can be used to purify mountain water and to keep stored water pure of coliform bacteria. Stabilized oxygen products can be taken with nutritional supplements, and enhance assimilation of some nutrients.

Stabilized oxygen solutions can be added to mouthwash, vaginal douches, enemas, and skin care products. They are also used in food preservation, water treatment, vegetable washes, and disinfectants.

Organ Cleansing

Two major organs that detoxify the body are the liver and colon. During times of stress and acute overload, cleansing procedures will help restore optimal function of these organs.

LIVER

The liver is a major organ of digestion and assimilation that processes fats with the bile it produces. It stores vitamins and minerals in order to have a reserve, storing enough vitamin A to last for four years, and enough vitamin D and B_{12} to last for four months. The liver is also the major organ for elimination of toxic wastes. It processes all the foreign chemicals to which we are increasingly exposed every day. Drugs, though they may be given for medicinal purposes, also stress the liver and must be detoxified by it.

Many foreign chemicals are lipid-soluble (soluble in fat). Liver cells have lipid membranes through which these foreign chemicals can enter. These cells can store toxins for months, even years. Using a complex system of enzymes, the liver transforms these toxic chemicals into water-soluble compounds. They can then be released and eliminated from the body through the kidneys and GI tract.

Hormones are metabolized by the liver. It processes both estrogen produced by the body as well as that taken in estrogen hormone therapy. If the liver cannot process the estrogen adequately, an excess results, leading to symptoms including endometriosis, high blood pressure, PMS, inflammation of blood vessels, and breast, uterine, and vaginal cancer. The liver also metabolizes testosterone. Excess testosterone affects levels of agressiveness, mood swings, and sexual energy. Dysfunction of reproductive cycles can result if the liver is unable to process hormones properly. The adrenalin produced in response to stress is also processed by the liver. Excess hormones add to emotional imbalances, as well as stressing the liver; anger and depession may indicate liver detoxification problems.

The liver also filters the blood. Its sinusoids (filtering channels) are lined with special cells that engulf foreign debris, bacteria, and toxic chemicals. An overburdened liver eliminates only part of the toxins. Other toxins are stored in its cells, eventually causing irreversible damage.

When the body has an excess of toxins and waste materials, it cannot metabolize and detoxify them all. This results in unmetabolized toxins throughout the body and can lead to disease. The liver will be overworked. Other organs involved in detoxification can help reduce the load for the liver. The good health of these organs helps the liver retain its own health and ability to function. (See chapter 5 for further discussion of the liver.)

An overworked or poorly functioning liver is indicated by:

- poor or painful digestion, and soreness in the liver area with moderate fingertip pressure
- gas, constipation, a feeling of fullness, loss of appetite
- nausea after fatty meals, oily taste in mouth or throat, revulsion to fatty foods
- frequent headaches not related to tension or eyestrain
- weak ligaments, tendons, and muscles
- skin problems, such as acne or psoriasis
- emotional excesses, moodiness

These factors influence liver health:

- Protein: Consume 30 to 60 grams a day. A low-protein diet is used for significant liver disease.

- Sulfur: To modulate enzymes, eat foods containing sulfur, such as garlic, onions and broccoli.
- Fats: Provide sources of energy but are hard to process. Small amounts of unsaturated fats are essential for health.
- Vitamins, minerals, herbs, amino acids, and flavonoids: Act as protectors.
- Refined sugars: Can lower enzyme activity.
- Phosphatidyl choline (part of lecithin): Can improve the health of membranes surrounding the microsomes, where enzymes are produced.
- Oxygen metabolism: High oxygen concentration is required for enzyme production as well as for detoxification.

The following suggestions will help to strengthen, support, and improve liver function.

- Drink roasted chicory and dandelion "coffee," and add ginger, cardamom, or fennel to taste.
- Avoid margarine and Crisco.
- Use virgin, cold-pressed olive oil in teaspoonful amounts over food; cold-pressed oil is resistant to oxidation.
- Lower fat intake; eat less food cooked in oils or fats.
- Take fruit pectin (powder): 1 to 3 tablespoons in water or fruit juice.
- Take bentonite clay: 1 teaspoon in a glass of water, stir, leave in the sun for a few hours, then stir and drink.
- Eat whole nuts and seeds.
- Eat small portions of light, easy-to-digest foods, such as steamed vegetables, raw salad greens, and semisweet fruits (apples and pears).
- Eat green, moderately bitter vegetables (endive, collard, dock, dandelion). A bitter taste activates the flow of bile.
- Eat sparingly, lightly, and early in the day.

- Allow at least 12 hours between the evening and morning meal.
- After 7 P.M. take only a little herb tea or a small amount of fruit.
- Drink lemon water: squeeze half a lemon into a quart of spring or distilled water (no honey). The sour taste cools and cleanses the liver.
- Use antioxidants (vitamins C and E, beta-carotene, zinc, and selenium).
- Exercise before breakfast to keep eliminative channels open (skin, bowels, lungs).
- Take a moderate walk after meals.
- Release worry and anger.

Liver Cleansing

LIVER MASSAGE Massage helps to cleanse the liver. While lying flat on your back, using your flat fingertips, *gently* massage the liver area with clockwise circular motions. If soreness persists or if there is marked tenderness, seek assistance from a qualified professional.

LIVER FLUSH Liver flushes stimulate the elimination of stored toxic wastes from the body, increase bile flow, and improve liver function. Christopher Hobbs, an herbalist from Santa Cruz, California, suggests this liver flush in his book, *Natural Liver Therapy*:

Mix fresh-squeezed orange, grapefruit, and lemon or lime juices to make 1 cup of liquid. The mixture should be sour. Add 1 to 2 cloves of fresh garlic and a small amount of fresh ginger juice. (Grate the ginger on a vegetable grater and squeeze the fibers in a garlic press.) Stir in 1 tablespoon of olive oil and drink.

Follow the liver flush mixture with the following tea:

1 part fennel	¼ part burdock
1 part fenugreek	¼ part licorice
1 part flax	

Using 1 ounce of herbs to 20 ounces of water,

simmer all the herbs for 20 minutes, then add 1 part peppermint. Steep for 10 more minutes. For additional soothing properties, add ½ part marshmallow root (cut and shredded) to the initial herb blend.

COFFEE ENEMA One of the best liver cleansers is a coffee enema. Coffee enemas were listed in the old medical literature for years as a method of helping the body rid itself of toxins and accumulated waste products. After pharmaceuticals became the main focus of medicine in the 1920s, coffee enemas were seldom used. Dr. Sherry Rogers has found that coffee enemas are an excellent detoxification method, and she discusses them in her book, *Wellness Against All Odds.*

A coffee enema is a low-volume enema that stays in the sigmoid colon, the s-shaped last part of the large intestine. There is a special circulatory system between the sigmoid colon and the liver called the entero-hepatic circulation system. When the stool reaches this point, it is full of putrefied material and toxins. These toxins are sent directly to the liver for detoxification rather than being circulated throughout the body.

A coffee enema:

- speeds up the emptying of the bowel, increasing the emptying speed of the liver ducts holding detoxified materials. This allows the detoxification process to proceed at a faster pace.
- makes the liver empty the toxins it has accumulated in the bile ducts. The caffeine that is absorbed into the entero-hepatic system causes this unloading of toxins, allowing other toxins in the body to filter into the liver to be detoxified.
- stimulates the production of the enzyme glutathione-S-transferase, which makes the liver detoxification pathways function. Alkaloids in the caffeine are responsible for this stimulation.

Coffee enemas do not wash out minerals and electrolytes. Important nutrients have already been absorbed higher in the bowel, long before the food residue reaches the sigmoid colon. Many people who are sensitive to coffee or do not tolerate caffeine are reluctant to try coffee enemas but, because the coffee stays in the sigmoid colon, and the caffeine goes only into the entero-hepatic circulation system, it is usually safe to use.

Materials Needed
- an enema bag
- if you have hemorrhoid problems, a soft rubber French catheter to fit over the hard plastic nozzle of the enema bag
- a large stainless-steel or glass pot
- a Pyrex one-quart measuring cup with handle and pour spout
- organic coffee, fully caffeinated drip grind
- unsulfured molasses
- tolerated water, as pure and chemical free as possible. Be certain you are using clean spring, well, or filtered water. Do not use treated tap water from a city water supply.

Preparing the Enema Bring 1 quart of tolerated water to a boil in the stainless-steel or glass pot. Add 2 flat tablespoons of coffee and continue to boil for five minutes. Turn off the heat and leave the pan on the burner. Add 1 tablespoon of unsulfured molasses. Cool to a tepid temperature that feels comfortable to the touch. *Never* use the coffee mixture hot or steaming.

Pour the coffee mixture into the Pyrex measuring cup, being careful not to let the coffee grounds go into the cup.

Put the enema bag in the sink and clamp off the tubing.

Pour half the coffee mixture into the enema bag and then release the clamp long enough to allow the liquid to run to the end of the enema tube.

Hang the enema bag at waist level. *Do not hang it any higher.* The enema solution should go only into the lower end of the sigmoid colon. Hanging the bag higher will force the fluid too high into the intestine.

Cover the area on which you are going to lie with old towels to prevent staining the floor covering or fabric with coffee.

Taking the Enema   First half:

Lie down on the floor and gently insert the nozzle or catheter. If you need lubrication, use only food-grade vegetable oil.

Release the clamp and let the coffee mixture flow slowly in. Clamp off the tubing as soon as there is any sensation of fullness. If you can do so, retain the enema for ten minutes. Do not force yourself to hold it if an uncomfortable feeling develops. Clamp the tubing and remove the nozzle or catheter, and empty your bowel.

Second half:

After emptying the bowel, repeat the procedure with the remaining half of the coffee mixture. If you cannot hold half of the enema mixture, take three or four small enemas.

When the bile duct empties, you will hear or feel the squirting under the right ribcage, or in that general area. Once you feel this, you do not need to take any more enemas that day.

If after a week of daily enemas you have not felt or heard the gallbladder release, you may need to:

- increase the strength of the coffee. Do not exceed 2 tablespoons per cup.
- take slightly larger volume enemas
- take three enemas of 2 cups each or less

Coffee enemas can be used without the unsulfured molasses if tolerance is a problem. However, after taking the enemas for several weeks, you will probably be able to safely add it. Molasses aids in retaining the enema and increases detoxification efficiency.

Most people do not feel "wired" or hyper as a result of coffee enemas. Should you feel this way, or if you have palpitations or irregular heartbeats after a coffee enema, reduce the amount of coffee by half for a few days to a week. Caffeine blood levels were non-detectable.

Use coffee enemas as often as needed; the usual frequency is around three times per week. They may be used at any time to clear chemical overloads and allergic reactions.

CAUTION: People who have gallstones should not take coffee enemas.

OTHER CLEANSING METHODS   Castor oil packs are extremely beneficial in cleansing the liver. For instructions on the use of a castor oil pack, see Packs, earlier in this chapter. There are several commercial prepared liver cleansing and support products. We have found complex homeopathic products, such as PHP Liver Liquesence, to be extremely helpful for liver support and repair.

GALLBLADDER

The liver creates bile that helps to emulsify fats, using bipolar molecules (one end of the molecule is water-soluble and the other end is fat-soluble) to make the globules more assimilable. The bile produced by the liver is stored in the gallbladder, a pear-shaped sac on the underside of the liver.

If the cholesterol content of the bile becomes too high for the amounts of phospholipid and bile salts, gallstones form. This happens when the liver secretes too much cholesterol or the bile becomes highly concentrated in the gallbladder. Gallstones affect not only the gallbladder, but also the liver when the bile does not move.

A diet favorable for the gallbladder is moderately high in protein and low in refined carbohydrates. Take a B-complex vitamin and lecithin along with a liberal amount of vitamin E. Soybeans and eggs are rich in lecithin.

Fat Digestion   Poor fat digestion may be accompanied by nausea and soreness in the gallbladder area. To help this condition, prepare as a tea:

1 part milk thistle seed
1 part artichoke leaves
1 part dandelion root
½ part mugwort
½ part skullcap

Use 1 ounce of herbal combination in 1 pint water. Simmer 20 minutes. Remove from heat and let stand 10 minutes. Dose: up to ½ cup three times a day.

Gallbladder Decongestion   Hanna Kroeger, an herbalist from Boulder, Colorado, uses a 17th-century Austrian physician's formula for gallbladder decongestion. It is widely used today by various practitioners.

Before you start the cleanse, your bowels must be clean. It is sometimes suggested that patients ingest 3 to 4 capsules of hydrangea or hyssop twice a day for about a week before this cleanse. Adjust the dosage according to the results you receive. To alleviate nausea created by ingesting a large amount of oil at one time, an enema may be necessary during the cleanse.

Fast for two days, then consume only the following:

Day 1: 8 A.M. 1 glass (8 ounces) pure, organic preservative-free apple juice

10 A.M.   2 glasses
12 P.M.   2 glasses
2 P.M.   2 glasses
4 P.M.   2 glasses
6 P.M.   2 glasses
8 P.M.   2 glasses

Do not eat on this day.

Day 2: Follow the same routine as on Day 1. Do not eat on this day. At bedtime drink 4 ounces of olive oil. (You may wash down the oil with hot lemon or apple juice.)

As a rule, this decongestion formula starts to work the second day. You may find small stones and/or green mud in the fecal matter. The malic acid in the apple juice breaks down stagnant bile. This flush may be repeated in two months.

COLON

Even though the colon contains beneficial bacteria, unfavorable strains can be introduced through overuse of antibiotics and improper diet. Often, it is not the bacteria themselves that do the harm, but their wastes, which lodge in surrounding tissues. This creates a breeding ground for harmful bacteria and viruses and causes an imbalance in bowel flora. Even the improper balance of beneficial bacteria can cause problems, known as bowel dysbiosis.

Supplementation with *Lactobacillus acidophilus,* the bacteria normally present in the colon, will help re-establish balance. See Beneficial Bacteria in chapter 14 for a discussion of acidophilus treatment. Allergy extracts for pathogenic bowel bacteria help to cleanse the colon. Extracts also relieve allergic symptoms caused by these organisms.

Homeopathic bowel nosodes are helpful for intestinal dysbiosis. A nosode is a remedy prepared from an organism or diseased tissue. Bowel nosodes are prepared from stool cultures. They are so dilute that the actual organism is not in the remedy. Bowel nosodes are prescribed based on the percentages of organisms found in the stools of patients or on clinical indications.

Colon Cleansing   Colon cleansing is a controversial method of detoxification/cleansing. There seems to be no middle viewpoint; people are either very much in favor of it or violently opposed to it. Those who favor colon cleansing feel that the health of the body reflects the health of the colon. They further believe that colon cleansing, either with enemas or colonics, is necessary for good health.

Those opposed to colon cleansing feel that

there is no medical reason to irrigate the colon. Homeopaths feel this method causes loss of vital body fluids. Opponents of colon cleansing believe that proper diet, sufficient water, and exercise should allow you to move your bowels regularly. When the bowels move regularly, their natural physiological action should keep them clean and working well.

Approach any cleansing method with caution, determining the appropriateness of each method for you. Certainly, sensitive people should be very careful if they try this method.

The information presented in this section reflects both views. You will have to make your own decision regarding this cleansing method.

Fasting is sometimes advocated before a colon cleanse. During a fast, your eliminative organs remove concentrated and old, hard wastes. If any wastes remain in the colon, toxins are reabsorbed into the system, causing fever, earache, sore throat, headache, and many other symptoms.

ENEMAS   Colon cleansing may be accomplished by administering enemas, which flush the lower intestines. Substances generally used in enemas include water, coffee, herbal tea, mild soap solution, meat broth, chicken soup, wheatgrass juice, barley juice, chlorophyll, oil, or other nutritional substances.

General instructions for enemas:

- Use warm distilled or other tolerated water in the enema bag.
- Some people follow the warm water enema with a cool water enema to stimulate peristaltic action and to soak off more material.
- Lying on a comfortable surface, assume a knee-chest position to help water go through the colon.
- Always lubricate the end of the rectal nozzle or French catheter tube with vitamin E, petroleum jelly, or K-Y jelly.

- Insert the tube or nozzle just inside the rectum. For a French catheter, as water flows, gently insert the tube further— never force it. The maximum tube insertion is 18 to 24 inches.
- At the first urge or cramp, remove the tube and allow elimination.
- Always take some form of acidophilus, yogurt, buttermilk, or kefir afterward to replace natural bacteria of the colon.
- The frequency of enema use depends on the person's philosophy. Some people take enemas once a month for preventive health maintenance. Others take a series of enemas seasonally.

The following enemas may be helpful for the indicated conditions:

- For stimulation of the liver, kidneys, spleen, and pancreas. It will also help stop bleeding that sometimes occurs with tissue irritation during rapid elimination: ½ teaspoon cayenne to an enema bag of water.
- As a general cleanser and to help eliminate parasites and Candida: Blend one or two crushed garlic buds in 1 quart of tolerated water. Strain. Add enough tepid water to fill the enema bag. Repeat this process three times.
- To clear allergic reactions: Use 60 grams (8 level tablespoons) of *buffered* vitamin C per quart of tolerated water. Allow the enema to run in very slowly and retain the fluid as long as you can comfortably do so.
    WARNING: *Never use ascorbic acid in an enema.* Use only *buffered* forms of vitamin C.

COLONICS   Some colon therapists advocate the use of high colonics. They use specialized equipment to deliver the solution into the colon, and this treatment cleans the entire colon. However, these therapists must take great care in cleaning the equipment between clients. If the equipment is not properly sterilized, parasites can be passed from one person to another.

CAUTION: Sensitive individuals may find colonics a shock to their bodies and minds.

CLAY AND FIBER CLEANSE A colon cleanse composed of a fibrous material and a clay can remove years of accumulated, caked-on materials. These materials can interfere with the absorption of nutrients. Psyllium is a good fibrous material to use, in conjunction with bentonite or other clay. The psyllium attracts moisture into the bowel, improving bowel function. The moisture causes the psyllium to expand, filling the intestine. As it passes through the intestines, it drags out the stored waste that is not ordinarily excreted. The clay absorbs toxins and helps carry them out of the colon. Do not exceed three colon cleanses per year, and wait at least two months between cleanses.

Materials needed:
- bentonite clay (liquid solution)
- psyllium husks
- pint jar

Preparing the Cleanse Mix 1 tablespoon of the liquid bentonite solution in the pint jar with 4 ounces of tolerated water. (If you cannot find a liquid bentonite solution, you may make your own by combining 2 ounces of bentonite to 1 quart of water. Shake well and allow to stand for 12 hours before using.) Add 1 tablespoon of psyllium husks. Cover and shake well.

Taking the Cleanse Drink the above mixture quickly after you shake it. The longer it stands, the more it will clump. Follow with 8 ounces of water. Drink this mixture three times a day, between meals, for 3 to 4 days. Take no food two hours before or for two hours afterward.

Drink at least eight 8-ounce glasses of water a day.

This mixture can be constipating. Should you become constipated, take extra vitamin C and magnesium. You may also need to use a plain water enema, or the coffee enema.

Some people feel abdominal discomfort the first day or two of the cleanse when the psyllium has expanded in the bowel. Many people pass various particles and substances of varying size and shape. Some report long casings that may be mucosal debris and dead cells covering the surface of the intestinal walls.

The colon cleanse will also remove organisms from the gut. This helps reduce the level of unwanted bacteria, yeast, and parasites. Take acidophilus powder for at least five days after the cleanse. See Beneficial Bacteria in chapter 14 for directions on taking acidophilus.

Exercise Movement during exercise creates a series of light shocks, thus creating reflexive movements of the colon. The active play of children is a perfect example of this concept. Skipping, hopping, and jumping movements are especially good. They initiate sudden, vigorous contractions of abdominal muscles and vigorous diaphragm movements, creating an accordian-like action in the intestines.

Many people who have constipation do not exercise. Researchers tell us that our bowels will not move unless we move. Exercise helps keep abdominal muscles healthy and muscle tone optimal. The following exercises are particularly helpful to combat constipation:

- hill climbing
- horseback riding
- climbing a ladder or stairs
- tennis
- rowing, with chest held high, and giving the trunk a strong backward movement
- medicine ball bouncing, so that the trunk muscles get vigorous action

- chopping, digging, swinging, mowing
- folk and square dancing

Fiber Fiber, sometimes called roughage or bulk, helps to relieve constipation. It absorbs water in the large intestine and makes stools larger, softer, and easier to pass. Food fiber is soluble and is best for your body. High-fiber foods include grains and bran, fresh fruits with skin on, dried fruit, raw vegetables, legumes, nuts, and seeds. Peeled, cooked, or puréed fruits and vegetables have less useful fiber than those consumed raw.

By increasing high-fiber food in your diet, fiber supplementation may not be necessary. Should you begin taking a fiber supplement, add it slowly and increase your water intake. You may have some cramping, diarrhea, or gas at first. Fiber supplements can cause dehydration, and minerals are lost with the water. They can also decrease the absorption of dietary protein.

Laxatives Commercial laxatives can make a constipation problem worse. They are addictive and overused. Frequent use can lead to vitamin and mineral deficiencies. Laxatives can weaken the muscles and damage the colon. If you need help, ground psyllium seeds are a concentrated source of fiber. Psyllium is available at health food stores.

If you take vitamin C to bowel tolerance every day, you will not be constipated. Even if you do not take vitamin C in this manner, extra doses of vitamin C help relieve constipation. For more discussion on vitamin C, see chapter 14.

Extra magnesium also relieves constipation. Magnesium is the active portion of Epsom salts and Milk of Magnesia. However, these laxatives are harsh. Just increasing your magnesium supplementation should clear constipation.

Fluid Many people are constipated or have difficult bowel movements because they do not consume enough liquid. Liquids, particularly water, keep the stools soft. Stools become small and hard when liquid intake is too low. Coffee and caffeinated soft drinks can deplete the body of water because caffeine acts a diuretic.

There is controversy over how much water you should drink. Some physicians say six to eight glasses per day. Some homeopaths feel that this much water overworks the kidneys. Certainly you should always drink when you are thirsty, and the bulk of your fluid intake should be water.

Breathing

We consider breathing an important cleansing method. It can help to cleanse the body physically as well as spiritually, mentally, and emotionally. If we learn to regulate our breathing and expand our usual capacities, it can be a master key to health.

Breathing is the only function of the body that we can perform both consciously and unconsciously. It is controlled by two sets of nerves, the involuntary (autonomic) nervous system, and the voluntary nervous system. Many illnesses and health problems come from an imbalance of the autonomic nervous system. By working with the breath, we can affect the autonomic nervous system and many of its involuntary functions.

Breathing also is directly connected to our emotions. Our emotional state affects the speed, depth, regularity, and noise level at which we breathe. Anger can be calmed by breathing slowly, deeply, quietly, and regularly. Clearing anger by changing breathing is in effect an emotional cleansing. In addition, the physical aftereffects of anger are prevented.

Dr. L. M. McEwen of London, England, reports that many people with environmental illness suffer from hyperventilation or dysventilation. Some of the most incapacitating symptoms experienced by these people are caused by the chronic cerebral lactic acidosis that follows hyperventilation. Once this pattern of breathing is established, it becomes self-perpetuating. Food and chemical allergies as well as candidiasis can contribute to hyperventilation, and asthmatics frequently hyperventilate. Hyperventilation encourages histamine release by the alterations it causes in the immune system. Learning appropriate breathing techniques can speed the recovery of many environmentally sensitive people.

The more air we move in and out of our lungs, the healthier we are. The delivery of oxygen and removal of carbon dioxide determines the efficiency of functioning for all body systems. The body cannot cleanse itself, heal itself, or maintain life without the oxygen supplied by breathing. (For more information on oxygen see Oxygen Therapy, earlier in this chapter.)

Breathing also affects the circulation of lymph. The motions of respiration mechanically pump lymphatic fluid and assist circulation. If breathing is restricted, fluid builds up, causing edema and the buildup of waste products from cellular metabolism.

YOGA

Yoga is a system of breathing movements and postures that has been practiced for over 6000 years. Many different forms of movement developed, in response to climate, culture, body constitution, lifestyle, and the physical environment. Each form of yoga has a particular emphasis, but will incorporate facets of other forms. Some of the more physical yoga forms are:

- *Hatha*: Concentration on postures and movement, stretching and toning the body.
- *Kundalini*: Concentration on the spinal column, strengthening and balancing the nervous system.
- *Pranayama*: Concentration on breathing, strengthening and balancing of the respiratory system.

The nerves that go to all parts of our body branch out from the spinal cord. Through postures and breathing, yoga focuses on this all-important area. Spine flexibility requires that the spine be stretched in all its six possible directions: bending forward, backward, to each side, and twisting to each side. Stretching is the key to relieving tension and releasing energy.

Yoga has been described as a methodical manipulation of the body. The postures and routines emphasize proper warm-up with gradual advancement of posture difficulty. Poses are sequenced so that both sides are worked adjunctively, providing a complementary balance.

Physical balance, relaxation, alertness, calm centeredness, and harmony are integral to the discipline of yoga. All movements are performed slowly, rhythmically, and with full attention from the center of one's being. A pose is assumed and then held while the practitioner "feels" the body and the energy generated by the position. Breathing fully, quietly, and calmly is also an integral part of holding the position.

One common yoga routine is the Complete Breath. This again supports the belief that the breath is our life force. It is intimately related to the amount of life energy we have, generate, and store. The breath must be deep, rhythmic, slow, and expansive. At the peak of the inhalation, there should be a slight pause before exhalation, which must also be slow, rhythmic, and deep. All yoga postures are practiced with this manner of breathing.

Yoga reverses the effects of gravity's downward pull on the vital organs and glands in the body. Inversion increases blood supply to organs and glands.

- The Head Stand affects the brain and pituitary gland.

- The Shoulder Stand involves the heart and thyroid.
- The Locust posture strengthens the reproductive organs and glands.
- The Cobra and the Bow postures stimulate the kidneys.
- The Abdominal Lift offers a type of natural massage for the stomach, colon, intestines, liver, kidneys, gall bladder, and pancreas.

Discipline in the practice of yoga is not limited to just setting aside a time to exercise. In addition to learning and coordinating the various body postures and breathing, patience with your own performance is necessary. The body experiences changes as each new posture creates the opportunity for growth and expansion. There will be days of practice when the body will not perform to the standard of the previous day. This apparent plateau is nothing more than the body preparing to take the next step forward to increased capabilities.

BREATHING EXERCISE

In his book *Natural Health, Natural Medicine,* Dr. Andrew Weil recommends the following simple exercise to relieve anxiety, stress, and emotional upset:

- Sit with your back straight.
- Place the tip of your tongue against the ridge of tissue behind your upper front teeth. Keep your tongue there for the entire exercise.
- Exhale completely through your mouth. You will make a noise as you do so.
- Close your mouth and inhale quietly through your nose to a count of four.
- Hold your breath for a count of seven.
- Exhale completely through your mouth to a count of eight, making a noise as you do so.
- This is one cycle. Repeat the cycle for three more times, making a total of four breaths.

Begin this exercise by doing it twice a day. As you become accustomed to it, you cannot do it too frequently. Always keep the ratio at 4:7:8, regardless of the speed with which you do the exercise.

Should you notice a shift in consciousness after four of these breaths, it is a sign that you are affecting your involuntary nervous system. Make this exercise a tool; you always have it available wherever you need it. Use it to help you in stressful situations, and to help you go to sleep.

18

Toxins and Cleansing in Children

Exposure Risks for Infants and Children

The fetus, newborn, and young child are unusually susceptible to chemicals from the environment. This is because of their larger surface area, rapid cell division, higher metabolic rate and oxygen consumption, and immature host defenses.

The fetus is especially susceptible to the effects of chemicals. Chemicals that can affect fetal development may not be toxic to the mother (for example, thalidomide). Developmental abnormalities and cancer occurring after birth can be caused by prenatal exposure (for example, alcohol). Fetal exposure to chemicals has been documented to cause abnormalities in growth, birth defects, or death.

The first trimester is the time of greatest vulnerability because of the formation and rapid growth of organs. Unfortunately, many women do not realize they are pregnant during this time and are not careful about exposures.

Relative to their weight, a child's body surface area is about three times larger than that of an adult. For this reason, children absorb a greater percentage of toxins from skin, respiratory, and gastrointestinal sources.

- Drugs applied to the skin are absorbed two and a half times as much on newborns as on adults.

- Children absorb more lead from the gastrointestinal tract than do adults.
- Children have a higher metabolic rate than adults, and they breathe twice as much air as an adult per body weight, causing higher exposure to air pollutants.

Host defenses, including the immune system, the organs of defense (lungs, skin, and gastrointestinal tract), and the detoxification systems, are immature in the fetus, newborns, and children. Newborns also have immature kidneys. Skin absorption of toxins can be increased by occlusion (prevention of skin breathing by plastic or similar substance) or when the skin is damaged. Diaper use causes skin occlusion, and diaper rashes are common in infants. Premature babies' skin is more permeable than that of adults.

The absorption of chemicals through the gastrointestinal tract is higher in children than in adults. Children have lower levels of the detoxification enzymes for Phase I and Phase II. Conjugation with glucuronic acid, a Phase II enzymatic reaction, has been documented to be slower in newborns than in adults. This conjugation capability does not become mature until about 3 months after birth. Hexachlorophene and PCBS are conjugated with glucuronic acid. Infants cannot detoxify these and other xenobiotics efficiently until their conjugation capability has matured. (See discussion on Phase I and Phase II detoxification in chapter 3.)

Children under five have a faster respiratory rate than adults, so they inhale more toxins. Children also tend to do more mouth breathing and bypass the nose, which can filter out some of the particles.

The immune system is not fully developed at birth, especially immunoglobulins. Adult levels of IgG occur by age five to six years. The levels of IgM reach those of an adult by one year of age. Children also tend to mouth objects, play in dirt, and spend more time on the ground than do adults. This results in greater exposure to metals, such as lead, solvents, and pesticides.

Children's cells divide more rapidly than adults'. They are more prone to cell mutations and the subsequent risk of cancer. The brain continues to grow after birth, so children are more at risk from neurotoxins than adults. The most rapid brain growth and most susceptible period is during the first two years of life, when nerve sheaths are becoming coated with a fatty substance called myelin. Myelination continues through adolescence.

TOXIC EXPOSURES

Foods and Plants Children may be sensitive to many foods, just as adults are. Children who are breast fed may receive food antigens in the breast milk.

Children are often more sensitive to food poisoning than adults, because they have higher exposure on a body weight basis. A recent outbreak of *Escherichia coli* infection from hamburger affected the children more seriously than the adults, and all the deaths were of children.

Healthy eating tips should be followed by children as well as adults. Children learn eating habits from adults. If adults eat in a healthy manner, their children are likely to eat in a healthy manner. See Healthy Eating Tips in chapter 5.

Calamine lotion and colloidal oatmeal can be used for children who have poison ivy, oak, or sumac rashes.

Water Children should use safe water. On trips to other countries, use bottled water. Avoid using ice cubes and brushing the teeth with water from the foreign country. Children may be more sensitive to intestinal parasites than are adults.

They can be become dehydrated more easily than adults, and the lower their body weight, the higher the risk of dehydration. Children who are dehydrated cry without tears, have a dry mouth, and have decreased urine output. Parents should give as much fluid as possible. If the child cannot or will not drink fluids, rehydrating intravenous treatment may be necessary.

Because children are more sensitive to lead, run the water for a few minutes in the morning to decrease the concentration of lead. Also run water from drinking fountains for a few minutes before allowing children to drink.

Air Because younger children have a higher respiratory rate and higher metabolic rate, they are more sensitive to the effects of air pollution. Asthma affects more than three million children in the United States. It is the leading cause of absenteeism from school and work. Between 1980 and 1987, the incidence of asthma went up 29% and deaths related to asthma increased 31%. In Canada, as well as in Japan, as many as one out of five children has asthma.

Asthmatic children may wheeze with exposure to such irritants as perfume, fireplace smoke, and cigarette smoke. Children exposed to cigarette smoke have 50% more respiratory infections and a lower rate of increase in lung function as they grow older. Infants with smoking parents are more likely to be hospitalized for bronchitis and pneumonia in the first year of life. Infants whose parents smoke are more likely to die from Sudden Infant Death Syndrome. Children of smokers have more chronic coughs, ear infections, and behavior problems.

A study reported by Dr. Marvin Boris of New York in 1985 has shown that children who live in homes with gas stoves have 15% more respiratory problems and ear infections than children who live in homes with electric stoves. Parents can decrease the use of gas and wood stoves and fireplaces, and strictly control wood burning in their homes.

To decrease allergens in a bedroom, do not use carpets. Do not allow pets to sleep in the bedroom. Stuffed animals should be washable in order to control dust accumulation. Use washable curtains, and keep clothes in closets with the doors shut. Remove dust catchers, such as pictures and books, from the bedroom. Cover the mattresses and pillows with barrier cloth for children who have severe dust mite sensitivities. Dust the bedroom every day.

Parents can use safe cleaning supplies and avoid using air fresheners, solvents, and pesticides. Air cleaners will help to remove chemicals, pollens, odors, dust, mold, bacteria, and viruses from the air.

Solvents   Children are more sensitive to solvents than adults because of their larger body surface area relative to their body weight. In addition, children may inhale more solvent fumes because of their higher respiratory rate. Whenever possible, use nontoxic substitutes instead of solvent-containing materials. Children should not be in the same area when solvent-containing sprays are used. Some furniture polishes contain mineral spirits, which can be very poisonous.

Keep solvents out of the reach of children, and never place them in a familiar container, such as a soft drink bottle. If a child swallows a solvent, do not induce vomiting because of the risk of pneumonia from aspiration. Call your physician or your state or provincial poison control center for advice.

Nurseries for newborn babies should not be freshly painted or have brand new carpet placed shortly before the baby is born or while the baby is still young. We have seen very sensitive infants who were born after their parents moved into a new mobile home or a new house. The mobile homes seem to be worse, but any new home can be dangerous for infants.

Children can use allergy extracts and homeopathic remedies for chemical sensitivities as needed.

Pesticides   Use nontoxic pest control methods. Follow the measures outlined in chapter 6 to help control insects and keep your home as pest-free as possible.

Organic gardening is recommended, both as a fun hobby for the child and for the health of the harvest. Recently, the U.S. National Academy of Science has recommended that changes be made to regulate pesticides used on food products to reflect the "unique characteristics of the diets of infants and children." Their report states that children may be uniquely sensitive to pesticide residues. Infants and children consume more calories per body weight and eat a smaller variety of foods than do adults.

The Academy also suggests that the Environmental Protection Agency should make decisions based on health issues rather than agricultural production. The Environmental Working Group, a nonprofit research organization, reports that most of a person's exposure to pesticides occurs by age five because children eat more fruits and vegetables in relation to their body weight than adults. The group states that the average child receives up to 35% of his or her entire lifetime dose of some carcinogenic pesticides by the age of five.

Metals   Lead poisoning is the most common type of metal poisoning in children. Lead causes potent central nervous system effects in children. Children are exposed to lead in air, food, and water. Intravenous EDTA and intramuscular BAL help remove lead from the kidneys. Succimer (DMSA) was approved for use in children in 1991, and it can be given orally. (See treatment for lead poisoning in chapter 6.) Extra vitamin C, thiamine, and zinc (15 to 20 mg a day) helps protect children against lead toxicity and deposition. Homeopathic remedies can be given to children for lead poisoning.

Children eating a diet high in whole grains and vegetables will ingest extra vitamin C, thiamine, and zinc, which decreases cadmium absorption and retention. They will also get adequate copper, fiber, and vitamin E. Because most children do not eat enough of these foods, a multivitamin is recommended. Pectin is found in fruits and helps protect against cadmium absorption. Homeopathic remedies can be used for children who have cadmium poisoning. For further discussion of cadmium, see chapter 6.

For mercury poisoning, children can be treated with BAL, penicillamine, and DMSA. Children can take extra nutrients, such as vitamin C, glutathione, calcium, magnesium, iron, zinc, and manganese. Homeopathic remedies can also be used for mercury poisoning. For more information on mercury and mercury poisoning, see chapter 6.

With aluminum poisoning, nutrients and homeopathic remedies can be used. When children are given selenium, doses have to be monitored closely and should not exceed 125 micrograms a day. See chapter 6 for more information on aluminum and aluminum poisoning.

Organisms Allergy extracts can be used for bacteria, parasites, and viruses in infants and children. Homeopathic medicines are well tolerated by infants and children. Acyclovir can be used for small children with severe viral infections, and it has been safely used for children with chicken pox. Steam inhalation can aid breathing during viral infections, if children are taken into a bathroom with a hot shower running. This method has been used for children with croup for years. The heat reduces the swellings and makes breathing easier. Breast feeding can give babies protection against viruses that cause diarrhea and vomiting. Breast-fed babies do not have to drink extra water, so they avoid ingesting contaminated water.

Hydrogen peroxide can be used for skin or nail fungal infections. Children can take caprystatin (if they can swallow pills or tablets), mycocidin, nystatin, diflucan, nizoral, germanium, Coenzyme Q_{10}, mathake and taheebo tea, garlic, and essential fatty acids.

Radiation Infants and children should not sunbathe. Suncreens are not recommended until infants are at least six months of age. Even then, it is better to use light-weight cotton clothes and a wide-brimmed hat as protection. This can minimize a child's exposure to sunscreen, to which some children are sensitive. Blistering sunburns in childhood are associated with melanoma, a skin cancer, in adults. For this reason, protect children's skin from the sun as much as possible.

Children should not sleep next to electrical appliances. If possible, a child's bed should face north or east. We have found some children who have awakened very irritable in the morning and who have improved with changing the position of their bed. Other children have improved when a magnet was placed under their pillow. Place the north side of the magnet toward the child. Children can wear diodes without problems. See Electromagnetic Fields in chapter 8 for more information.

Natural Body Functions Older children who exercise frequently may experience muscle pain from excess lactic acid. Homeopathic remedies can be used for these children.

Children with a congenital defect in their urea cycle enzymes may develop an excess of ammonia. A low protein diet is necessary for these children.

Children can develop an excess of free radicals by the same mechanisms that occur in adults. Antioxidant vitamins can be used safely in proper doses in children to combat excess free radicals (see below).

CLEANSING, BALANCING, AND PREVENTIVE TECHNIQUES

We recommend that parents consult a qualified health practitioner to confirm a confusing or unclear diagnosis, to rule out complications, to investigate any sudden or unexpected change in a child's condition, and to deal with any life-threatening emergency. Parents who learn about natural medicines are more involved in their children's health and become more sensitive to their child's physical and emotional temperament. A parent will become more attuned to the early warning signs of illness in their child.

Homeopathy Homeopathy can be used safely in newborns, infants, and children. In babies, a poppy-seed-sized pellet can be placed in the mouth and will rapidly dissolve. Even if a child spits out a homeopathic remedy, if it touched his mouth he has received a dose. Usually a 6X dose is recommended for infants and children. In acute conditions, 30C doses may be used. However, for an acute condition or an emergency, any available strength would be acceptable.

Allergy Extracts Allergy extracts have been used safely in infants. Neutralizing doses of allergy extracts can be given sublingually or by injection. Food, pollen, and chemical extracts can be used for infants and children, and are very safe. The traditional injectable allergy extracts, with the same doses and build-up for each patient, must be administered in a physician's office as there is a risk of anaphylaxis. These shots are usually not tolerated well by children until age five or older because of the frequency of the injections.

Detox Baths and Saunas Detox baths can be used safely by children and adolescents. Plain water baths, Epsom salt baths, and apple cider vinegar baths have all been used safely by children. Children have used saunas safely in Sweden and Finland for hundreds of years, with shorter times and lower temperatures than are used by adults. If a child does sauna, monitor the heart rate.

Hydrotherapy Baths, other than cold baths, can be used for children. A plain hot-water detoxification bath is a form of hydrotherapy. Cold and hot compresses can be applied. A full-body cold pack is not recommended for children.

Organ Cleansing Neither organ cleansing nor enemas are recommended for children. They are considered too harsh and invasive. Grated flaxseeds can be added to a drink or given as a purée to help with constipation. Flaxseeds are essentially tasteless, whereas flax oil has a definite taste.

Fasting Complete fasting should not be used for small children. Older children can tolerate the fasting drinks. A child will self-select a diet of from one to three puréed fruits or vegetables from cleansing diet choices offered by the parent. Older children have fasted for religious reasons without adverse effects. This type of fast is usually from sunrise to sundown. Children who have insulin-dependent diabetes or any serious disease should not fast.

Macrobiotics Children can safely eat a macrobiotic diet. The diet will be natural, wholesome, free from chemicals, simple sugars, saturated fats, and processed food. On the macrobiotic diet, children will:

- Eat more complex carbohydrates and fewer simple sugars.
- Eat more vegetable protein than animal protein.
- Reduce the intake of fat.
- Have less saturated fat in their diet.
- Have a better balance between vitamins, minerals, and other nutrients.
- Use fewer artificially processed and chemically treated foods.
- Use more foods in whole form than in refined or partial form.
- Increase the amount of foods eaten with natural fiber.

Studies show that children on a balanced vegetarian diet grow adequately and are healthy.

Herbs   Many herbs can be used safely for children, but should be chosen with care. For the untrained person, consultation with an expert in herbs is recommended. Some herbs have a very narrow range of safety. In many cases, these herbs have also been prepared as homeopathic remedies, and for children the homeopathic remedies are recommended.

Rarely, a child may be sensitive or allergic to a particular herb. If a child shows an unusual reactions after taking an herb, stop the treatment and consult an expert in herbs for advice. For children, the standard dose of a dried herb is one-quarter to one-half the adult dose of one heaping teaspoon of dried herbs. The dose for infants is one teaspoon of infusion (tea) or decoction. For chronic conditions, the dose is three times a day, and for acute conditions the herbs may be taken every two to four hours.

For herbal tinctures, the dose for children is two to four drops three times a day. For infants, one drop three times a day is recommended. The tinctures should be mixed in 2 to 3 ounces of water, stirred, and then the child can sip it. The tinctures should never be given undiluted because the alcohol can burn the mouth.

There are other ways to give herbs to children or babies. The tincture can be rubbed into the skin of the abdomen at three times the dose recommended above. It can be rubbed on the bottoms of the feet at the recommended dose. The herbal preparation may also be put in the bath water at 10 to 20 times the normal dose. Because a child's skin is more porous than an adult's, the herbs can be absorbed this way.

Aromatic herbs, which contain volatile oils that give them an agreeable odor and stimulating qualities, can be put in a vaporizer for inhalation. They will also cross the breast milk, and an infant can be given a dose this way.

When choosing herbs for children, taste is important. Use the sweeter tasting herbs. Once a child tastes a strong herb, he or she will be reluctant to take another dose. Onion and garlic syrups and glycerin have been used as herbal vehicles to improve the taste.

Nutrients   Children may take extra nutrients. For children, no more than 5000 to 10,000 units a day of vitamin A are recommended. Vitamin A can be toxic if used in excess doses. Beta-carotene is the precursor of vitamin A, and it is not toxic at all. The only side effect from beta-carotene is a yellow color to the skin, known as carotenemia. Carotenemia does not cause any clinical symptoms and can be reversed by reducing or stopping the excess intake of beta-carotene. Babies who eat large amounts of carrots, squash, and sweet potatoes have a tendency to develop carotenemia.

Excess amounts of vitamin D (over 400 IU in nondeficient states) can cause excessive calcification of bones or organs of the body, but rickets (a vitamin D deficiency) is more common in children. Premature babies are prone to develop rickets, and various diseases of calcium metabolism can also cause rickets.

No more than 400 IU of vitamin E should be given to children.

Vitamin B$_3$ may cause transient tingling or flushing if taken in excess amounts. A small dose, such as 100 mg, can be used and built up as tolerated (see Hubbard Method of Detoxification in chapter 2). If children take larger doses of vitamin B$_3$, levels of liver enzymes should be monitored. Vitamin B$_6$ has been reported to cause peripheral neuropathy when used in huge doses, such as 1200 to 2000 mg a day for extended periods of time. Vitamin B$_6$ is safe for children in doses from 25 to 100 mg.

Vitamin C has been recommended in doses of 20 mg per pound of body weight per day, but can be taken by children in doses close to bowel tolerance. Vitamin doses are usually recommended at one-third to one-half the adult dosages, depending on the child's body weight. This can be estimated using an adult typical body weight of 120 to 140 pounds.

Bodywork Bodywork can be done safely on children. Children should be comfortable with the practitioner. Sometimes they show nervousness by giggling and acting silly. Gentle stroking massage techniques are recommended for children and infants. Some of these techniques can be done by the parents. The physical contact of this gentle massage is beneficial to both the parents and the child.

Massage techniques have been used safely with premature babies, resulting in better neurological development and weight gain. Massage has positive benefits for many hormone levels, promotes bonding, and eases the discomforts of the baby.

Massage releases tension and stimulates the skin, which is necessary for adequate organic and psychological development. Skin stimulation increases cardiac output, promotes respiration, and develops the efficiency of the GI tract of infants. Massage also teaches babies ways to relax their bodies when stressed.

Use natural cold-pressed fruit and/or vegetable oils for massage in infants and children. Baby oils have a petroleum base (mineral oil), which is distilled from crude petroleum. Apricot kernel and almond oil are two oils recommended. Parents who massage their children must be relaxed as they massage.

Reflexology can be very relaxing for children, especially if they are too excited to fall asleep at bedtime. Acupressure can be safely done on children. For acupuncture, the children should be old enough not to be frightened by the acupuncture needle. Rolfing is not recommended for children until they are older. Meridian bodywork and shiatsu can be done safely on children.

Exercise Children can do walking, running, swimming, bike riding, aerobic dancing, and cross-country skiing. Those as young as four to five years of age are able to cross-country ski. Some children are able to swim at an even younger age.

Children should not be forced into exercise. They seem to be motivated if their parents exercise and serve as role models. They should be encouraged in the aerobic exercises that they enjoy, not what the parents want them to enjoy.

Dr. Kenneth Cooper of Dallas, Texas, recommends that children do *not* begin a disciplined long-distance aerobic program until age ten. This allows time for their bones and muscles to become fairly well developed. He recommends that children should be tested for physical fitness in fourth grade, and by seventh grade an aerobic exercise program should be a part of a child's lifestyle.

Plasters/Packs/Poultices Plasters, packs, and poultices can be used safely by children. Children may not need to use the plaster or poultice as long as adults. For example, garlic poultices (garlic crushed and mixed with oil) can be used overnight on the sole of the foot for coughs.

Oxygen   Hyperbaric oxygen therapy has been used for children with carbon monoxide poisoning. Carbon monoxide poisoning has occurred in children who ride in the back end of a pickup truck. Hyperbaric oxygen may be used for older children who have decompression sickness (the "bends"). It may also be used for other conditions at the discretion of the treating physician.

Hydrogen peroxide should not be taken orally by children or given intravenously to children. It can be used topically on small areas of skin, and as a diluted mouthwash when children are old enough to be able to gargle. Ozone can be used topically on children in a bath, but should not be used in any other manner. Stabilized oxygen therapy can be used for localized skin care in children, but should not be given internally.

Breathing Exercises   Breathing exercises are safe and effective, and can be used with all age groups when children are old enough to understand the directions. Infants automatically do abdominal breathing, which is said to be the ideal way to breathe. Yoga can be performed by children old enough to understand the directions.

Chelation Therapy   Chelation therapy for atherosclerosis is not used in children. Chelation therapy has been used in children for lead poisoning, and EDTA and BAL have been used intravenously and intramuscularly, respectively. DMSA has been used as an oral chelation agent.

Dental Work   Dental hygiene should begin as soon as teeth erupt. Until children are six to seven years of age, their tooth brushing should be monitored and/or done by an adult. If children are not too chemically sensitive, they may have their molars sealed with a dental sealant. You may request that your dentist not use amalgam fillings in your child's teeth.

The amount of toothpaste shown on toothbrushes in advertisements contains enough fluoride to be toxic to young children. Use only a very small amount of fluoride-containing toothpaste. Other toothpastes, available at health food stores, are preferable to a fluoride-containing toothpaste. Baking soda on a damp toothbrush makes a good toothpowder.

Some dentists use fluoride treatments for children to prevent tooth decay. There is controversy over the safety of these treatments and whether they are of benefit after age 11.

19

Current Medical Treatments and Detoxification

Surgery

Many health problems can be prevented by proper diet, nutrition, exercise, and early noninvasive treatment.

Too many surgeries are the result of ignoring early signs and symptoms of disease, with nothing being done to help the situation until it is too late.

However, there are circumstances under which surgery not only is necessary, but unavoidable. Broken bones must be set, and more complicated breaks may require surgical procedures. A ruptured appendix must be removed before the person develops peritonitis. Some congenital defects must be surgically repaired. Intestinal blockages must be opened or removed, and hernias must be repaired. Detached retinas must be reattached, and cataracts must be removed.

Regardless of the medical condition and the reason for the surgery, you will encounter toxins both in the hospital and the operating room. If properly approached, exposures to these toxins can be minimized and the toxic after-effects of the surgery and medications can be cleansed.

HOSPITAL ARRANGEMENTS

Many preparations and requests can be made before surgery that can lower your toxic expo-sures. Although most U.S. hospitals are non-smoking, many allow patients to smoke in their rooms and have special smoking areas for both patients and visitors. If at all possible, insist on a "no smoking" private room. If you have to share a room, insist that your roommate be a nonsmoker. In Canada, smoking is only permitted in outdoor areas of hospitals.

You will have no control over the gifts, flowers, or books your roommate may receive, but request that no scented products be used.

Talk to the surgeon and anesthesiologist and advise them of any medication sensitivities you may have. Also discuss any other medical problems you have, such as asthma or diabetes. Find out what medications and anesthetic they plan to use. If testing is available to you, have these substances tested before your surgery to determine which ones are safe for you and to find safe alternatives.

Discuss any medications you are taking, including allergy extracts. You will be unable to take these substances while you are in the hospital unless the surgeon specifically puts an order in your chart for you to do so. Ask the surgeon to write this order and have him or her also include any vitamin and mineral supplements you might need. Request that oxygen be available to you in your hospital room, along with an order in your chart that you may use it when you feel it necessary. Oxygen helps clear allergic reactions and helps your body cleanse itself of toxins.

Talk to the hospital dietitian and discuss any food allergies or dietary requirements that you may have. Do not cause confusion by giving too many restrictions; just list the major problems. Suggest that whole, unprocessed foods be served, and ask that your snacks be fresh fruit. Inspect each meal to be sure it does not contain foods you must avoid.

If cleaning supplies are a problem for you, schedule a talk with the housekeeping department of the hospital. Request that they do not use bleach, disinfectants, detergents, soaps, or room deodorizers in your room while you are in the hospital. Request that hot water and baking soda be used instead. If they are willing, you could provide a cleaner that is safe for you.

An air cleaner is helpful in maintaining the purity of the air in a hospital room. If you want to use an air cleaner, ask if it needs to be inspected by anyone before you use it. Some hospitals require that the plug and wiring of any electrical appliance used in a hospital room be inspected first. Also, if you want to use your own bedding, you must discuss it with housekeeping and laundry.

If you have allergies to flowers, plants, or molds, talk to the nurses on the floor where your room will be. They can ensure that live plants will not be placed in your room. Extremely sensitive people may need to request that nurses and aides not wear perfumes, scented hand lotion, scented deodorant, or scented hair spray.

Your admitting physician or an environmental physician can assist if you experience difficulty having your requests met.

PREPARING FOR SURGERY

For several weeks before your surgery, avoid all substances to which you are allergic, as well as toxic exposures. You want to be as strong as possible when you enter the hospital. Increase your intake of vitamin C. It will strengthen your immune system, promote healing, and lessen pain. However, do not take it the night before surgery as vitamin C can lessen the effects of anesthesia. Resume taking it after surgery as soon as approved by your surgeon.

Stop vitamin E two days before the surgery and do not take it for five to six days afterward. High amounts of vitamin E could potentially contribute to excessive bleeding during and after surgery. Be certain you are taking Coenzyme Q_{10} and GeOxy 132. Both these supplements act as buffers against the effects of hypoxia (oxygen deficiency) during surgery. They also combat the free radicals released by damaged tissue.

Arrange for family or friends to sit with you during the first two days and nights after your surgery. Their support is very important, and they can watch for and prevent exposures while you are unable to be vigilant. Be certain they are aware of all the foods and substances you need to avoid.

RECOVERING FROM SURGERY

After surgery, move around as soon as your surgeon gives you permission. This will prevent fluid from collecting in your lungs, which can cause such complications as pneumonia. Muscles, nerves, bones, and body functions can suffer even after short periods of inactivity. Begin walking slowly, and increase the speed and the length of your walks as your strength permits. Most hospital halls have rails on the walls. You can hold on to these if necessary while you take your strolls.

Be careful of your diet after surgery. Avoid empty calorie foods, and eat quality food. Avoid prepared foods and concentrate on fresh fruits, vegetables, meats, and fish. Eat several smaller meals throughout the day, avoiding large meals at one sitting. Your digestive organs require large amounts of energy to digest large meals. Your energy needs to be available for healing your body. Eating smaller meals reduces the energy requirement of your digestive organs while still providing nourishment for your body.

Allow yourself to rest. Our bodies heal while we sleep and rest. Do not push yourself to recover too quickly. Everyone has his or her own speed of recovery. Give your body and your immune system the time needed to recover from the stress and exposures of surgery.

CLEANSING, BALANCING, AND PREVENTIVE TECHNIQUES

Exercise, GeOxy 132, Coenzyme Q_{10}, and increased water intake will help to detoxify the anesthetic and medications in your body. Vitamin C taken orally or intravenously will also help cleanse your body of anesthetic and medications. Vitamin E taken orally and applied topically helps to prevent scars after surgery. Pantothenic acid (B_5) helps regain intestinal motility after intestinal surgery.

Several homeopathic remedies help cleanse the body of anesthetics. *Phosphorus* and *Aceticum acidum* both help with anesthetic poisoning. *Phosphorus* is of particular value when there is weakness, emaciation, anemia, and vertigo after surgery.

Other homeopathic remedies help with various problems that may be encountered after surgery.

- *Graphites*: prevents keloids after surgery
- *Strontium carbonicum*: for surgical shock, post-operative problems, exhaustion after surgery, bone pain, and never well since surgery.
- *Pyrogenium*: for fever after surgery
- *Carbo vegetabilis* or *Carbo animalis*: for coma after surgery
- *China*: for post-operative gas
- *Staphysagria*: for severe pain after breast surgery
- *Arnica*: for discomfort of bedridden patient, trauma of respirator
- *Ledum*: for hematomas from intravenous sites and bedsores
- *Hypericum*: helps healing after pelvic surgery

Post-surgery trauma is helped by the following herbal combination, using equal amounts of each herb. For those who tolerate herbs, this blend provides therapeutic support during recuperation. It can be used as a tea or taken in capsules.

Red clover	Burdock root
Licorice root	Cascara sagrada bark
Oregon grape root	Sarsaparilla root
Stillingia	Prickly ash bark
Kelp	Buckthorn bark

Radiation Treatment

Radiation is used both for diagnostic and therapeutic procedures. Treatment includes the administration of radioactive substances in the body as well as X-rays.

X-rays, radioactive cobalt, or radium are employed to treat cancer. The radiation must be directed at the cancerous cells and offshoots so that the tumor is destroyed, but there is minimal damage to normal cells. Normal tissue should survive and recover from the treatment.

Debate continues over whether there is a dose of radiation small enough to be safe. For this reason, do not let a health professional X-ray you without good reason. Medical and dental X-rays and fluoroscopic examinations are excellent diagnostic tools when they are needed. Unfortunately, they are greatly overused in both the medical and dental professions. Be certain that your medical or dental care cannot proceed without an X-ray before you agree to one.

The one exception to this is mammograms. The benefits of early detection of breast cancer probably outweigh the dangers of exposure for women at risk for this disease. Be certain that the equipment used for your mammogram delivers low-dose radiation. Ask the technician or radiologist how many millirads of radiation are being delivered to the center of your breast. The amount should be in the range of 1000 millirads. If it is more than this, do not have the mammogram done on that equipment.

CLEANSING, BALANCING, AND PREVENTIVE TECHNIQUES

To prevent damage to the immune system during diagnostic X-rays to the head and neck, be certain that the technician covers your thymus with a lead shield. The thymus is behind the breast bone and is an important part of the immune system. If the technician will not provide the lead shield, consider refusing the X-ray.

While diagnostic tests and treatments involving radiation are sometimes necessary, cleansing afterward is very important for the body. Several methods can help remove the harmful effects of exposure.

Salt and soda baths are a very important cleansing method to remove the harmful effects of radiation. For details on how to take these baths, refer to chapter 13, Detoxification Baths.

Nutritional therapy is helpful in cleansing the body after radiation therapy. It also helps repair tissues. Antioxidant vitamins are particularly important because they combat the free radicals released by damaged tissue.

- Vitamin A aids in repair and growth of all body tissues. It protects the cell membranes from oxidation.
- B$_5$ helps protect against radiation injury and is helpful after radiation treatment. It is necessary to cell metabolism and is heavily used by the body in times of stress.
- B$_{15}$ provides extra oxygen to the cells and has antioxidant properties.
- Vitamin C acts as an antistress factor.

During stress vitamin C is depleted from the tissues. It is also an antioxidant and a free-radical scavenger. Taken either orally or intravenously, vitamin C helps cleanse the body from the toxic effects of radiation.

- Vitamin E is a free-radical scavenger that improves oxygen transportation by the red blood cells, and decreases radiation damage to the chromosomes and DNA.
- Selenium is an antioxidant that enhances the action of vitamin E. It is necessary to the production of glutathione peroxidase, which is also an antioxidant.
- GeOxy 132 (organic germanium) increases oxygen utilization by the body and helps to prevent radiation sickness.
- Coenzyme Q$_{10}$ acts as an antioxidant to protect cell membranes.
- N-acetyl cysteine helps to prevent side effects from radiation therapy. (An ointment of N-acetyl cysteine will prevent hair loss, decrease skin burns, and protect the eyes.)
- Cysteine prevents inflammation of the intestinal lining caused by radiation.
- Glutathione, given *before* radiation therapy, helps protect cells.
- Methionine protects against toxic effects of radiation because it is converted to glutathione.

Several homeopathic remedies provide cleansing and balancing after radiation exposures.

- *Nux vomica* helps with nausea after radiation.
- *Radium bromatum* antidotes the effects of radiation poisoning and helps with radiation burns and eczema after X-ray.
- *Sol* antidotes radiation poisoning and helps with X-ray burns and weakness after X-rays.
- *Ipecac* helps with nausea of radiation

therapy.

- *Cadmium iodatum* helps with nausea after radiation and antidotes radiation poisoning.
- *Cadmium sulphuratum* also antidotes radiation and helps people never well since X-rays.
- *Phosphorus* helps people weak, emaciated, anemic, and with vertigo since radiation.
- *Fluoricum acidum* for radiation burns.
- *Ferrum metallicum* for anemia after radiation.
- *Iodium* helps with recovery from exposure to radioactive iodine.
- *X-ray* (homeopathic potentized X-ray) antidotes radiation sickness; helps X-ray burns, weakness after X-rays, bone damage, and people who are worse after X-rays.

There are also herbs that help cleanse the body from the effects of radiation.

- Algin prevents tissue from absorbing radioactive material.
- Celery seed is an antioxidant.
- Echinacea promotes white blood cell formation.

Chemotherapy

The term chemotherapy as it is used today refers to the treatment of malignant disease with cytotoxic drugs. Cytotoxic drugs are general cellular poisons that have a toxic effect on cancer cells and, hopefully, minimal effect on normal cells. Cancer chemotherapy is always a compromise between toxic and therapeutic effects.

Excellent results have been obtained with chemotherapy for a few cancers, including Hodgkin's disease, lymphomas, leukemias, and gestational choriocarcinoma. However, in most malignant disease, response to chemotherapy alone is poor. Chemotherapy can be a valuable adjunct to radiation therapy in some cases.

Chemotherapeutic drugs are given in combination because of resistance of the cancer cells, to reduce the size of the individual drug doses, and to combine different drug actions. Cumulative drug and organ toxicity must be considered. There are sometimes side effects to chemotherapy, one of which is nausea. Some people may lose their hair, and many get sores in their mouths. Blood counts are affected, and the bone marrow may also be affected, putting the person at risk for infection.

CLEANSING, BALANCING, AND PREVENTIVE TECHNIQUES

Preventing cancer is the best defense, and early detection is the next best defense. Lifestyle changes may be necessary. For example, a diet high in fiber and cruciferous vegetables exerts a protective effect. Decreasing intake of fats, meats, carcinogenic chemicals in foods, smoked foods, coffee, and tea can decrease the risk of cancer.

Should you develop cancer and chemotherapy becomes necessary, homeopathic remedies can alleviate side effects and help to cleanse and rebalance the body. *Hydrastis* is a good stomach tonic after chemotherapy. *Nux vomica, Ipecac, Cadmium sulphuratum,* and *Opium* can relieve nausea. *Ferrum metallicum* helps acute anemia.

Nutritional supplements can also help combat the effects of chemotherapy. Several nutrients, particularly the antioxidant nutrients, help to combat the free radicals released by damaged tissue.

- Vitamin A protects cell membranes from oxidation.
- Beta-carotene converts to vitamin A and prevents damage to cellular components, especially DNA and cell membranes.
- Vitamin B_1 works with other antioxi-

dants, vitamin C, and cysteine to combat free radicals.

- Vitamin E protects against free radicals that damage DNA.
- Vitamin C is a powerful antioxidant.
- Germanium is a free-radical scavenger and aids in oxygen utilization. Cancer cells are anaerobic, and increasing oxygen in the body helps prevent their growth.
- Selenium is an antioxidant that protects cell membranes. It also enhances the action of vitamin E.
- Coenzyme Q_{10} is an antioxidant that protects cell membranes.
- N-acetyl cysteine helps to prevent liver and heart toxicity. It also prevents bleeding and inflammation of the bladder and increases survival time of the patient if given before cyclophosphamide, a chemotherapeutic agent.

Coffee enemas are an excellent method for helping the body cope with chemotherapy and its side effects, many of which are caused by a toxic overload from the destruction of cells during chemotherapy. The body is unable to process the toxins produced. Coffee enemas help the body detoxify more rapidly so that it is able to handle the toxic load. See Colon in chapter 17 for instructions on taking a coffee enema.

Medications

The French satirist Voltaire (1694–1778) wrote these words: "Physicians pour drugs of which they know little, to cure diseases of which they know less, into humans of which they know nothing." While Voltaire was speaking of the physicians of his time, there is still some truth in his words today. Pharmaceuticals, commonly called drugs or medications, are the main allopathic treatment for most health problems. A drug is any compound that modifies the way the body works, and can be used for prevention, diagnosis, or treatment of a disease. Because of the problem with "recreational drugs" and drug abuse, the word drug now has a negative connotation.

All drugs can become poisonous in high doses, but in low doses some poisons are useful drugs. The only difference between a drug and a poison is the dose. Drug toxicity is a problem, and there have been many adverse drug reactions to prescription drugs. Some drug reactions are caused by an allergic reactions. Others are caused by a wrong dosage or from combining drugs.

Certainly, there are many times when drugs are the indicated therapy and they may be lifesaving. The administration of adrenalin for anaphylactic shock and antibiotics for serious infections has allowed many people to recover and continue their lives. Many cardiovascular accidents have been prevented with blood pressure medication. Judicious and skilful prescribing of drugs has a justified place in medicine. However, the practice of treating with drugs is so universal that many people expect always to leave their physician's office with a prescription for some type of medication.

Drugs produce a rapid effect on the body. The magnitude of the effect of a drug depends on how fast it reaches high concentration in the bloodstream and target organs. When the blood concentration of a drug rises quickly, its effects are fast, intense, and usually last a short time. Under these circumstances, the effects are usually more toxic than therapeutic. Even if taken orally, soluble drugs are in high concentration in the stomach and diffuse into the blood very quickly. Most drugs are either extracted from plants or manufactured with synthetic compounds. Modern pharmacologists tend to believe that all the desired medicinal properties of the plant are specific to one compound. They consider the other contents of the plant as inactive. Unfortunately, the drugs refined from plants are more toxic than the plant source. They do not have the natural safeguards that are in the plants and that modify the action of the medicinal portion of the plant. The active portion of the medicinal plant is more dilute and less soluble.

No drug has just one effect. Side effects accompany the medicinal effects of all drugs. The toxic effects of the drug must be weighed against the clinical benefits for the patient. Drug toxicity is rated by a therapeutic ratio: the ratio of the minimum dose producing toxic effects to the minimum dose producing desired effects. Most allopathic drugs have a therapeutic ratio between 10 and 20. The smaller the number, the smaller the margin of safety. Many drugs have quite small margins of safety. For example, digitalis has a therapeutic ratio of 2.

New drugs are developed at research institutes and at the research laboratories of pharmaceutical companies. The price of drugs is formulated to allow the drug company to recoup its research and marketing expenses before the patent expires.

In the United States and Canada, new drugs are patentable. A patent expires 20 years after the patent application filing date. If the manufacturer registers a brand name as a trademark, that name cannot be used by anyone else, even after the patent has expired. Once a patent expires, any company can make the drug if it uses the generic (chemical) name and does not violate protected doses, colors, or shapes. Most generic drugs are chemically equivalent to the proprietary drug. However, inert additives may differ, altering the availability of the drug to the body.

In addition to the toxicity of the drug and its possible side effects, drug interactions must be considered. Many people have more than one prescription that they take daily. These drugs may have been prescribed by more than one physician. Drugs may interact, and each may influence the metabolism and absorption of the other. The interaction may make them less effective and less long-acting, or more toxic with intensified action. A pharmacist can give constructive advice regarding drug interactions.

Diet may also play a role in the effectiveness of drugs. For example, milk, calcium, and iron products inactivate tetracycline. It becomes an insoluble product when exposed to calcium and iron, and cannot be absorbed by the body. Anti-inflammatory drugs and narcotics must be taken with food or milk to reduce stomach upset. Alcoholic beverages must be avoided with many medications.

Some drugs are phototoxic. Over 60 common medications may cause photosensitivity, which is a skin reaction similar to sunburn. Prolonged or excessive exposure to direct or artificial sunlight must be avoided while taking these drugs. They include some diuretics, antidepressants, birth control pills, antihistamines, blood pressure medications, diabetes medications, anticancer drugs, sulfa drugs, and topical antiseptic creams.

Many drugs can cause drowsiness or dizziness and may impair a person's ability to drive or operate machinery. Activities may have to be curtailed while taking drugs causing this type of side effect.

Some drugs may cause symptoms of chronic toxicity if taken in excess over long periods of times. This is called a drug-induced disease. Reversing these effects is very difficult and frequently impossible.

An illness caused from the actions of a physician is called an iatrogenic illness, and drugs are frequently involved. Drug reaction, drug interaction, the incorrect dosage, or even the incorrect drug may cause iatrogenic illness. Hospitalization is sometimes necessary.

Iatrogenic illness may be caused during a hospitalization. A series of "wrongs" sets up the illness:

- wrong patient
- wrong drug
- wrong dosage
- wrong time

Because of the nature of the drugs commonly prescribed, adverse reactions are inevitable. Drug reactions may include the following symptoms:

- skin rashes
- allergic reaction
- anaphylactic shock
- overgrowth of bacteria or yeast
- organ damage
- dizziness
- headache
- joint pain
- eye damage
- lung disease
- kidney stones
- seizures
- neurological symptoms

Some problems with drugs are caused by the people who take them. Some people will try every drug in sight: they take their own prescriptions, plus those of their family, or those loaned to them by a friend. They may take a drug because it was a bargain or because it was a free sample. Some people may even take double doses because they think "One of anything never does me any good!"

As mentioned earlier, there are times when the use of drugs is indicated, and in many instances they are life-saving. However, frequently they provide the "easy way out"; they control symptoms with the least amount of effort on the part of the patient. They seem to be a "magic bullet," but are not. Symptoms may be controlled, but the underlying problem is not corrected.

Before you take a drug, investigate whether it is for symptom relief only, or if it will correct your basic problem. Also, investigate any alternative treatments that might be effective. For

example, blood pressure can be controlled with a specific nutritional regimen. Heart disease improves with Coenzyme Q_{10}; exercise can strengthen the cardiovascular system; bodywork can reduce edema and relax tight muscles causing pain; and vitamin C can often clear a headache. Homeopathic remedies will relieve and cure many conditions, as will herbs.

CLEANSING, BALANCING, AND PREVENTIVE TECHNIQUES

The best action is to live a healthy lifestyle so that illnesses and the need to take medications do not occur too frequently. With proper diet, exercise, and sufficient rest, many health problems can be avoided.

When you do have to take a medication, be certain your physician knows of any other medications you may be taking before writing your prescription. In addition, be certain to mention any nonprescription drugs or products you take. Also ask about possible side effects of the medication.

As a double check, ask the pharmacist filling your prescription about possible interaction with any other prescriptions or nonprescription products you may be taking. Also ask the pharmacist about possible side effects of the new medication.

Take the prescription according to the directions. The directions may indicate that you are not to take the drug with meals. This usually means that less of the drug will be absorbed if it is taken when you have just eaten. Take the prescription for the prescribed number of days. Stopping too soon may cause a relapse.

When your health problems necessitate treatment, investigate other possibilities. For example, excellent homeopathic remedies are available for many different health problems. Herbs may be a treatment possibility for some people. Check with alternative health practitioners to see if they have a suggestion or a treatment for you. While results are sometimes slower from alternative treatments, they can be effective.

If you do take pharmaceuticals and have problems afterward, homeopathic remedies can help. For example, *Nitricum acidum* will help with diarrhea after antibiotics.

Vaccinations

A vaccination is an injection of a killed or attenuated organism as a means of producing immunity against that organism. Exposure to the vaccine causes the body to produce antibodies that will protect the person if he or she is exposed to the disease.

The first vaccinations routinely done were for smallpox. Since that time, vaccinations for measles, mumps, yellow fever, cholera, tetanus, typhoid fever, diphtheria, whooping cough, polio, and influenza have been developed. However, many of these diseases had essentially disappeared by the time the vaccines appeared. Improved sanitation, sewage disposal, water purification, and safe food distribution were instrumental in the decline of these diseases.

Vaccines and vaccination were presented as the only way to prevent and control the diseases. For example, it was thought that vaccination would eradicate smallpox. However, data from England give a different story. After smallpox vaccination became compulsory in England in 1853, there were many cases of smallpox that caused death among the vaccinated. After the law was repealed and vaccinations stopped, the disease all but disappeared. The death rate from smallpox dropped to zero.

The end of the polio epidemic in the United States and Canada was credited to the polio vaccine. However, the epidemic stopped in Europe at approximately the same time, with no vaccination program for polio in Europe. Cases of polio actually went up in the United States after mass inoculations began in 1954. When the live virus vaccine is used, the virus remains in the throat for one to two weeks and in the feces for approximately two months. The recipients of the vaccine are at risk, and they are potentially contagious as long as the virus is in the feces.

Similar statistics exist for nearly all the vaccines commonly used in the U.S. The diseases were declining and almost gone when vaccinations began. For example, the measles death rate had decreased by 95% before the measles vaccine was introduced in 1963. In 1981, an outbreak of measles occurred in Pecos, New Mexico. Seventy-five percent of those who contracted measles had been fully vaccinated, but the vaccinations did not protect the children. In other epidemics, a high percentage of the victims had been vaccinated for the disease.

Vaccinations may also cause side effects. Fevers, rashes, soreness at the injection site, allergic reactions, and neurological symptoms have all been reported following vaccinations. In some rare instances brain damage and death have occurred.

Proponents feel that vaccinations have reduced the incidence of disease to its present low levels. They further feel that vaccinations are essential for the continued health of our children. This is an issue that all parents have to decide for themselves. We have presented some of the negative aspects of vaccination because most people are unaware of these facts. Both views need to be known in order to make an informed decision.

CLEANSING, BALANCING, AND PREVENTIVE TECHNIQUES

Should you decide to proceed with vaccination, a combination of allergy extracts and homeopathy can help avoid problems with vaccinations. If an extract is given the day before the vaccination and for a week afterward, many problems and side effects can be avoided.

The following homeopathic remedies can help with side effects that may occur:

- *Pulsatilla*: problems after MMR
- *Diphtherinum*: worse since DPT
- *Sulphur*: never well since vaccination
- *Thuja occidentalis*: problems after vaccination
- *Vaccininum*: antidotes vaccination symptoms
- *Variolinum*: problems after smallpox vaccination. However, smallpox vaccinations are no longer given in the United States or Canada.
- *Ledum*: acute antidote for vaccination. Helps also with the puncture wound caused by the injection. Can be given beforehand as a preventative for side effects.
- *Hypericum*: painful injection site. Can be given beforehand as a preventative for side effects.
- *Carcinosum*: worse since vaccination
- *Silicea terra*: worse since vaccination
- *Mezereum*: skin eruptions after vaccination
- *Malandrinum*: ill effects of vaccination

Dental Work

Although needed regularly for good dental health, dental work can be a toxic exposure. The materials used in the mouth can be a problem, and the dental office itself may present a chemical exposure. With careful investigation, it is possible to find a dentist whose office contains a minimum of chemical odors and contamination. In addition, there are dentists who specialize in helping their patients determine safe and compatible dental materials.

EXPOSURES IN DENTAL OFFICES

Office supplies, cleaning supplies, room deodorizers, and office furnishings can be toxic to some people. Formaldehyde, acrylic, phenol, nitrous oxide, and mercury are indigenous to most dental offices. Even low levels of these chemicals can be a problem, but mercury is the most toxic.

Personal care products of the dental staff and other patients can cause problems for some people. Beware of tobacco odors on the hands of the dentist and/or assistants. Even if faint, the odor can amount to a sizable tobacco exposure during the time you are in the dental chair.

Today, most dentists and their assistants wear rubber gloves. Some dentists also use rubber dams in the mouth for various procedures. The gloves and rubber dams are made of latex and are a toxic exposure for the latex-sensitive person.

X-rays are another possible toxic exposure. However, today's X-ray equipment is relatively safe. For more information on X-rays and radiation, see Radiation Treatment, earlier in this chapter.

Regular prophylaxis, or professional cleaning, by a dentist or hygienist is important to good dental care. These professionals are able to remove plaque that has hardened to calculus. Removing calculus is impossible with home dental care methods. However, the polishing material used in the final step of prophylaxis is a paste of pumice, water, flavoring, and colorings. The flavoring and coloring can be a toxic exposure to some sensitive people.

If you must have a crown, bridge, or dentures, study models have to be made. An impression of your teeth or gums must be taken to prepare the study models. The materials used to make the impression of your teeth contain alginate, flavorings, and colorings, which are a problem for some people.

Local anesthetics are a chemical exposure for all people, but may be a particular problem for chemically sensitive individuals. There are two chemical classes of local anesthetics. If a person is sensitive to an anesthetic in one of the groups, he or she is usually sensitive to all of the anesthetics in that group.

DENTAL RESTORATIONS

Restoration materials present the largest toxic exposure in dental work because they become a relatively permanent part of the tooth. The amalgam filling is the most common, but controversial, restoration material used. An amalgam filling contains approximately 50% mercury and 20% to 30% silver. Zinc, copper, and tin make up the balance.

Amalgam fillings release mercury in minute amounts, particularly when a person is chewing, brushing, or drinking hot liquids. Mercury is also released when an amalgam filling is polished as the final step in prophylaxis.

For many people, mercury itself causes problems. For others, it may contribute to an overload phenomenon. Studies have demonstrated that mercury does leach out of amalgam fillings. In one study at the University of Calgary Faculty of Medicine, mercury appeared in the organs and tissues of test animals within 29 days after amalgam fillings were placed in their teeth. High concentrations of the mercury were found in the kidneys and liver of the sheep used in the study.

The American Dental Association (ADA), Canadian Dental Association (CDA), and many dentists believe that amalgam fillings are safe. The ADA and CDA do admit that mercury leaches out of the amalgam fillings, but maintain that the mercury levels are too low to be dangerous. However, mercury is considered a hazardous waste before it is put into the mouth. When amalgams are removed, the dentist must dispose of them as hazardous waste. Mercury adversely affects every system in the body. It accumulates in the body, suppressing the immune system and damaging hormones and enzymes. It also damages the brain, thyroid, pituitary, adrenal glands, heart, lungs, and nervous system.

When dissimilar metals are in the mouth, such as both gold and amalgam fillings, electric charges build up on the fillings. These charges are a result of the "battery effect" produced between the saliva and the different metals. Continuous exposure to these small currents stresses the endocrine glands and further depresses the immune system.

The usual alternative for amalgam fillings is composite fillings. They bond well with the tooth enamel and can be used for both front and back teeth. The composition of composite fillings varies with the manufacturer, but they are basically ground glass powder with quartz fillers in a plastic binder. They may also contain methylmethacrylate or aromatic dimethacrylates with additives of urethane, diacrylate, vinyl silane, benzoyl peroxide, and benzophenone ether. Composites are either light or chemically cured, depending on their formulation. The light-cured forms are generally tolerated better by sensitive people.

Temporary fillings contain zinc oxide, eugenol, and trace amounts of alcohol, acetic acid, and silica. These fillings are used while crowns and bridgework are being prepared. The materials in these fillings are toxic to some people.

Gold alloy is used in cast restorations. Other metals in the alloy include palladium, silver, and trace amounts of copper, iron, indium, tin, and zinc. Some metals cause problems in sensitive individuals. Crowns, inlays, and bridges are cast restorations. Nonprecious metals can be used, but nickel should not be a part of the alloy. The cement used to secure cast restorations in the mouth can also be toxic for some people.

Root canals may also cause problems. Recent studies by Dr. Hal Huggins of Colorado Springs, Colorado, as well as studies done in the 1920s by an American dentist, Dr. Weston Price, provide much evidence for concern. Bacteria remaining in the tubules of the tooth are anaerobic and produce toxins. If these toxins seep out of the tooth and into the body, a variety of symptoms and seemingly unrelated health problems can result, including immune system suppression.

In young people and in teeth that have been killed by trauma, the chances of a successful root canal are higher. Those performed on abscessed or infected teeth have much lower success rates. It is a difficult choice because the only alternative to a root canal at present is the extraction of the tooth.

Cavitations can be another source of dental problems that are sometimes difficult to diagnose. Cavitations are literally a hole in the jaw bone, containing necrotic bone, and frequently resulting from an extraction that did not heal properly. Cavitations are also found around root canal teeth. A thin, hard layer of bone over the area frequently prevents the cavitations from being visible on X-ray. EAV testing is the best diagnostic tool for cavitations. At present, surgical intervention is the only treatment available for cavitations, although other methods are being researched.

The braces used to straighten teeth can be a problem for some people, regardless of age. The bands used on the teeth and the wires attached to them are usually metal, and may contain iron, manganese, nickel, chromium, molybdenum, and titanium. Sometimes special rubber bands are used to help exert pressure on the teeth in order to move them, causing problems for people with latex allergy. Even the pressure exerted by the braces on the teeth can affect people. Vision care professionals report changes in eyeglass prescriptions after braces have been placed.

FLUORIDE TREATMENTS

Many dentists use fluoride treatments for both children and adults as a decay preventative. This is a controversial treatment. Some authorities feel it has no benefit after age 11, and others feel it benefits people of all ages. A growing number of scientists regard fluoride treatment as the administration of a poison because of the extreme toxicity of fluoride.

Solutions used for the fluoride treatment contain coloring agents as well as flavoring agents to mask the flavor of the fluoride compound. These agents may also be toxic to some sensitive individuals. Those sensitive to fluoride should avoid this treatment.

CLEANSING, BALANCING, AND PREVENTIVE TECHNIQUES

Prevention is probably the most important technique to practice in order to avoid dental problems and thus the toxic exposures that some types of dental work involve. Brushing and flossing after each meal and at bedtime are musts.

Most commercial toothpastes contain glycerine and corn syrup or saccharine. These substances are a problem for some sensitive individuals. Acceptable substitute toothpastes are available at health food stores. Baking soda also makes a good substitute for commercial toothpaste. Sodium lauryl sulfate, contained in most toothpastes, causes canker sores for some people and may not be listed on the toothpaste label.

A capful of a 3% dilution of 35% food-grade hydrogen peroxide and several pinches of baking soda combined with a little water make a good mouthwash (see Hydrogen Peroxide in chapter 17). Vitamin C (ascorbic acid) dissolved in water also makes a good mouth wash. Follow with a water rinse to prevent damage to tooth enamel.

Proper nutrition will not only contribute to your general health, but will also aid in maintaining good tooth and gum quality. Calcium and magnesium contribute to healthy tooth enamel and strong root and bone structure. Vitamin C, organic germanium (GeOxy 132), and Coenzyme Q_{10} are important both in restoring and maintaining gum integrity. However, do not take vitamin C for 24 hours before a dental appointment. It can reduce the effectiveness of dental anesthetics.

For latex-sensitive people, gloves made of vinyl are an alternative. Make arrangements several weeks before your appointment for the dentist to use these gloves while working on your teeth.

Do not allow any more X-rays than are absolutely necessary. Be certain a lead apron is placed over your vital organs, particularly the thymus, which is under the breast bone. If the vinyl-wrapped X-ray film is a problem, request paper-wrapped film.

You may request a substitute polish of pumice and water when having your teeth cleaned. This will allow you to avoid the colorings and flavorings in the standard polishes.

Avoid having study models made if possible. There are no problem-free alternatives for the impression materials. Minimizing your exposures to these compounds is the only way of reducing this toxic exposure.

There are numerous dental materials from which the dentist may choose. If testing is available to you, have these materials and local anesthetics tested to determine those you tolerate best.

Hypnosis and acupuncture may be used as an alternative to local anesthetic. Acupuncture anesthesia is generally accomplished by placing one needle in the foot, two needles in each hand, two in each ear, and two or three in one cheek. The needles are inserted just below the surface of the skin, and there is little or no sensation with the insertion. This should be done 15 to 20 minutes before your dental appointment.

Hypnosis requires a few practice trials with a hypnotist. The hypnotist will work with you 15 to 20 minutes before your dental appointment so that you will be prepared before the dental procedures are begun.

For many people, having amalgam fillings removed is a positive step toward improving their health. Some people feel better as each amalgam is removed and replaced with a compatible filling material. Others feel better with time, as their bodies detoxify the mercury. Still others experience little or no improvement.

Charges, both positive and negative, build up on the amalgam fillings. Dentists can measure these charges with a special instrument. It is important that amalgams be removed in the proper order, depending on the charges and their magnitude. Those with higher charges, whether positive or negative, should be removed first. The use of a rubber dam and oxygen during the removal phase will greatly reduce inhalation of mercury vapors.

It may take several months, or even a year, for the body to detoxify after amalgams have been removed and replaced. Nutrients are helpful in reducing the effects of the mercury that is released when these fillings are removed. Take these nutrients for several weeks before and several months after the amalgams are removed: vitamin C; vitamins B_1 and B_2; vitamin E; glutathione, cysteine, or methionone; selenium; beta-carotene; zinc; magnesium; and manganese all aid in detoxification. Dry sauna treatments or detoxification baths will aid in speeding the detoxification process (see chapter 13).

Homeopathy offers several remedies that cleanse and balance after dental work.

- *Arnica*: Use routinely after any dental procedure in which there is a chance of pain. *Arnica* helps following tooth extractions, gum surgery, and pain from drilling. It can also be used for sore gums and to control toothache pain until a visit to the dentist can be arranged.
- *Calendula*: Used as a mouthwash. It also helps to relieve gum pain after dental procedures. It can be used on any oral lesion.
- *Hypericum*: Take for any procedure involving nerve injury. It helps relieve the pain from drilling, extractions, or root canal preparation.

- *Ruta*: Helps a "dry socket," a healing problem that sometimes occurs after an extraction.
- *Kreosotum*: Helps with dry sockets where there is a bad taste in the mouth. It also helps with decayed teeth.
- *Ledum*: Helps with the trauma of root canals.
- *Plantago major*: Helps with a toothache when there is also earache and salivation. It is also a major teething remedy and helps with TMJ pain and bruxism (grinding the teeth).
- *Rhododendrum*: Take for toothache.
- *Magnesia phosphorica*: Helps a toothache that is better with warm water.
- *Mercurious solubilis*: Use for periodontal disease.
- *Spigelia*: Helps a toothache that is worse with cold.
- *Mezereum*: Use in cases of tooth decay.

Herbs are also useful for cleansing in dentistry, but some individuals sensitize to herbs very rapidly.

For canker sores, infected gums, sore tongue, or tonsillitis, a goldenseal mouth rinse is helpful. Combine:

    1 cup of warm water
    ¼ teaspoon of salt
    ½ teaspoon goldenseal powder

For people who tolerate it, a little cayenne pepper in this mixture is also helpful. Use as needed to control pain and soothe the tissues.

Chamomile will reduce swelling and pain if used on the gums.

The following herbs are useful for toothache:

- Clove: takes away pain and disinfects
- Hops: acts as a sedative, reduces fever
- Myrrh: use for periodontal problems and canker sores

Aniseed, mint leaves, and parsley can be chewed to freshen the breath. They may also be made into a tea. For directions on making an herb tea or infusion, see Herbs in chapter 15. If soaked in alcohol (ethanol) for a week and then diluted, the herbs make an effective mouthwash.

AFTERWORD

In this book we have tried to present a broad overview of toxins as well as cleansing, balancing, and preventive techniques for each toxin. Space does not permit us to discuss other toxins, and certainly not all preventive and treatment methods. For example, Bach Flower remedies, aromatherapy, color therapy, gem therapy, and other types of bodywork can be helpful. In addition, attention to the spiritual quality of life is important for complete recovery or the fullest enjoyment of life.

With your new awareness of toxins, as well as treatment possibilities, you can now increase your quality of health and life. Simple precautions enable you to avoid or minimize exposures to toxins and prevent further damage to your body. Treatment methods allow you to detoxify your body of the toxins to which you have already had exposure. Armed with your new knowledge, you can regain or enhance your health. We wish you joy and success in your journey.

RECOMMENDED SOURCES
AND ORGANIZATIONS

AABD
American Academy of Biological Dentistry
P.O. Box 856
Carmel Valley, CA   93942
(408) 659-5385

AAEM
American Academy of Environmental Medicine
4510 W. 89th Street, Suite 110
Prairie Village, KS   66207-2282
(913) 642-6062
Fax: (913) 341-6912

AAOA
American Academy of Otolaryngic Allergy
8455 Colesville Road, Suite 745
Silver Springs, MD   20910
(310) 588-1800

Acupuncture Foundation of Canada
P.O. Box 93688, Shopper's World Postal Outlet
3003 Danforth Ave.
Toronto, ON   M4C 5R5
(416) 752-3988

American Association of Naturopathic Physicians
2366 Eastlake Ave. E., Suite 322
Seattle, WA   98102
(206) 323-7610
Fax: (206) 323-7612

American Chiropractic Association
1701 Clarendon Blvd.
Arlington, VA   22209
(703) 276-8800

ACAM
American College for Advancement in Medicine
23121 Verdugo Drive, Suite 204
Laguna Hills, CA   92653
(714) 583-7666

American Osteopathic Association
142 E. Ontario Street
Chicago, IL   60611
(800) 621-1773

Canadian Chiropractic Association
1396 Eglinton Ave. W.
Toronto, ON   M6C 2E4
(416) 781-5656

Canadian College of Naturopathic Medicine
2300 Yonge Street, 18th Floor
P.O. Box 2431
Toronto, ON   M4P 1E4
(416) 486-8584

Canadian Massage Therapist Association
950 Yonge Street, Suite 1007
Toronto, ON   M4W 2J4
(416) 968-6487
1-800-668-2022

Canadian Memorial Chiropractic College
1900 Bayview Ave.
Toronto, ON   M4G 3E6
(416) 482-2340

Canadian Network of Toxicology Centres
Bovey Building, Gordon Street
University of Guelph
Guelph, ON   N1G 2W1
(519) 837-3320

Chinese Medical Clinic
411 St. Michael's Drive
Santa Fe, NM 87505
(505) 988-2592

IFH
International Foundation for Homeopathy
P.O. Box 7
Edmonds, WA   98020
(206) 776-4147

Institute of Chinese Herbology
3871 Piedmont Ave., Suite 363
Oakland, CA   94611
(510) 428-2061

International Institute of Chinese Medicine
P.O. Box 4991
Santa Fe, NM   87502
(505) 473-5233
(800) 377-4561

National Center for Homeopathy
801 N. Fairfax Street, Suite 306
Alexandria, VA   22314
(703) 548-7790
Fax: (703) 548-7792

National Commission for Certification of
   Acupuncturists, Inc.
1424 16th Street, N.W., Suite 501
Washington, DC   20036-2211
(202) 232-1404

New Mexico Academy of Healing Arts
P.O. Box 932

Santa Fe, NM   87504
(505) 982-6271

Ontario Massage Therapist Association
365 Bloor Street E., Suite 1807
Toronto, ON   M4W 3L4
(416) 968-6487
(800) 668-2022

Ontario Naturopathic Association
60 Berl Ave.
Etobicoke, ON   M8Y 3C7
(416) 503-9554

The Rolf Institute
205 Canyon Blvd.
Boulder, CO   80302
(800) 530-8875

Shiatsu School of Canada
547 College Street
Toronto, ON   M6G 1A9
(416) 323-1818
1-800-263-1703

Southwest Acupuncture College
325 Paseo de Peralta
Santa Fe, NM   87501
(505) 988-3538

DETOXIFICATION UNITS

Bio-Ethics Medical Center
Dr. Tano Lucero
10752 N. 89th Place, Suite 102
Scottsdale, AZ   85260
(602) 860-0490
Fax: (602) 860-0631

Center for Environmental Medicine
Dr. Allan Lieberman
7510 Northforest Drive
North Charleston, SC   29420
(803) 572-1600

Environmental Health Center
Dr. William Rea
8345 Walnut Hill Lane, Suite 205

Dallas, TX 75231
(214) 368-4132

Health Med
Frank A. Damiata
5501 Power Inn Road, Suite 140
Sacramento, CA 95820
(800) 451-0116

The Northwest Healing Arts Center
Dr. Walter Crinnion
1200 112th Ave. N.E., Suite A100
Bellevue, WA 98005
(206) 747-9200

Robbins Environmental Medicine Clinic
Dr. Albert Robbins
400 S. Dixie Highway, Building 2, Suite 210
Boca Raton, FL 33432
(561) 395-3282
Fax (561) 395-3304

SUPPLIES

Air Cleaners

AllerMed Corporation
31 Steel Road
Wylie, TX 75098
(214) 422-4311

Allerx Air Cleaners
P.O. Box 239
Fate, TX 75123
(800) 477-1100

Foust Air Purifiers
E. L. Foust Company, Inc.
P.O. Box 105
Elmhurst, IL 60126
(312) 834-4952

Ceramic Oxygen Masks

American Environmental Health Foundation
8345 Walnut Hill Lane, Suite 200
Dallas, TX 75231-4262
(214) 361-9515
(800) 428-2343
Fax: (214) 691-8432

Environmental Purification Systems
P.O. Box 191
Concord, CA 94522
(510) 284-2129

Electromagnetic

ELF Teslar (watches)
State Route 1, Box 21
St. Francisville, IL 62460
(618) 948-2393
Fax: (618) 948-2650

Ener-G Polari-T (diodes)
P.O. Box 2449
Prescott, AZ 86302-2449
(520) 778-5039
Fax: (520) 771-0611

EnviroTech (magnets)
17167 S.E. 29th Street
Choctaw, OK 73020
(405) 390-3499

Essentia (EMF meters, full-spectrum lights, air
  systems)
100 Bronson, Suite 1001
Ottawa, ON K1R 6G8
(613) 238-4437

Radon Environmental Monitoring, Inc.
3334 Commercial Ave.
Northbrook, IL 60062
(847) 205-0110
Fax: (847) 205-0114

Tachyon Energy Research, Inc. (tachyon
  beads)
2200 Pacific Coast Highway, Suite 304
Hermosa Beach, CA 90254
(310) 374-8777
Fax: (310) 374-1138

Herbal

Eclectic Institute
14385 S.E. Lusted Rd.
Sandy, OR 97055
(503) 668-4120

(800) 332-4372
Fax: (503) 668-3227

Home Saunas

Heavenly Heat
1106 Second Street
Encinitas, CA   92024
(619) 942-0401
(800) MY SAUNA

Homeopathic

BHI Homeopathic Products
11600 Cochiti, S.E.
Albuquerque, NM   87123
(505) 293-3843
(800) 621-7644
Fax: (505) 275-1642

Dolisos America, Inc.
3014 Rigel Ave.
Las Vegas, NV   89102
(702) 871-7153
(800) 365-4767
Fax: (702) 871-9670

Homeopathic Educational Services
2124 Kittredge Street
Berkeley, CA   94704
(510) 649-0294
(800) 359-9051 to place orders

PHP Professional Health Products, Ltd.
Homeopathic Division
79 N. Industrial Park
211 Overlook Drive, Bay 5
Sewickley, PA 15143
(800) 929-4132

Mold Testing (mold plates)

American Environmental Health Foundation
8345 Walnut Hill Lane

Dallas, TX   75231-4262
(214) 361-9515

Mold Survey Service
Dr. Sherry A. Rogers
P.O. Box 2716
Syracuse, NY   13220
(315) 488-2856

NeoLife Products

Neolife
3500 Gateway Blvd.
Fremont, CA 94538
(510) 651-0405
(800) 432-5848

Oral Chelation Formulas

AMNI
Advanced Medical Nutrition, Inc.
P.O. Box 5012
Hayward, CA   94540-5012
(510) 783-6969
(800) 437-8888

Shower Filters

American Environmental Health Foundation
8345 Walnut Hill Lane, Suite 200
Dallas, TX   75231-4262
(214) 361-9515
(800) 428-2343
Fax: (214) 691-8432

Environmental Purification Systems
P.O. Box 191
Concord, CA   94522
(510) 284-2129

Purebasics
1903 Blake Drive
Richardson, TX   75081
(214) 231-2555

SUGGESTED READING

Alternative Healing, Mark Kastner and Hugh Burroughs. Halcyon Publishing, La Mesa, CA, 1996.

This very informative book discusses over 160 different alternative therapies. It allows the reader to understand other methods that help fight disease, maintain good health, and promote happiness, naturally.

The Chelation Way, Morton Walker. Avery Publishing Group, Garden City Park, NY, 1990.

The full scope of chelation therapy is covered in this easy-to-read book. Dr. Walker has been very thorough, and a partial list of physicians using chelation in the United States, England, Mexico, Holland, New Zealand, and West Germany is included.

Chemical Sensitivity, volumes 1–4, William J. Rea. Lewis Publishers, Boca Raton, FL, 1992–96.

A knowledge of chemistry is helpful when reading these very scholarly and well-researched books on chemical sensitivity. Mechanisms of chemical sensitivity are presented, including biochemical pathways. Discussion includes the role of nutrients in sensitivity as well as treatment.

Desktop Guide to Keynotes and Confirmatory Symptoms, Roger Morrison. Hahnemann Clinic Publishing, Albany, CA, 1993.

Keynotes and confirmatory symptoms for homeopathic remedies are presented with accuracy and clarity, making this a very usable and helpful reference book. Both newcomers to homeopathy, as well as the experienced homeopath, will find this book valuable.

Earl Mindell's Vitamin Bible, Earl Mindell. Warner Books, New York, 1991.

Earl Mindell, a pharmacist and nutritionist, discusses the full scope of vitamins and nutritional supplements, and their effect on your health.

Health and Healing, Andrew Weil. Darling-Kindersley, New York, 1995.

Alternative medicine, its merits and treatments are discussed, as is traditional or standard medicine. The reader can gain a true understanding of the options for treatment of many different conditions.

Industrial Toxicology: Safety and Health, Phillip L. Williams and James L. Burson. Van Nostrand Reinhold, New York, 1989.

This book discusses various toxins, their effects on the body, and the systems affected. Toxicological cases are presented as detective stories. This book is relatively easy to read for the lay person.

Job's Body, Deane Juhan. Station Hill Press, Barrytown, NY, 1987.

All systems of the body are discussed in relation to function and bodywork. A very informative book for all readers.

Root Canal Cover-up, George Meinig. Bion Publishing, Ojai, CA, 1994.

A founder of the Association of Root Canal Specialists discusses the damage root canals can do to your health.

Scientific Validation of Herbal Medicine, Daniel B. Mowrey. Keats Publishing, New Canaan, CT, 1990.

Herbal medicine is related to clinical medicine in this excellent book. The action of the herbs is presented, conditions for use are described, and methods for administration are discussed.

Tired or Toxic?, Sherry A. Rogers. Prestige Publishing, Syracuse, NY, 1990.

Dr. Rogers discusses the effects toxins may have on the body. Many people may not be simply tired; they may be toxic. Detoxification methods for both the body and environment are presented. Although much valuable information is presented, it is difficult to find because the index is not comprehensive.

Toxicological Chemistry, Stancy E. Manahan. Lewis Publishers, Boca Raton, FL, 1992.

The chemistry of substances toxic to man are presented with simplicity and clarity. A knowledge of chemistry is helpful, but not necessary.

Vibrational Medicine, Richard Gerber. Bear & Company, Santa Fe, NM, 1988.

This excellent book on energetic medicine covers many alternative methods for diagnosis and healing. By enlightening the reader regarding these therapies, choices for treatment and health are greatly increased.

Wellness Against All Odds, Sherry A. Rogers. Prestige Publishing, Syracuse, NY, 1994.

Dr. Rogers discusses treatment and defense against toxic insults from the environment. She also includes dietary and nutritional information.

The Whole Way to Allergy Relief and Prevention, Jacqueline A. Krohn, Frances A. Taylor, and Erla Mae Larson. Hartley & Marks, Point Roberts, WA, 1996.

The full gamut of allergies, allergy treatments, and allergy prevention is presented. Book includes a complete discussion of the body and systems in relation to allergy. Treatment, both by self and by professionals, is discussed in detail, including nutritional and natural therapies.

BIBLIOGRAPHY

Ackerknecht, Erwin H. *A Short History of Medicine*. New York: The Ronald Press Company, 1968.

Alvarado, Donna. "Too Much Sun May Suppress the Immune System." *Albuquerque Journal*. June 19, 1993: A-1, A-11.

Anshutz, E. P. *New, Old, and Forgotten Remedies*. New Delhi, India: B. Jain Publishers Pvt. Ltd., 1989.

Asai, Kazuhiko. *Miracle Cure—Organic Germanium*. Tokyo, Japan: Japan Publications, 1980.

Bardswell, Frances A. *The Herb Garden*. Brattleboro, VT: Practical Press, 1987.

Bartusiak, Marcia. "The Sunspot Syndrome." *Discover*. Nov. 1989: 45–52.

Beaver, Paul Chester, Rodney Clifton Jung, and Eddie Wayne Cupp. *Clinical Parasitology*. Philadelphia, PA: Lea & Febiger, 1984.

Becker, Robert O. *Cross Currents*. Los Angeles, CA: Jeremy P. Tarcher, 1990.

Beverly, Cal, ed. *Natural Health Secrets Encyclopedia*. Peachtree City, GA: F.C. & A. Publishing, 1991.

BHI. "A Modern Approach to Homeopathy." Pamphlet. Albuquerque, NM: Menaco Publishing Co., n.d.

Bianchi, Ivo. *Principles of Homotoxicology*, vol. I. Baden-Baden, Germany: Aurelia-Verlag, 1989.

Blake, Michael. *The Natural Healer's Acupressure Handbook*, vol. I: Basic G–Jo. Fort Lauderdale, FL: Falkynor Books, 1983.

Bland, Jeffrey. "Functional Testing of Detoxification Pathways in Chemical Sensitivities." Presented at the American Academy of Environmental Medicine, 28th Annual Meeting, Reno, NV, Oct. 10, 1993.

Bland, Jeffrey. "Antioxidants, Co-factors, et al. in Maximizing the Functioning of the Detoxification Pathways." Presented at the American Academy of Environmental Medicine, 28th Annual Meeting, Reno, NV, Oct. 10, 1993.

Boericke, William. *Materia Medica with Repertory*. New Delhi, India: Homeopathic Publications, Indian ed., originally published 1927.

Booklet. "The Purifying Program™." Beverly Hills, CA: Eden's Secrets Corp., n.d.

Borneman, John A. "Homeopathy and Naturopathy—Gentle Partners for Healing." *Let's Live*. April 1993: 16–25.

Boyd, Hamish. *Introduction to Homeopathic Medicine*. Beaconsfield, Bucks, England: Beaconsfield Publishers, 1981.

Braverman, Eric R., with Carl Pfeiffer. *The Healing Nutrients Within*. New Canaan, CT: Keats Publishing, 1987.

Briggs, Shirley A., and the staff of the Rachel Carson Council. *Basic Guide to Pesticides—Their Characteristics and Hazards*. Washington, D.C.: Taylor and Francis, 1992.

Brody, Jane E. *Jane Brody's Nutrition Book*. New York: W.W. Norton & Co., 1981.

Brostoff, Jonathon, and Stephen J. Challacombe, eds. *Food Allergy and Intolerance*. London, England: Bailliere Tindall, 1987.

Brown, Harold W., and Franklin A. Neva. *Basic Clinical Parasitology*. Norwalk, CT: Appleton-Century-Crofts, 1983.

Brown, Michael. "Can You Detox Your Body?" *American Health*. September 1986: 53–58.

Browne, Malcolm. "High Cost of Noise." *Albuquerque Journal*. March 11, 1990: B-14.

Burger, Alfred. *Drugs and People*. Charlottesville, VA: University Press of Virginia, 1988.

Campion, Margaret Reid. *Hydrotherapy in Pediatrics*. Rockville, MD: An Aspen Publication, 1985.

Cardiovascular Research. "Clinical Uses of Coenzyme Q$_{10}$." Pamphlet. Concord, CA: Cardiovascular Research, 1983.

Carlson, Robert. "Aloe Vera versus Atherosclerosis." *Medical Gazette*, vol. 6 (50): 1 (Dec. 13, 1984).

Carter, Stephen K., Marie T. Bakowdki, and Kurt Hellman. *Chemotherapy of Cancer*. New York: John Wiley & Sons, 1977.

Castleman, Michael. *The Healing Herbs*. Emmaus, PA: Rodale Press, 1991.

Cathcart, Robert F. "The Method for Determining Proper Doses of Vitamin C by Titrating to Bowel Tolerance." *Journal of Orthomolecular Psychiatry* 10: 125–32 (1991).

Cathcart, Robert F. "Vitamin C: The Nontoxic, Non-role Limited, Antioxidant Free Radical Scavenger." *Medical Hypothesis* 18: 61–77 (1985).

Cathcart, Robert F. "The Vitamin C Treatment of Allergy and the Normally Unprimed State of Antibodies." *Medical Hypothesis* 21: 307–21 (1986).

Chabner, Bruce A., and Jerry M. Collins. *Cancer Chemotherapy*. Philadelphia, PA: J. B. Lippincott Co., 1990.

Chaitow, Leon. *Amino Acids in Therapy*. Rochester, VT: Healing Arts Press, 1988.

Cheraskin, Emanuel, Marshall W. Ringsdorf, Jr., and Emily L. Sisley. *The Vitamin C Connection*. New York: Harper and Row, 1983.

Choi, Steve. "Oxygen and Life." *Health World*. March/April 1990: 14–17.

Chopra, Deepak. *Perfect Health—The Complete Mind/Body Guide*. New York: Harmony Books, 1991.

Christopher, John R. *Dr. Christopher's Three-Day Cleansing Program, Mucusless Diet and Herbal Combinations*. Springville, UT: John R. Christopher, 1991.

Christopher, John R. *Herbal Home Health Care* (formerly *Childhood Diseases*). Springville, UT: Christopher Publications, 1976.

Clarke, John Henry. *A Dictionary of Practical Materia Medica*. New Delhi, India: Aggarwal Book Centre, originally published 1900.

Claussen, C. F. "Homotoxicology: The Basis of a Probiotic, Holistic Practice of Medicine." *Biological Therapy*. VIII (2): 37–39. April 1989.

Clearwater, Susan. "Herbal Cleansing and Detoxification." *Enlightenments*. June 1993: 20.

Clendening, Logan. *Source Book of Medical History*. New York: Dover Publications, 1942.

Coats, Bill. "The Versatility of Whole Leaf Aloe Vera." *Dermascope Magazine*. Sep./Oct. 1991: 54, 56.

"Coenzyme Q$_{10}$: Animal-Vegetable-Mineral." *American Institute of Health and Nutrition News*. 1 (1993):1–4.

Coffel, Steve, and Karyn Feiden. *Indoor Pollution*. New York: Ballantine Books, 1990.

Collins, Jonathan. "Carpet Toxicity." *Townsend Letter for Doctors*. April 1989: 197.

Cooper, Kenneth H. *The Aerobics Program for Total Well-Being*. New York: Bantam Books, 1982.

Costello, Mike, and Sarah Thurbes. "Bruised Faces and Broken Hearts: Violence in the Home." *Family Safety and Health*. 51(4): 23–27 (winter 1992–93).

Cott, Allan. *Fasting As A Way Of Life*. New York: Bantam Books, 1977.

Cridland, Marion D. *Fundamentals of Cancer Chemotherapy*. Baltimore, MD: University Park Press, 1978.

Crompton, Paul. *The T'ai Chi Workbook*. Boston, MA: Shambhala, 1987.

Cross, Mercer. "Lighting Up Your Life May Help Winter Depression." *Albuquerque Journal*. Feb. 14, 1988: F-6.

Davis, Jefferson C., and Thomas K. Hunt, eds. *Problem Wounds—The Role of Oxygen*. New York: Elsevier Science Publishing Co., 1988.

Donciger, Elizabeth. *Homeopathy—From Alchemy to Medicine*. Rochester, VT: Healing Arts Press, 1988.

Donegan, Jane B. *Hydropathic Highway to Health*. New York: Greenwood Press, 1986.

Dong, Paul, and Aristide H. Esser. *Chi Gong*. New York: Paragon House, 1990.

Ebner, Maria. *Connective Tissue Massage*. Huntington, NY: Robert E. Krieger Publishing Co., 1962.

Ecological Formulas. "Intestinal Microflora and Persistent Illness." Research Perspective in Gastroenterology. Concord, CA: Ecological Formulas, n.d.

Edelstein, Ludwig. *Ancient Medicine*. Baltimore, MD: The Johns Hopkins Press, 1967.

Environmental Protection Agency. "The Inside Story: A Guide to Indoor Air Quality." United States Environmental Protection Agency, Washington, D.C., Sept. 1988.

Environmental Protection Agency. "Radon Reduction Methods: A Homeowner's Guide."

United States Environmental Protection Agency, Washington, D.C., Sept. 1987.

Evelyn, Nancy. *Herbal Medicine Chest.* Freedom, CA: Crossing Press, 1986.

"Exercise is Good for the Brain." *East West.* April 1990: 13.

Faelton, Sharon, and the editors of Prevention Magazine. *The Complete Book of Minerals for Health.* Emmaus, PA: Rodale Press, 1981.

Fasciana, Guy S. "The E. I. Dentist—Dental Materials Part I." *The Human Ecologist* (25): 9–11 (spring 1984).

Fasciana, Guy S. "The E. I. Dentist—Dental Materials Part II." *The Human Ecologist* (26): 11–12 (summer 1984).

Feltman, John, ed. *Prevention How To Dictionary of Healing Remedies and Techniques.* Emmaus, PA: Rodale Press, 1992.

Feinstein, Alice. *Training the Body to Cure Itself.* Emmaus, PA: Rodale Press, 1992.

Fischer, B., and others. *Handbook of Hyperbaric Oxygen Therapy.* New York: Springer-Verlag, 1988.

Flodin, Kim C. "Now Hear This." *American Health.* Jan./Feb. 1992: 59–62.

"Food Irradiation." *East West.* April 1990: 14.

Foote, Clara Kroeger, and Jerald Foote. *How to Counteract Environmental Poisons.* Boulder, CO: Chapel of Miracles, 1990.

Fritzgerald, Susan. "Sunlight on Winter Days Lifts Depression for Some." *Albuquerque Journal.* Dec. 11, 1986: B-8.

Gach, Michael Reed. *Acupressure's Potent Points.* New York: Bantam Books, 1990.

Gard, Zane R., and Erma Jean Brown. "The Bio-Toxic Reduction Program: Eliminating Body Pollution." *Townsend Letter for Doctors.* April 1987: 49, 56–60.

Gard, Zane R. "Literature Review and Comparison Studies of Sauna/Hyperthermia in Detoxification." *Townsend Letter for Doctors.* July 1992: 1–50.

Gardner, Joy. *Healing Yourself.* Seattle, WA: Healing Yourself, 1982.

Garrison, Fielding H. *An Introduction to the History of Medicine.* Philadelphia, PA: W. B. Saunders Company, 1914.

Gerber, Richard. *Vibrational Medicine.* Santa Fe, NM: Bear and Company, 1988.

Gerras, Charles, Joseph Golant, and E. John Hanna, eds. *The Complete Book of Vitamins.* Emmaus, PA: Rodale Press, 1977.

Goodenough, Josephus, compiler and ed. *Dr. Goodenough's Home Cures and Herbal Remedies.* New York: Avenel Books; Crown Publishers, 1982.

Gordon, Benjamin Lee. *Medicine Throughout Antiquity.* Phildelphia, PA: F.A. Davis Co., 1949.

Green, James. *Herbal Medicine Maker's Handbook.* Forestville, CA: Simplers Botanical Co., 1990.

Green, Nancy Sokol. "America's Toxic Schools." *The Environmental Magazine.* N.d.: 30–37.

Green, Nancy Sokol. *Poisoning Our Children.* Chicago, IL: The Noble Press, 1991.

Greenberg, Robert. "Modification of Biological Terrain in Preventive and Restorative Therapeutics." Presented at Mountain States Health Care Products Seminar, Westminster, CO, Dec. 11, 1993.

Grieve, Mrs. M. *A Modern Herbal,* vol. I and II. Mineola, NY: Dover Publications, 1971.

Hallenbeck, W. H., and K. M. Cunningham-Burns. *Pesticides and Human Health.* New York: Springer-Verlag, 1985.

Hallowell, Christopher. "Clearing the Air." *Earthwise.* March 1993: 52–54.

Harte, John, and others. *Toxics A to Z: A Guide to Everyday Pollution Hazards.* Berkeley, CA: University of California Press, 1991.

Heine, Kathy. "Hearing Loss More Likely at Play Than at Work." *Albuquerque Journal.* Nov. 12, 1989: D-4.

Hittleman, Richard. *Yoga 28 Day Exercise Plan.* New York: Workman Publishing, 1969.

Hobbs, Christopher. *Natural Liver Therapy.* Capitola, CA: Botanica Press, 1988.

Hobbs, Christopher. *Super Immunity—Herbs and Other Natural Remedies for a Healthy Immune System.* Capitola, CA: Botanica Press, 1985.

Hobbs, Christopher. *Usnea—Herbal Antibiotic.* Capitola, CA: Botanica Press, 1984.

Hoffer, Abram. *Orthomolecular Medicine for Physicians.* New Canaan, CT: Keats Publishing, 1989.

Hoffman, David. *The Herbal Handbook: A User's Guide to Medical Herbalism.* Rochester, VT: Healing Arts Press, 1987.

Hoffman, David. "Herbs and Children." *Let's Live.* June 1993: 70–71.

Hoffman, David. *The Holistic Herbal.* Shaftesbury, Dorset, England: Element Books, 1988.

Hoffman, Matthew, William LeGro, and editors of *Prevention Magazine. Disease Free.* Emmaus, PA: Rodale Press, 1993.

Hoffman, Ronald L. *Tired All The Time.* New York: Poseidon Press, 1993.

Hubbard, L. Ron. *Clear Body, Clear Mind.* Los Angeles, CA: Bridge Publications, 1990.

Huggins, Hal A., and Sharon A. Huggins. *It's All in Your Head.* Colorado Springs, CO: Huggins, 1985.

Huggins, Hal A. "Root Canals." *Let's Live.* Nov. 1990: 71.

Hylton, William H., ed. *The Rodale Herb Book.* Emmaus, PA: Rodale Press Book Division, 1974.

Inlander, Charles B., and Ed Weiner. *Take This Book to the Hospital With You.* Emmaus, PA: Rodale Press, 1985.

Jaffe, Russell. "Occurrence of Xenobiotic Hypersensitivity in an Autoimmune/ Multiple Chemical Sensitivity (AI-MCS) Cohort Compared with an Ambulatory Control Population." Presented at the American Academy of Environmental Medicine, 28th Annual Meeting, Reno, NV, Oct. 11, 1993.

Jensen, Bernard. *Nature Has A Remedy.* Escondido, CA: Dr. Bernard Jensen, 1978.

Joklik, Wolfgang K., and others. *Zinsser Microbiology.* Norwalk, CT: Appleton and Lange, 1988.

Jones, Marjorie Hurt. "Working at Wellness." *Mastering Food Allergies.* VIII(6): 1–8 (Nov.–Dec. 1993).

Jones-Smith, Jacqueline. "Safety from the Ground Up." *Home.* Feb. 1993: 27.

Jouanny, Jacques. *The Essentials of Homeopathic Materia Medica.* Boiron S.A., France: Editions Boiron, 1984.

Juhan, Deane. *Job's Body—A Handbook For Body-work.* Barrytown, NY: Station Hill Press, 1987.

Justice, Blair. *Who Gets Sick: Thinking and Health.* Houston, TX: Peak Press, 1987.

Kahn, Farrol S. *Why Flying Endangers Your Health: Hidden Health Hazards of Airline Travel.* Santa Fe, NM: Aurora Press, 1992.

Kale, W. S. *Your Health, Your Moods, and the Weather.* New York: Doubleday, 1982.

Kastner, Mark, and Hugh Burroughs. *Alternative Healing.* La Mesa, CA: Halcyon Publishing, 1996.

Kent, John Tyler. *Repertory of Homeopathic Materia Medica.* New Delhi, India: Homeopathic Publications, Indian edition. Reprinted from the Sixth American Edition, n.d.

Kime, Zane R. *Sunlight Could Save Your Life.* Penryn, CA: World Health Publications, 1980.

Kisner, Carolyn, and Lynn Allen Colby. *Therapeutic Exercise Foundations and Techniques.* Philadelphia, PA: F. A. Davis Company, 1990.

Klaire Laboratories. "Myths About Microbial Supplementation Dispelled." Technical bulletin. San Marcos, CA: Klaire Laboratories, 1988.

Klaire Laboratories. "Vital Plex." Pamphlet. San Marcos, CA: Klaire Laboratories, n.d.

Kostias, John. *The Essential Movements of T'ai Chi.* Bookline, MA: Paradigm Publications, 1989.

Krieger, Dolores. *Accepting Your Power to Heal.* Santa Fe, NM: Bear and Company, 1993.

Kroeger, Hanna. *Instant Herbal Locator.* Boulder, CO: Hanna Kroeger, 1979.

Krohn, Jacqueline, and others. *A Guide to the Identification and Treatment of Biocatalyst and Biochemical Intolerances.* Los Alamos, NM: J. Krohn, 1989.

Krohn, Jacqueline, Frances Taylor, and Erla Mae Larson. *The Whole Way To Allergy Relief and Prevention.* Point Roberts, WA: Hartley & Marks, 1996.

Krohn, Jacqueline. "Lead Poisoning." Presented at the American Adacemy of Environmental Medicine, 27th Annual Meeting, Lincolnshire, IL, Oct. 27, 1992.

Krueger, Albert Paul. "On Air Ions—and Your Health, Moods, and Efficiency." *Executive Health.* 17(2): (Nov. 1980).

Krueger, Albert Paul, and Eddie James Reed. "Biological Impact of Small Air Ions." *Science.* 19: 1209–13 (Sept. 1976).

Kushi, Michio. *The Macrobiotic Way. The Complete Macrobiotic Diet and Exercise Book.* Wayne, NJ: Avery Publishing Group, 1985.

LaDou, Joseph. *Occupational Medicine.* Norwalk, CT: Appleton and Lange, 1990.

Lanpher, Katherine, and Kathryn Keller. "Turn Down That Noise!" *Redbook.* April 1991: 58–64.

Lappe, Marc. *Chemical Deception.* San Francisco, CA: Sierra Club, 1991.

Larson, E. M., J. Krohn, and F. Taylor. "The Emotional and Psychological Impact of Environmental Illness." Presented at the American Academy of Environmental Medicine, 26th Annual Meeting, Jacksonville, FL, Oct. 29, 1991.

Larson, E. M., J. Krohn, and F. Taylor. "Clinical Manifestations of Nutrient Deficiencies." Presented at the American Academy of Environmental Medicine, 27th Annual Meeting, Lincolnshire, IL, Oct. 27, 1992.

Larson, E. M., J. Krohn, and F. Taylor. "Abuse as a Contributing Factor in Environmental Illness." Presented at the American Academy of Environmental Medicine, 28th Annual Meeting, Reno, NV, Oct. 11, 1993.

Levine, Stephen, and Parris M. Kidd. *Antioxidant Adaptation.* San Leandro, CA: Biocurrents Division, Allergy Research Group, 1986.

Leviton, Richard. "How the Weather Affects Your Health." *East West*. Sept. 1989: 64–68, 112–13.

Leviton, Richard. "Can the Earth's Stress Spots Make You Sick?" *East West*. June 1989: 48–52, 83–85.

Leviton, Richard. "The Ley Lines of Seattle." *East West*. March 1989: 54–57.

Lewis, Alan. "Coenzyme Q_{10}: A Review." Pamphlet, Karuna, n.d.

Licht, Sidney Herman, ed. *Massage, Manipulation and Traction*. New Haven, CT: Elizabeth Licht, 1960.

Lieberman, Allan. "The Role of Sauna Detoxification in the Treatment of Chemical Sensitivities." Presented at the American Academy of Environmental Medicine, 28th Annual Meeting, Reno, NV, Oct. 10, 1993.

Liles, Necia Dixon, and Allan Liles. "This Mercury Is Not the Gods' Messenger-II." *Let's Live*. Dec. 1992: 66–67.

Lin, David. "Antioxidants, Free Radicals, and Health." *Health Consciousness*. 14(3): 58–59 (1993).

Litt, Jerome Z., ed. "Phytodermatis." *Cross Section*. 16(4): 11 (1991).

Loddeke, Leslie. "Aloe Vera to be Tried as AIDS Treatment." *The Houston Post*. Oct. 4, 1992: n.p.

Ludlum, David M. *The Audubon Society Field Guide to North American Weather*. New York: Alfred A. Knopf, 1991.

Lust, John, and Michael Tierra. *The Natural Remedy Bible*. New York: Pocket Books, 1990.

Mairesse, Michelle. *Health Secrets of Medicinal Herbs*. New York: Arco Publishing, 1981.

Majno, Guido. *The Healing Hand. A Commonwealth Fund Book*. Cambridge, MA: Harvard University Press, 1975.

Makower, Joel. *Office Hazards: How Your Job Can Make You Sick*. Washington, D.C.: Tilden Press, 1981.

Male, David. *Immunology—An Illustrated Outline*. St. Louis, MO: The C. V. Mosby Company, 1986.

Manahan, Stanley E. *Toxicological Chemistry*. Chelsea, MI: Lewis Publishers, 1992.

Manning, Clark A., and Louis J. Vanrenen. *Bioenergetic Medicines East and West: Acupuncture and Homeopathy*. Berkeley, CA: North Atlantic Books, 1988.

Martin, Eric W. *Hazards of Medication*. Philadelphia, PA: J. B. Lippincott Co., 1978.

Martina, Roy. *Endogenous Detoxification—Seminar Notes*. Los Angeles, CA: Apex Energetics, 1992.

Mayer, Jack L., and Sophie J. Balle. "A Pediatrician's Guide to Environmental Toxins." *Contemporary Pediatrics*. Aug. 1988: 63–76.

McCabe, Ed. "People." *Health Consciousness*. 14(3): 81–82 (1993).

McGilvery, Robert W., and Gerald W. Goldstein. *Biochemistry—A Functional Approach*. Philadelphia, PA: W. B. Saunders Company, 1983.

McGrew, Roderick Erle. *Encyclopedia of Medical History*. New York: McGraw Hill, 1985.

McWilliams, Charles. "Electrobiology, Homotoxicology, Overview of Homeopathy, and Today's Miasmatic Terrain." Eclectic Remedy Seminar, Nevis, West Indies, Nov. 21–24, 1992.

Meinig, George. *Root Canal Cover-up*. Ojai, CA: Bion Publishing, 1994.

Metametrix Laboratory. "Liver Detoxification Functions." Pamphlet. Norcross, GA: Metametrix Laboratory, n.d.

Miller, Neil Z. *Vaccines: Are They Really Safe and Effective?* Santa Fe, NM: New Atlantean Press, 1992.

Mindell, Earl. *Earl Mindell's Vitamin Bible*. New York: Warner Books, 1979.

Morrison, Roger. *Desktop Guide to Keynotes and Confirmatory Symptoms*. Albany, CA: Hahnemann Clinic Publishing, 1993.

Mowrey, Daniel B. *The Scientific Validation of Herbal Medicine*. New Canaan, CT: Keats Publishing, 1986.

Mowrey, Daniel B. *Next Generation Herbal Medicine*. New Canaan, CT: Keats Publishing, 1990.

Murphy, Robin. *Fundamentals of Materia Medica*. Santa Fe, NM: R. Murphy, 1988.

Murphy, Robin. "H.A.N.A. Certificate Homeopathy Classes 1–18." Santa Fe, NM: Hahnemann Academy of North America, 1991–92.

Murphy, Robin. "H.A.N.A. Certificate Class Home Study Tapes 1–21." Santa Fe, NM: Hahnemann Academy of North America, 1991–92.

Murphy, Robin. *Homeopathic Medical Repertory*. Pagosa Springs, CO: Hahnemann Academy of North America, 1993.

Namikoshi, Toru. *Shiatsu + Stretching*. Tokyo, Japan: Japan Publications, 1985.

Niaz, Sarfaraz K. *The Omega Connection*. Oak Brook, IL: Esquire Books, 1987.

NIH Consensus Development Conference. "Noise and Hearing Loss." *JAMA*. 263(23): 3185–90 (June 20, 1990).

Nutritional Enzyme Support System. Ness Product

Update—Ness Formula 3. Pamphlet. Forsyth, MO: Nutritional Enzyme Support System, April 1992.

Nuzzi, Debra. *Pocket Herbal Reference Guide.* Freedom, CA: Crossing Press, 1992.

1,001 Home Health Remedies. Peachtree City, GA: FC & A Publishing, 1993.

Osborn, Carl D. "Treatment of Spider Bites by High Voltage Direct Current." *Journal of the Oklahoma State Medical Association.* 84: 257–60 (June 1991).

Pangborn, Jon B. *Nutrition, Amino Acids, and Human Metabolism.* Lisle, IL: Bionostics, n.d.

Pauling, Linus. *Vitamin C, the Common Cold, and the Flu.* San Francisco, CA: W. H. Freeman and Co., 1976.

Pelletier, Kenneth R. *Holistic Medicine—From Stress to Optimum Health.* New York: Dell Publishing, 1979.

Pennisi, E. "Free-Radical Scavenger Gene Tied to ALS." *Science News.* 143: 148 (1993).

Philpott, William H., with Shawn Taplin. *Biomagnetic Handbook: A Guide to Medical Magnets—The Energy Medicine of Tomorrow.* Choctaw, OK: Envirotech Products, 1990.

Pischinger, Alfred. Edited by Hortmut Heine. *Matrix and Matrix Regulation: Basis for a Holistic Theory in Medicine.* Brussels, Belgium: Haug Internationals, 1991.

"Preliminary Evidence Points to Affective Disorder Triggered by Summer Weather." *JAMA.* 295(7): 958 (1988).

Professional Health Products. "Heavy Metal Intoxication and Detoxification." Pamphlet. Sewickley, PA: Professional Health Products, 1992.

Purdom, Walton, ed. *Environmental Health.* San Deigo, CA: Academic Press, 1980.

Randolph, Theron G., and R. Michael Wisner. "Detoxification: Personal Survival in a Chemical World." Pamphlet. Sacramento, CA: Healthmed, 1988., n.p.

Rea, William J. *Chemical Sensitivity*, vol. 1–4. Boca Raton, FL: Lewis Publishers, 1992–96.

Rea, William J. "The Environmental Control Unit (ECU) as a Tool in the Diagnosis and Treatment of Chemical Sensitivities." Presented at the American Academy of Environmental Medicine, 28th Annual Meeting, Reno, NV, Oct. 10, 1993.

Rea, William. "The Non-Immunologic Mechanisms of Chemical Sensitivity." Presented at the American Academy of Environmental Medicine, 28th Annual Meeting, Reno, NV, Oct. 9, 1993.

Reader's Digest Magic and Medicine of Plants. Pleasantville, NY: The Reader's Digest Association, 1986.

Reckeweg, Hans-Heinrich. *Homotoxicology: Illness and Healing Through Anti-homotoxic Therapy.* Albuquerque, NM: Menaco Publishing Co., 1989.

Riggs, Maribeth. *Natural Child Care: A Complete Guide to Safe and Effective Herbal Remedies and Holistic Health Strategies for Infants and Children.* New York: Harmony Books, 1989.

Rippon, John Willard. *Medical Mycology.* Philadelphia, PA: W. B. Saunders Company, 1982.

Rogers, Sherry A. *You Are What You Ate. An R_x for the Resistant Diseases of the 21st Century.* Syracuse, NY: Prestige Publishing, 1988.

Rogers, Sherry A. *Tired or Toxic?* Syracuse, NY: Prestige Publishing, 1990.

Rogers, Sherry A. *Wellness Against All Odds.* Syracuse, NY: Prestige Publishing, 1994.

Root, David, and Michael Wisner. "Detecting and Treating Chemical Exposure." *LA Weekly.* 1989.

Ross, A.C., Gordon, M.B., and Hom, M.F. *The Amazing Healer Arnica.* Wellingborough, Northamptonshire, England: Thorsons Publishers Limited, 1977.

Rousseau, David. *Creating a Healthy Home.* Point Roberts, WA: Hartley & Marks, 1996.

"Rx: Don't Mix Medications and the Sun." *Parade Magazine.* Aug. 22, 1993: 13.

"Rx for Laughter: Cancer Patients Find Fun on the Road to Recovery." *American Institute for Cancer Research Newsletter.* 41: 10 (fall 1993).

Saifer, Phyllis, and Merla Zellerbach. *Detox.* Los Angeles, CA: Jeremy P. Tarcher, 1984.

Samet, Jonathan M., Marian C. Marbury, and John D. Spengler. "Respiratory Effects of Indoor Air Pollution." *Journal of Allergy and Clinical Immunology.* 79: 685–700 (1987).

Samet Jonathan M., and John D. Spengler. *Indoor Air Pollution: A Health Perspective.* Baltimore, MD: The Johns Hopkins University Press, 1991.

Schause, Alexander G. *Aloe Vera.* Tacoma, WA: American Institute for Biochemical Research, 1990.

Schechter, Steven R. "That Cad, Cadmium." *Let's Live.* Jan. 1993: 88.

Seba, Douglas B. "Thermal Chamber Depuration— A Perspective on Man in the Sauna." *Clinical Ecology.* 7(1): 1–12. 1989.

Sherris, John C., and others. *Medical Microbiology.* New York: Elsevier Science Publishing Co., 1984.

Sigerist, Henry E. *A History of Medicine*, vol. I and II. New York: Oxford University Press, 1951.

"Skin Hormone, Melatonin May Work Together." *Brain/Mind Bulletin*. Oct. 1989: 2.

Smith, Cyril, and Simon Best. *Electromagnetic Man*. New York: St. Martin's Press, 1989.

Smits, Tinus. *Practical Materia Medica for the Consulting Room*. 5581 J M Waalre, Holland: Tinus Smits, 1993.

Stone, Irwin. *The Healing Factor: Vitamin C Against Disease*. New York: Perigee Books, 1982.

Stryer, Lubert. *Biochemistry*. New York: W. H. Freeman and Co., 1988.

Sullivan, John B. Jr., and Gary P. Krieger. *Hazardous Materials Toxicology: Clinical Principles of Environmental Health*. Baltimore, MD: Williams and Wilkins, 1992.

Tappan, Frances. *Healing Massage Techniques*. Norwalk, CT: Appleton & Lange, 1988.

Tarcher, Alyce Bezman, ed. *Principles and Practice of Environmental Medicine*. New York: Plenum Medical Book Co., 1992.

Taylor, Frances, Jacqueline Krohn, and Erla Mae Larson. "Allergic Implications of Viral Infections." Presented at the American Academy of Environmental Medicine, 27th Annual Meeting, Lincolnshire, IL, Oct. 27, 1992.

Taylor, Frances, and Jacqueline Krohn. "Expanded Chemical Testing: Utilization of New Chemicals for More Complete Relief for the Chemically Susceptible Patient." Presented at the American Academy of Environmental Medicine, 28th Annual Meeting, Reno, NV, Oct. 11, 1993.

Tenney, Louise. *Today's Herbal Health*. Provo, UT: Woodland Books, 1983.

Thomson, Bill. "Rejuvenate Yourself in Three Weeks." *Natural Healing*. Jan./Feb. 1993: 2–7.

Thrash, Agatha, and Calvin Thrash. *Home Remedies*. Seale, AL: Thrash Publications, 1981.

Tierra, Michael. Edited and supplemented by Dr. David Frawley. *Planetary Herbology*. Santa Fe, NM: Lotus Press, 1989.

Trattler, Ross. *Better Health Through Natural Healing*. New York: McGraw-Hill Book Co., 1985.

Ullman, Dana. *Discovering Homeopathy*. Berkley, CA: North Atlantic Books, 1991.

Ullman, Dana. *Homeopathic Medicine for Children and Infants*. New York: Jeremy P. Tarcher/Perigee Books, 1992.

Vander, Arthur J., James H. Sherman, and Dorothy S. Luciano. *Human Physiology*. New York: McGraw-Hill Book Co., 1985.

Wade, Carlson. *Inner Cleansing*. West Nyack, NY: Parker Publishing Co., 1992.

Walker, J. Frederic. *Formaldehyde*. New York: Reinhold Publishing, 1964.

Walker, Morton. *The Chelation Way*. Garden City Park, NY: Avery Publishing Group, 1990.

Walsh, James Joseph. *Medieval Medicine*. London, England: A. & C. Black, 1920.

Wartik, Nancy. "A Question of Abuse." *American Health*. May 1993: 62–67.

Weaver, Daniel C. "Heavy Metal." *Discover*. April 1993: 76–78.

Weil, Andrew. *Health and Healing—Understanding Conventional and Alternative Medicine*. New York: Darling-Kindersly, 1995.

Weil, Andrew. *Natural Health, Natural Medicine—A Comprehensive Manual for Wellness and Self-Care*. New York: Darling-Kindersley, 1995.

Werbach, Melvyn R. *Third Line Medicine*. New York: Arkana, 1986.

Werner, David. *Where There Is No Doctor*. Palo Alto, CA: The Hesperian Foundation, 1977.

Whitaker, Julian. "Clean Up Indoor Pollution With Plants." *Health and Healing*. 3(10): 1–3 (Oct. 1993).

Whitaker, Julian. "EDTA Chelation Therapy: Your Safe Alternative to Surgery." *Health and Healing*. 2 (4): 1–4 (April 1992).

Whitney, Eleanor Noss, and Eva May Nunnelley Hamilton. *Understanding Nutrition*. St. Paul, MN: WestPublishing Co., 1984.

Williams, David G. "Cleaning House." *Alternatives for the Health Conscious Individual*. 4: 97–100 (1992).

Williams, Phillip L., and James L. Burson, eds. *Industrial Toxicology: Safety and Health Applications in the Workplace*. New York: Van Nostrand Reinhold, 1985.

Williams, Sid. "Bones of Contention." *Health*. July/Aug. 1993: 44–53.

Witlin, Barbara, and Roy Witlin. "Our Lives: Artist Finds Nontoxic Paints and Methods." *The Human Ecologist*. Winter 1991: 13–15.

Wooster, Sarah M. "Geopathogenic Stress and Cancer." *Townsend Letter for Doctors*. Nov. 1988: 482–86.

Yudkin, Marcia. "The Forecast for Tomorrow is Headaches." *Natural Health*. Jan./Feb. 1993: 40–41.

Zucker, Norman. "Hubbard's Purification Rundown: A Workable Detox Program." *Townsend Letter for Doctors* Jan. 1990: 54–55.

INDEX

JACQUELINE A. KROHN received her MD from Washington University and an MPH from Medical College of Wisconsin. She is board certified in Pediatrics and Environmental Medicine, and is board eligible in Occupational Medicine. She is the co-author of *The Whole Way to Natural Allergy Relief and Prevention*, *Rotation Isn't Just for Tires* (a rotation diet cookbook), and *A Guide to the Identification and Treatment of Biocatalyst and Biochemical Intolerances*. Dr. Krohn practices in Los Alamos, New Mexico.

FRANCES A. TAYLOR has a BS in chemistry, biology and math. Her MA is in microbiology and biochemistry. She is Dr. Krohn's Head Allergy Technician, and is the co-author of *The Whole Way to Allergy Relief and Prevention*, *Rotation Isn't Just for Tires*, and *A Guide to the Identification and Treatment of Biocatalyst and Biochemical Intolerances*.

JINGER PROSSER is a licensed massage therapist whose specialties are reflexology and orthobionomy TM.

Answers

- Toxins can enter the body through the skin, inhalation through the respiratory tract into the lungs, and ingestion through the mouth into the gastrointestinal tract.
- The skin, lungs, gastrointestinal tract, and the liver are our major organs of detoxification. They try to eliminate foreign chemicals, drugs, and compounds produced by the body, such as hormones, cholesterol, and fatty acids.
- Water flushes toxins and waste material from the cells. Nutrients must be kept in solution, available for cell nutrition and repair, and adequate fluid levels are necessary for ions in the body to flow and maintain electrical equilibrium.
- An electromagnetic imbalance may cause electrical equipment to malfunction when you are near and may make it difficult to find a watch that keeps the correct time. Symptoms may occur when near fluorescent lights, transformers or high-powered electric lines and may worsen before a storm.
- The most important part of any diet is chewing food well. Food should be chewed until you can feel the saliva break up the foods.